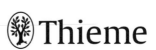

Neurosurgery Rounds

Questions and Answers

Second Edition

Mark R. Shaya, MD, FACS
Founder and President
Neurosurgical Institute of Florida
Coral Gables, Florida

Cristian Gragnaniello, MD, PhD, MSurg, MAdvSurg, FICS
Surgical Director
Harvey H. Ammerman Microsurgical Laboratory
Department of Neurosurgery
George Washington University
Washington, DC

Remi Nader, MD, CM, FRCSC, FACS, FAANS
Founder and President
Texas Center for Neurosciences
Houston, Texas;
Adjunct Clinical Professor of Neurosurgery
University of Texas Medical Branch
Galveston, Texas;
Affiliate Clinical Professor
William Carey University
Hattiesburg, Mississippi;
Clinical Assistant Professor of Neurosurgery
Tulane University
New Orleans, Louisiana

Section Editor (Spine, Peripheral Nerve, Neuroradiology)
Hussam Abou-Al-Shaar, MD
Postdoctoral Research Fellow
Department of Neurosurgery
Clinical Neurosciences Center
University of Utah Hospital
Salt Lake City, Utah

160 illustrations

Thieme
New York • Stuttgart • Delhi • Rio de Janeiro

Executive Editor: Timothy Y. Hiscock
Managing Editor: Sarah Landis
Director, Editorial Services: Mary Jo Casey
Editorial Assistant: Nikole Connors
Production Editor: Naamah Schwartz
International Production Director:
Andreas Schabert
Editorial Director: Sue Hodgson
International Marketing Director:
Fiona Henderson
International Sales Director: Louisa Turrell
Director of Sales, North America:
Mike Roseman
Senior Vice President and Chief Operating
Officer: Sarah Vanderbilt
President: Brian D. Scanlan

Library of Congress Cataloging-in-Publication Data

Names: Shaya, Mark, author. | Gragnaniello, Cristian, author. | Nader, Remi, author.

Title: Neurosurgery rounds : questions and answers / Mark R. Shaya, Cristian Gragnaniello, Remi Nader.

Description: Second edition. | New York : Thieme, [2018] | Preceded by Neurosurgery rounds : questions and answers / Mark R. Shaya ... [et al.]. 1st ed. 2011. | Includes bibliographical references and index.

Identifiers: LCCN 2017030297| ISBN 9781626233461 | ISBN 9781626233638 (e-book)

Subjects: | MESH: Neurosurgical Procedures | Neurosciences—methods | Examination Questions | Handbooks

Classification: LCC RD593 | NLM WL 18.2 | DDC 617.4/8—dc23 LC record available at https://lccn.loc.gov/2017030297

© 2018 Thieme Medical Publishers, Inc.

Thieme Publishers New York
333 Seventh Avenue, New York, NY 10001 USA
+1 800 782 3488, customerservice@thieme.com

Thieme Publishers Stuttgart
Rüdigerstrasse 14, 70469 Stuttgart, Germany
+49 [0]711 8931 421, customerservice@thieme.de

Thieme Publishers Delhi
A-12, Second Floor, Sector-2, Noida-201301
Uttar Pradesh, India
+91 120 45 566 00, customerservice@thieme.in

Thieme Publishers Rio de Janeiro,
Thieme Publicações Ltda.
Edifício Rodolpho de Paoli, 25° andar
Av. Nilo Peçanha, 50 – Sala 2508,
Rio de Janeiro 20020-906 Brasil
+55 21 3172-2297 / +55 21 3172-1896

Cover design: Thieme Publishing Group
Typesetting by DiTech Process Solutions

Printed in The United States of America by
Sheridan Press 5 4 3 2 1

ISBN 978-1-62623-346-1

Also available as an e-book:
eISBN 978-1-62623-363-8

Important note: Medicine is an ever-cha ing science undergoing continual developme Research and clinical experience are contin ly expanding our knowledge, in particular knowledge of proper treatment and drug the py. Insofar as this book mentions any dosage application, readers may rest assured that authors, editors, and publishers have made ery effort to ensure that such references are accordance with **the state of knowledge at t time of production of the book.**

Nevertheless, this does not involve, imply, express any guarantee or responsibility on part of the publishers in respect to any dos instructions and forms of applications state the book. **Every user is requested to exam carefully** the manufacturers' leaflets acco panying each drug and to check, if necess in consultation with a physician or specia whether the dosage schedules mentio therein or the contraindications stated by manufacturers differ from the stateme made in the present book. Such examinat is particularly important with drugs that either rarely used or have been newly relea on the market. Every dosage schedule or ev form of application used is entirely at the us own risk and responsibility. The authors a publishers request every user to report to publishers any discrepancies or inaccurac noticed. If errors in this work are found af publication, errata will be posted at ww thieme.com on the product description page

Some of the product names, patents, and reg tered designs referred to in this book are in f registered trademarks or proprietary nam even though specific reference to this fact is always made in the text. Therefore, the appe ance of a name without designation as prop etary is not to be construed as a representat by the publisher that it is in the public doma

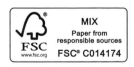

Contents

Preface

Whether you are taking the neurosurgery written board examination, the oral boards, or participating in Maintenance of Certification, this book will provide a diverse coverage of the multiple disciplines that are involved and intertwined in the understanding, care, and treatment of the neurosurgical patient. Important updates are included in this second edition. The book is divided into two sections including basic and clinical neurosciences. There are also subsections which include neuroanatomy, neurophysiology, spine, peripheral nerves, neurology, and neuroradiology.

The differences in the board examinations in neurosurgery are worth mentioning. The written board exam will test certain items that one will not necessarily see on the oral board exam. As you are probably aware, more neuroscience is seen on the written board examination and more clinical situations are seen in the oral boards. Most importantly, the oral board examination involves interaction with the examiners, and passing this exam is heavily dependent on your ability to communicate succinctly and precisely what to do in a particular clinical situation. One cannot hope to pass such an exam relying only on attending large lectures from the oral board preparation courses given by the national organizations. For the oral board exam it is best to identify neurosurgeons in your geographical area and also your previous training program, and ask interested neurosurgeons to prepare some cases for you and have them examine you. Those taking the exam must practice communicating neurosurgical ideas in a pressure situation and this cannot be rehearsed in a large lecture hall with hundreds of people. Maintenance of Certification (MOC) is offered though the American Board (abns.org) or through the National Board of Physicians and Surgeons (nbpas.org). It is important to select a path of MOC that best fits your practice situation, whether it is academic or private practice.

Neurosurgery is an ever-changing field. There is certainly a growing phenomenon among insurance companies, the legal profession, and administrators of putting pressure on neurosurgeons that at times may delay, confuse, or conflict with the standard of care we learned during training. Now more than ever we must be true to our profession, and we as neurosurgeons must be the ones to define the stimulating and privileged profession of neurosurgery.

Mark R. Shaya, MD

Acknowledgments

The following individuals contributed to the first edition of this book, and their efforts are gratefully acknowledged by the editors of this second edition:

Editors
Jonathan S. Citow, MD
Hamad I. Farhat, MD
Abdulrahman J. Sabbagh, MD

Contributors
Nazek Ahmad, MD *(Cranial Neurosurgery–Pediatric)*
Mohammd Alfawareh, MD *(Spine)*
Aisha Nassr Al-Hajjaj, MD *(Neuroradiology)*
Tamer Altay, MD *(Neuroradiology)*
Gmaan Alzahrani, MD *(Cranial Neurosurgery–Pediatric)*
Walid I. Attia, MD, MSc, PhD *(Spine)*
Eman Bakhsh, MD *(Neuroradiology)*
Leonardo Rangel Castillia, MD *(Neuropharmacology)*
Cristian Gragnaniello, MD *(General)*
Nazer Qureshi, MD *(Cranium)*
Ali Raja, MD *(Cranium)*
Bahauddin I. Sallout, MD *(Cranial Neurosurgery – Pediatric)*
Michael Zwillman, MD *(Neuropharmacology)*

Reviewers
Neuroradiology
Ayman A. Albanyan, MBBS, FRCSC
Khaled N. Almusrea, MBBS, FRCSC
Neuropathology
Manuel B. Graeber, MD *(Neurology)*
Referencing
Irish L. Grant, RN *(Neurology)*
Spine
Milan G. Mody, MD

Content Reviewer
Jaime Gasco, MD

1 Neuroanatomy

Cranial

■ Vasculature

1. How can one distinguish the internal carotid artery (ICA) from the external carotid artery (ECA) in the neck?

The ICA has no branches in the neck, whereas the ECA has multiple branches.[1] The common carotid artery (CCA) splits into the ECA and ICA in the neck.

2. What are the major branches of the ECA?

The mnemonic SALFOPSI is very useful in remembering the branches of the ECA in ascending order (proximal to distal) (**Fig. 1.1**)[1]:

1. Superior thyroid artery.
2. Ascending pharyngeal artery.
3. Lingual artery.

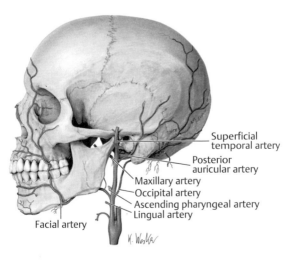

Fig. 1.1 External carotid artery and branches. (Reproduced with permission from Schuenke et al. Illustration by Karl Wesker.[2])

4. *F*acial artery.
5. *O*ccipital artery.
6. *P*osterior auricular artery.
7. *S*uperficial temporal artery.
8. (*I*nternal) maxillary artery.

3. From where do the CCAs arise?

Normally, the right CCA comes off the brachiocephalic trunk, whereas the left CCA comes off straight from the aortic arch.[3]

4. What is referred to as the carotid siphon?

The intracavernous and the supraclinoid segments of the ICA make up the carotid siphon. The carotid siphon is the S-shaped part of the ICA which begins at the posterior bend of the cavernous ICA and ends at the ICA bifurcation.

5. What classical clinical findings occur in an occlusion of the anterior choroidal artery?

Hemiparesis, hemianesthesia, and hemianopsia.

6. The posterior cerebral artery divides into what two terminal branches?

The parietooccipital artery and calcarine artery (**Fig. 1.2**).[4]

7. What artery supplies the choroid plexus of the temporal horn and atrium?

The posterior cerebral artery supplies both (**Fig. 1.2**).[4]

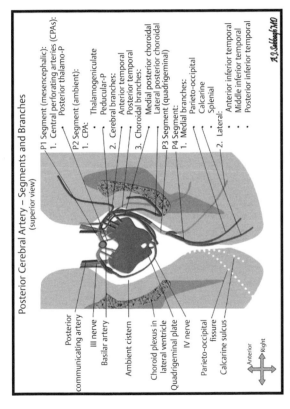

Fig. 1.2 Posterior cerebral artery—segments and branches.

8. What are Virchow-Robin spaces?

The spaces between the blood vessels and the arachnoid and pia layers within the brain and spinal cord. Rudolf Virchow was a German pathologist and Charles Robin was a French anatomist. The perivascular spaces of the brain are known as Virchow-Robin spaces.

9. Which sinus courses within the attachment of the tentorium to the petrous ridge?

The superior petrosal sinus.[4]

10. Which large anastomotic vein joins the superior sagittal sinus?

The vein of Trolard (also called the superior anastomotic vein) (**Fig. 1.3**).[4]

Paulin Trolard (1842–1910) was a French anatomist who described venous drainage of the brain.

11. Which large anastomotic vein joins the veins of the sylvian fissure with the transverse sinus?

The vein of Labbé.[4]

12. What is the largest branch of the intracavernous portion of the carotid artery?

The meningohypophyseal trunk (**Fig. 1.4**).[5]

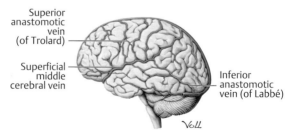

Fig. 1.3 Superficial venous anatomy of the brain. (Reproduced with permission from Schuenke et al. Illustration by Markus Voll.[2])

13. What is the most constant branch of the meningohypophyseal trunk?

The tentorial artery. It passes forward to the roof of the cavernous sinus and then posterolaterally along the free edge of the tentorium. It sends branches to cranial nerves (CNs) III and IV. Bernasconi and Cassinari first reported this artery angiographically in 1957 (**Fig. 1.4**).[5]

14. Which branch of the intracavernous carotid artery passes between CN VI and the ophthalmic division of the trigeminal nerve?

The inferolateral trunk.[5]

15. What is the venous angle as seen on a lateral view of a cerebral angiogram?

The angle is formed by the junction of the thalamostriate vein and the internal cerebral veins at the thalamic tubercle. This area approximates the site of the foramen of Monro. Alexander Monro (1733–1817) was a Scottish anatomist. The interventricular foramen between the lateral and third ventricles is known as the foramen of Monro.

16. What are the three main superficial cerebral veins?[6]

1. The superior anastomotic vein of Trolard.
2. The inferior anastomotic vein of Labbé.
3. The superficial middle cerebral vein.

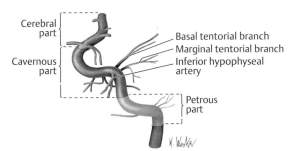

Fig. 1.4 Internal carotid artery and branches. (Reproduced with permission from Schuenke et al. Illustration by Karl Wesker.[2])

17. What is the most likely clinical symptom in a patient with a large unruptured cavernous sinus carotid aneurysm?

Ipsilateral sixth nerve palsy. The cavernous sinus contains CNs III, IV, V1 and V2 as well as CN VI. The abducens nerve has the most proximal spatial relationship to the carotid artery.[7]

18. Which artery is the most common cause of lateral medullary syndrome?

Also known as Wallenberg's syndrome, it is most commonly due to occlusion of the vertebral artery on the ipsilateral side. This syndrome results from infarct in the region supplied by the posterior inferior cerebellar artery (PICA), which is a branch of the vertebral artery (**Fig. 1.5**).[8]

19. What is the arterial supply of the thalamus?

Branches of the posterior communicating arteries and the perimesencephalic portion of the posterior cerebral arteries (**Fig. 1.6**).[4]

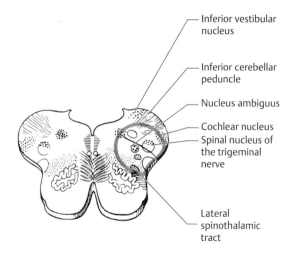

Fig. 1.5 Cross-section of the medulla with outlined blood supply of the vertebral artery. (Reproduced with permission from Mumenthaler and Mattle.[9])

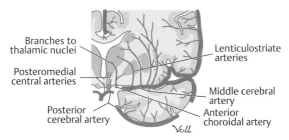

Fig. 1.6 Blood supply to internal capsule and basal ganglia. (Reproduced with permission from Schuenke et al. Illustration by Markus Voll.[2])

20. What is the arterial supply of the lateral geniculate nucleus (LGN)?

The LGN has a dual arterial supply. Laterally, it receives supply from the anterior choroidal artery, and medially from the lateral posterior choroidal artery. Hence, infarcts are relatively uncommon in this area.[10]

21. Which artery is most commonly involved in trigeminal neuralgia?

The superior cerebellar artery (SCA) (**Figs. 1.7** and **1.8**).[11] Oftentimes, no artery can be identified on imaging studies of patients with trigeminal neuralgia.

22. Which artery is most commonly involved in hemifacial spasm?

The anterior inferior cerebellar artery (AICA) (**Figs. 1.7** and **1.8**).[13]

23. What is the most common artery involved in glossopharyngeal neuralgia?

The PICA (**Figs. 1.7** and **1.8**).[14]

24. What is the main arterial supply of the internal capsule?

This is derived from several sources. The lateral lenticulostriate branches from the middle carotid artery, the medial striate artery from the *anterior cerebral artery* (ACA), and the direct branches from the ICA. The anterior choroidal artery comes off the ICA (**Fig. 1.6**).[10]

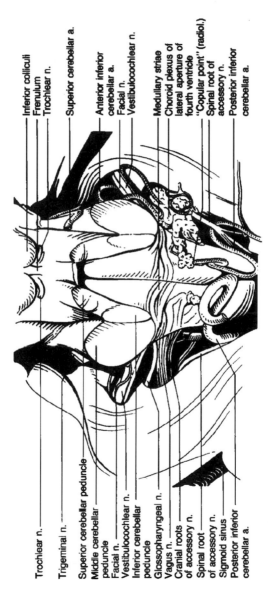

Trochlear n.

Trigeminal n.

Superior cerebellar peduncle

Middle cerebellar peduncle

Facial n.

Vestibulocochlear n.

Inferior cerebellar peduncle

Glossopharyngeal n.

Vagus n.

Cranial roots of accessory n.

Spinal root of accessory n.

Sigmoid sinus

Posterior inferior cerebellar a.

Inferior colliculi

Frenulum

Trochlear n.

Superior cerebellar a.

Anterior inferior cerebellar a.

Facial n.

Vestibulocochlear n.

Medullary striae

Choroid plexus of lateral aperture of fourth ventricle

"Copular point" (radiol.)

Spinal root of accessory n.

Posterior inferior cerebellar a.

Fig. 1.7 Topographic anatomy of dorsal brainstem and tectum. (Reproduced with permission from Koos et al.[12])

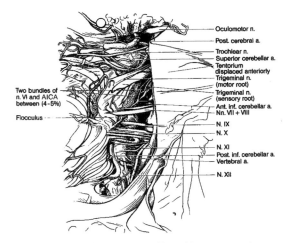

Oculomotor n.
Post. cerebral a.
Trochlear n.
Superior cerebellar a.
Tentorium displaced anteriorly
Trigeminal n. (motor root)
Trigeminal n. (sensory root)
Ant. inf. cerebellar a.
Nn. VII + VIII
N. IX
N. X
N. XI
Post. inf. cerebellar a.
Vertebral a.
N. XII

Two bundles of n. VI and AICA between (4–5%)

Flocculus

Fig. 1.8 Topographic anatomy of lateral brainstem and cerebellum. (Reproduced with permission from Koos et al.[12])

25. Which vessel has the highest risk of injury in a Chiari decompression surgery?

The PICA.[14] Hans Chiari (1851–1916) was a Austrian physician.

26. Which vessels supply the superior, middle, and inferior cerebellar peduncles?

The SCA, AICA, and PICA, respectively.[15]

■ Skull

27. Where is the motor strip located in relation to the skull?

It is located 4 to 5.5 cm behind the coronal suture (**Fig. 1.9**).[16]

28. What external landmark on the skull marks the lateral margin of the sphenoid ridge and sylvian fissure?

The pterion (**Fig. 1.10**).[16]

29. What part of the mandible does the temporalis muscle attach to?

The coronoid process of the mandible.[1]

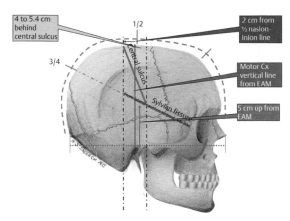

Fig. 1.9 Coronal and rolandic fissure locations. EAM, external auditory meatus.

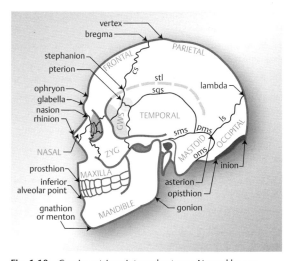

Fig. 1.10 Craniometric points and sutures. Named bones appear in all uppercase letters. GWS, greater wing of sphenoid bone; stl, superior temporal line; ZYG, zygomatic. Sutures: cs, coronal; ls, lambdoid; oms, occipitomastoid; pms, parietomastoid; sms, squamomastoid; sqs, squamosal. (Reproduced with permission from Greenberg.[16])

30. What muscle of mastication does the parotid duct cross?

The masseter muscle.[1] The masseter muscle can become enlarged in patients who clench or grind their teeth.

31. Which cranial fossa is the largest?

The posterior cranial fossa. It is also the deepest of the three cranial fossae (**Fig. 1.11**).

32. What are the boundaries of the suboccipital triangle?[17]

The suboccipital triangle is a region bounded by the following three muscles:

1. Above and medially by the rectus capitis posterior major.
2. Above and laterally by the superior oblique.
3. Below and laterally by the inferior oblique.

33. In a far lateral approach, it is helpful to palpate and know the location of the transverse process of the atlas. Between what landmarks can the transverse process of the atlas be palpated?

Through the skin between the mastoid process and the mandibular angle.[17]

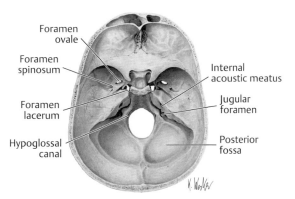

Fig. 1.11 Interior view of the skull base. (Reproduced with permission from Schuenke et al. Illustration by Karl Wesker.[2])

34. What sutures make up the asterion?

The lambdoid, parietomastoid, and occipitomastoid sutures. It is an important landmark to define the lower half of the junction of the transverse and sigmoid sinuses (**Fig. 1.10**).[16] In the adult, it lies 4 cm behind and 12 mm above the center of the entrance of the ear canal.

35. Which bones make up the osseous nasal septum?

The perpendicular plate of the ethmoid and the vomer (**Fig. 1.12**).[1]

36. What are the compartments of the jugular foramen?

Pars venosa (posterolateral), which contains the sigmoid sinus, jugular bulb, and CNs X and XI.

Pars nervosa (anteromedial), which contains CN IX and Jacobson's nerve (**Fig. 1.13**).[18]

37. What structure does the abducens nerve go through to enter the cavernous sinus?

Dorello's canal.[5]

38. What structures go through the internal acoustic meatus?

The facial nerve (VII), the vestibulocochlear nerve (VIII), and the labyrinthine artery (**Fig. 1.13**).[19]

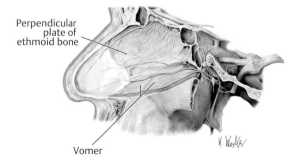

Perpendicular plate of ethmoid bone

Vomer

Fig. 1.12   Nasal septum innervation. (Reproduced with permission from Schuenke et al. Illustration by Karl Wesker.[2])

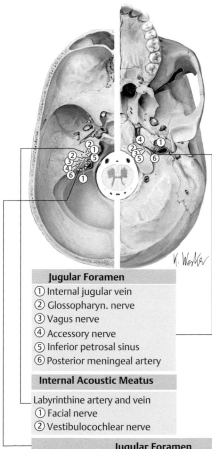

Jugular Foramen

1. Internal jugular vein
2. Glossopharyn. nerve
3. Vagus nerve
4. Accessory nerve
5. Inferior petrosal sinus
6. Posterior meningeal artery

Internal Acoustic Meatus

Labyrinthine artery and vein
1. Facial nerve
2. Vestibulocochlear nerve

Jugular Foramen

1. Internal jugular vein
2. Glossopharyn-
   geal nerve
3. Vagus nerve

4. Accessory nerve
5. Inferior petrosal sinus
6. Posterior meningeal
   artery

Fig. 1.13 Foramina of the skull base with exiting structures. (Reproduced with permission from Schuenke et al. Illustration by Karl Wesker.[2])

39. What are the major parts of the temporal bone?

Squamous and petrous parts.[1]

40. The cribriform plate is part of what bone?

The ethmoid bone. The ethmoid bone separates the nasal cavity from the brain. It contributes to the medial wall of the orbit.

41. What are the bones that form the walls of the orbit (Fig. 1.14)?[20]

1. Frontal.
2. Zygomatic.
3. Maxilla.
4. Sphenoid.
5. Lacrimal.
6. Ethmoid.
7. Palatine.

42. What structures pass through the annulus of Zinn?

The optic nerve, ophthalmic artery, oculomotor nerve, abducens nerve, and nasociliary nerve (**Fig. 1.14**).[20]

43. What are the structures in the pterygopalatine fossa?

The maxillary artery, maxillary nerve, and pterygopalatine ganglion.[22]

44. What passes through the inferior orbital fissure?

The infraorbital nerve and zygomatic nerve.[20]

45. What bones are approximated at the pterion?

The frontal, parietal, temporal, and sphenoid bones.[16]

46. The clivus is formed by which bones?

The occipital and the sphenoid bones.

47. What structure separates the optic canal from the superior orbital fissure?

The optic strut.[20]

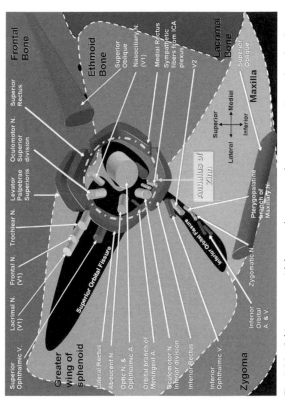

Fig. 1.14 Orbit anatomy with bony and neurovascular structures. (Reproduced with permission from Nader and Sabbagh.[21])

■ Ventricles

48. What are the five parts of the lateral ventricle (Fig. 1.15)?[23]

1. Frontal horn.
2. Temporal horn.
3. Occipital horn.
4. Body.
5. Atrium.

49. Choroid plexus and flocculus protrude from which foramen?

The foramen of Luschka.[24] Hubert von Luschka (1820–1875) was a German anatomist. The lateral apertures of the fourth ventricle are named after him.

50. Which CN nuclei are positioned in the lateral recess near the foramen of Luschka?

The dorsal and ventral cochlear nuclei of CN VIII.[24]

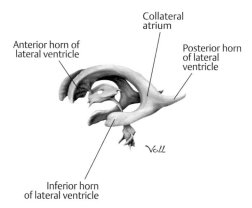

Collateral atrium

Anterior horn of lateral ventricle

Posterior horn of lateral ventricle

Inferior horn of lateral ventricle

Fig. 1.15 Ventricular anatomy. (Reproduced with permission from Schuenke et al. Illustration by Markus Voll.[2])

51. The choroid plexus of the lateral ventricle is attached along the choroidal fissure, which is the cleft between which two structures?

The fornix and thalamus (**Fig. 1.16**).[23]

52. What are the circumventricular organs?

These are areas where the blood–brain barrier is absent. Seven different such areas have been identified (**Fig. 1.17**):

1. Pineal gland.
2. Subfornical organ.
3. Organum vasculosum of the lamina terminalis.
4. Median eminence of the hypothalamus.
5. Neurohypophysis.
6. Area postrema.
7. Subcommissural organ.

53. What is the corresponding intraventricular structure at the calcarine sulcus?

The calcarine sulcus forms a prominence, the calcar avis, in the medial wall of the atrium.[23]

54. The atrium is deep to which cortical structure?

Supramarginal gyrus (area 40).[23]

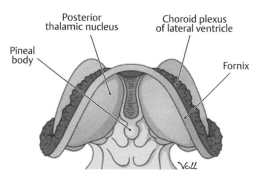

Fig. 1.16 Lateral ventricle and choroid plexus location. (Reproduced with permission from Schuenke et al. Illustration by Markus Voll.[2])

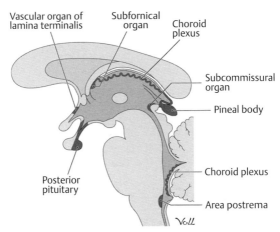

Vascular organ of lamina terminalis

Subfornical organ

Choroid plexus

Subcommissural organ

Pineal body

Choroid plexus

Area postrema

Posterior pituitary

Voll

Fig. 1.17 Circumventricular organs. (Reproduced with permission from Schuenke et al. Illustration by Markus Voll.[2])

55. What form the lateral walls, medial wall, and roof of the frontal horns of the lateral ventricles?

The caudate nucleus, septum pellucidum, and corpus callosum, respectively.[23]

56. Two pairs of small swellings can be seen in the floor of the fourth ventricle, the lateral and medial ridges. What do these structures represent?

The lateral ridges constitute the vagal trigone and indicate the location of the underlying dorsal motor nucleus of the vagus. The medial ridges constitute the hypoglossal trigone and indicate the location of the underlying hypoglossal nucleus (**Fig. 1.18**).[24]

57. What is the outlet of the fourth ventricle?

There are two laterally located foramina of Luschka and there is one single medial foramen of Magendie.[24]

58. Which structure separates the chiasmatic cistern from the interpeduncular cistern?

The Liliequist membrane.[25]

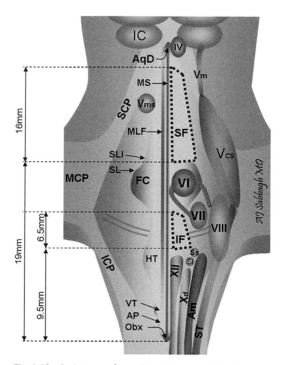

Fig. 1.18 Brainstem schematic anatomy, posterior view. Am, N. ambiguus of 9th and 10th cranial nerves with parasympathetics on its medial border; AP, area postrema; AqD, aqueduct of Sylvius; FC, facial colliculus; HT, hypoglossal triangle; IC, inferior colliculus; ICP, MCP, and SCP, inferior, middle, and superior cerebellar peduncle; IF, intrafacial triangle; IV, trochlear nucleus; MLF, medial longitudinal fascicle; MS, median sulcus; Obx, obex; SF, superfacial triangle; Si and Ss, inferior and superior salivatory Nn.; SL, sulcus limitans; SLI, sulcus limitans incisure; ST, spinal trigeminal tract; Vcs, chief (sensory) nucleus of V; VI, abducent nerve; VII, facial N. and fiber tracks and nerve; VIII, vestibular N.; Vm, mesencephalic nucleus of the fifth cranial nerve (V); Vms, motor (mastication) nucleus of V; VT, vagal triangle; Xd, dorsal vagal N.; XII, hypoglossal N. (Reproduced with permission from Nader and Sabbagh.[21])

■ Autonomic System

59. Where do the sympathetic fibers of the head originate from?

The hypothalamus. They descend through the brainstem and cervical spinal cord to the T1–L2 level, where they exit and go back up to the head (**Fig. 1.19**).[26]

60. Where in the brain are the cholinergic neurons found?

The basal nucleus of Meynert. Abnormalities of this area have been found in patients with Alzheimer's disease.[27] Theodor Hermann Meynert (1833–1892) was an Austrian neuropsychiatrist.

61. Where are the norepinephrine-containing neurons found in the brain?

The locus coeruleus.[28]

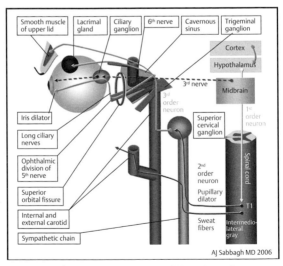

Fig. 1.19 Schematic representation of Horner's syndrome. (Reproduced with permission from Nader and Sabbagh.[21])

62. What supplies the sympathetic innervation to the head and neck?

The stellate ganglion.[26]

63. What ganglions form the stellate ganglion?

The inferior cervical ganglion fuses with the first thoracic ganglion to form the cervical thoracic (stellate) ganglion (**Fig. 1.19**).[26]

64. What type of nerve fibers does the vidian nerve carry?

Parasympathetic fibers from the greater superficial petrosal nerve and sympathetic fibers from the deep petrosal nerve around the ICA. The nerve passes in the pterygoid canal with the vidian artery.

65. What kind of fibers does the intermediate nerve (nervus intermedius) carry?

This is the sensory and parasympathetic division of the facial nerve. The intermediate nerve carries preganglionic parasympathetic fibers from the superior salivary nucleus that synapse in the pterygopalatine and submandibular ganglia. It also carries taste sensation from the anterior two-thirds of the tongue (**Fig. 1.20**).[29]

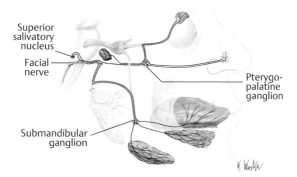

Superior salivatory nucleus

Facial nerve

Pterygo-palatine ganglion

Submandibular ganglion

Fig. 1.20   Parasympathetic visceral innervation of the facial. (Reproduced with permission from Schuenke et al. Illustration by Karl Wesker.[2])

66. What provides the parasympathetics of the parotid glands?

The glossopharyngeal nerve. These parasympathetic fibers originate from the inferior salivatory nucleus and travel via CN IX. These fibers synapse in the otic ganglion before reaching the parotid gland (**Fig. 1.21**).[30]

■ The Meninges

67. What are the leptomeninges?

The arachnoid and pia mater. The pia and arachnoid layers have a common embryologic origin (ectoderm), whereas the dura is formed by the mesoderm (**Fig. 1.22**).

68. How much cerebrospinal fluid (CSF) is produced each day?

About 450 mL. CSF is continuously reabsorbed and secreted. There is only approximately 150 mL of CSF in an average body at any one time; 75% of the CSF is produced by the choroid plexus.[31] CSF pressure gradients produced by cervical stenosis and disks are thought to contribute to cervicogenic headaches.

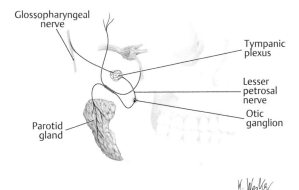

Fig. 1.21 Parasympathetic visceral innervation of the glossopharyngeal nerve. (Reproduced with permission from Schuenke et al. Illustration by Karl Wesker.[2])

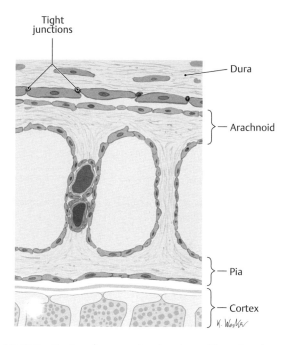

Fig. 1.22 Meningeal cross-sectional anatomy. (Reproduced with permission from Schuenke et al. Illustration by Karl Wesker.[2])

69. What separates the interpeduncular cistern from the chiasmatic cistern?

The Liliequist membrane. The Liliequist membrane is an arachnoidal sheet extending from the dorsum sellae to the anterior edge of the mamillary bodies.[25]

■ Cortex

70. Which Brodmann area corresponds to Broca's area, Wernicke's area, and primary auditory cortex?

Area 44, area 22, and area 41, respectively (**Fig. 1.23**).[32] Korbinian Brodmann (1868–1918) was a German neuropsychiatrist who devised the cytoarchitectural map of the cerebral cortex.

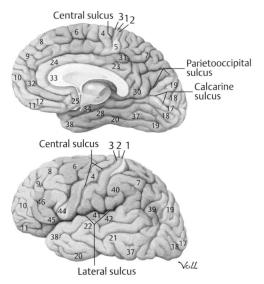

Fig. 1.23 Brodmann areas of the cortex. (Reproduced with permission from Schuenke et al. Illustration by Markus Voll.[2])

71. Which area of the hippocampus is most vulnerable to hypoxia?

CA1, also called Sommer's sector. The CA3 area is relatively resistant to hypoxia (**Fig. 1.24**).

72. What is the indusium griseum?

The remnant of the hippocampus that courses over the dorsal surface of the corpus callosum (the supracallosal gyrus). It contains two longitudinally directed strands of fibers termed the medial and lateral longitudinal striae (**Fig. 1.25**).[33]

73. What makes up the neostriatum?

The caudate and putamen.[34]

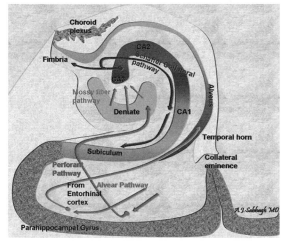

Fig. 1.24 Cross-sectional anatomy of the hippocampus.

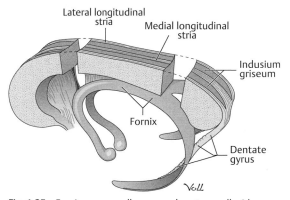

Fig. 1.25 Fornix, corpus callosum, and septum pellucidum. (Reproduced with permission from Schuenke et al. Illustration by Markus Voll.[2])

74. What is the name of the white matter tract that projects from Wernicke's area to the inferior frontal lobe in Broca's region?

The arcuate fasciculus.[35]

75. The gustatory area receives input from which nucleus?

The ipsilateral nucleus solitarius.

76. What is the ischemic penumbra?

An area where there is decreased blood flow of 8 to 23 mL/100 mg/min. Normal blood flow is around 50 mL/100 mg/min. At this decreased blood flow level, neurons survive, but do not function; below this level, neurons die. Gray matter requires more blood supply than white matter.

77. What deficit would result from a lesion of the right Meyer's loop?

Left upper quadrantanopia.[36]

78. What clinical finding is seen when there is a lesion of the posterior part of the middle frontal gyrus?

Conjugate eye deviation toward the ipsilateral side. This is area 8, the cortical lateral conjugate gaze center. Stimulation of this area results in eye deviation toward the contralateral side.

79. The hypothalamus receives fibers from the amygdala via which bundle?

Stria terminalis.[26]

80. What classical syndrome may result from a dominant parietal lobe lesion?

Gerstmann's syndrome. This syndrome includes agraphia without alexia, left–right confusion, finger agnosia, and acalculia.[37]

81. Where is the lesion in a patient with hemineglect?

Posterior parietal association cortex. Hemineglect may affect attention, motor skills, sensation, and cognition.

82. Where in the internal capsule do the corticobulbar fibers run?

The genu of the internal capsule (**Fig. 1.26**).[23] Genu is a Latin word for "knee."

83. Where in the internal capsule is the corticospinal tract located?

The posterior limb of the internal capsule (**Fig. 1.26**).[23]

84. What is the main neurotransmitter of the corticothalamic tracts?

Glutamate.[28]

85. Where is the satiety center?

In the medial hypothalamus. Stimulation of this area results in decreased food intake. Its counterpart, the hunger center, is located in the lateral hypothalamus (**Fig. 1.27**).[26]

86. Where is vasopressin synthesized?

In the supraoptic and paraventricular nuclei of the hypothalamus (**Fig. 1.27**).[26]

Vasopressin is also known as antidiuretic hormone. Its functions are to constrict blood vessels and retain water in the body.

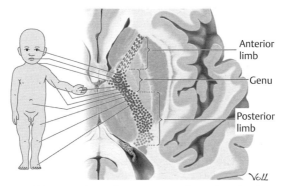

Fig. 1.26 Internal capsule organization. (Reproduced with permission from Schuenke et al. Illustration by Markus Voll.[2])

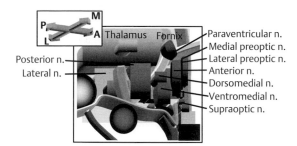

A.J. Sabbagh MD

Fig. 1.27 Hypothalamic nuclei. A, anterior; L, lateral; M, medial; n, nucleus; P, posterior. (Reproduced with permission from Nader and Sabbagh.[21])

87. Which part of the hypothalamus acts to lower the body temperature?

The anterior part. Stimulation of this area causes dilatation of the blood vessels and sweating, which lower body temperature (**Fig. 1.27**).[26]

88. Where does the corticospinal tract originate?

The corticospinal tract originates from layer V of the cerebral cortex. It passes through the corona radiata and posterior limb of the internal capsule. This tract then runs in the cerebral peduncles and the pyramids of the medulla; it terminates at lamina VII in the spinal cord.[35]

89. What makes up the inferior parietal lobule?

The angular and supramarginal gyri. The parietal lobe is divided into superior and inferior parietal lobules by the interparietal sulcus.

90. Damage to which part of the brain causes prosopagnosia?

The temporal association cortex. Prosopagnosia is the inability to recognize familiar faces; it is caused by the impairment of pathways involved in visual processing. The patients usually can still recognize the voice of their family and friends as the auditory pathways are not affected.[38]

91. What makes up the inferior frontal gyrus?

The pars orbitalis, pars opercularis, and pars triangularis.

92. What is the Papez circuit of the brain?

This pathway was described by James Papez in 1937. He injected the rabies virus into a cat's hippocampus and followed its progress through the brain. This circuit is one of the major pathways of the limbic system; it is mainly involved in the cortical control of emotions and storage of memories. The initial pathway was hippocampus → fornix → mammillary bodies → mammillothalamic tract → anterior thalamic nucleus → cingulate gyrus → parahippocampal gyrus → entorhinal gyrus → hippocampus (**Fig. 1.28**).[33]

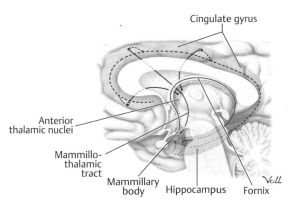

Fig. 1.28 Papez's circuit. (Reproduced with permission from Schuenke et al. Illustration by Markus Voll.[2])

93. Afferent fibers of the pupillary light reflex cross to the contralateral Edinger-Westphal nucleus via which structure?

The posterior commissure.

94. Sensation from the face is received by which thalamic nucleus?

Ventroposteromedial (VPM) nucleus. The ventroposterolateral (VPL) nucleus receives sensory input from the body (**Fig. 1.29**).[35]

95. Which layer of the cerebral cortex receives the thalamocortical afferents?

Layer IV (the internal granular layer) is the principal receiving station of the cerebral cortex (**Fig. 1.30**).[35]

96. Which layer of the cerebral cortex has the main efferent neurons?

Layer V (the internal pyramidal layer). This layer contains pyramidal cells that send their axons through the white matter to the internal capsule. The efferent corticothalamic fibers originate from layer VI (**Fig. 1.30**).[35]

97. What are the layers of the cerebral neocortex?

It is divided into six layers. Layer I, the molecular layer, is the most superficial layer and is primarily a synaptic area. Layer II, the external granular layer, is characterized by an abundance of densely packed neurons whose dendrites project to layer I and whose axons project to deeper layers. Layer III, the external pyramidal layer, has medium-sized pyramidal cells and granule cells. Layer IV, the internal granular layer, is the primary receiving station of the cerebral cortex. Layer V, the internal pyramidal layer, contains pyramidal cells that send their axons to the internal capsule. Layer VI, the fusiform layer, contains fusiform and pyramidal cells, which are the primary origin of the corticothalamic fibers (**Fig. 1.30**).

98. What is the reason for macular sparing in occipital cortex lesions?

Macular sparing is due to the dual blood supply from middle cerebral and posterior cerebral arteries to the occipital poles.

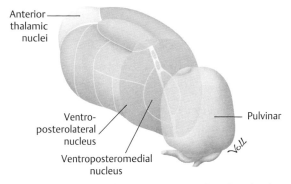

Fig. 1.29 Thalamic nuclear organization. (Reproduced with permission from Schuenke et al. Illustration by Markus Voll.[2])

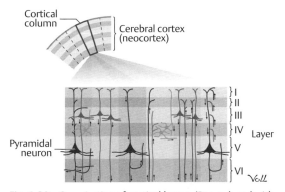

Fig. 1.30 Organization of cortical layers. (Reproduced with permission from Schuenke et al. Illustration by Markus Voll.[2])

99. The occipital (striate) cortex has dominance columns, except in which two regions?

1. The region where the blind spot is located.
2. The cortical region representing the monocular temporal crescent of both eyes.

■ Cerebellum

100. How many cortical layers does the cerebellum have?

Unlike the cerebral cortex, the cerebellar cortex has three layers (**Fig. 1.31**).[24] They are:

1. Molecular (most superficial).
2. Purkinje.
3. Granular.

101. Which cells give rise to the only output of the cerebellar cortex?

Purkinje cells. Their signal is inhibitory (**Fig. 1.31**).[39] Purkinje cells are some of the largest neurons in the human brain with numerous dendritic spines. Purkinje cells send inhibitory (GABAergic) projections to the deep cerebellar nuclei and constitute the sole output of all motor coordination in the cerebral cortex.

102. What do the cerebellar glomeruli consist of?

Synaptic connections consisting of mossy fiber rosettes, axons of Golgi type II neurons, and dendrites of granule cells. The mossy fibers stimulate the granule cells, whereas the Golgi type II cells inhibit them (**Fig. 1.31**).[39]

103. Where do climbing fibers originate from?

The contralateral inferior olive. These olivocerebellar fibers cross to the inferior cerebellar peduncle and ascend to the molecular layer, where they directly stimulate the dendrites of Purkinje cells. They are excitatory and use glutamate as their transmitter (**Fig. 1.31**).[39]

104. Which cerebellar peduncle contains only afferent fibers?

The middle cerebellar peduncle. The superior and inferior cerebellar peduncles contain both afferent and efferent fibers (**Fig. 1.32**).[15]

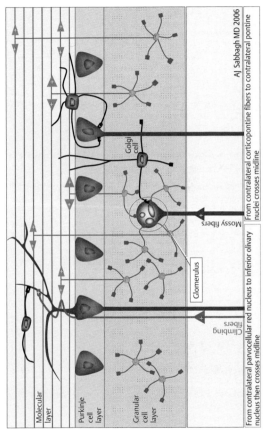

Fig. 1.31 Connections of the cerebellar cortex.

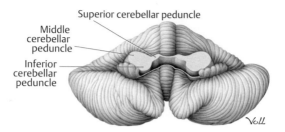

Fig. 1.32 Cerebellum, superior view. (Reproduced with permission from Schuenke et al. Illustration by Markus Voll.[2])

105. What are the middle cerebellar peduncle and the superior cerebellar peduncle also called?

Brachium pontis and brachium conjunctiva, respectively.[24]

106. What is the other name of the inferior cerebellar peduncle?

Restiform body.[24]

107. What is the only afferent tract that runs through the superior cerebellar peduncle?

The ventral spinocerebellar tract. The superior cerebellar peduncle consists mostly of efferent fibers from the cerebellum; however, it also contains this one afferent tract, which carries proprioceptive information to the cerebellum from the lower extremities and trunk.[39]

■ **Brainstem**

108. What are the second-order neurons of the olfactory pathway?

Mitral cells that project to the lateral olfactory area and the tufted cells that project to the lateral, intermediate, and medial olfactory areas. These neurons are located in the olfactory bulb.[40]

109. What syndrome can be caused by a pineal region tumor?

Parinaud's syndrome. This consists of upper gaze palsy, dissociated light-near response, retraction nystagmus, and an absence of convergence.[41]

110. What is Weber's syndrome?

CN III palsy and contralateral hemiparesis. This is due to an infarct in the medial midbrain (**Fig. 1.33**).[42]

111. Where is the lesion located in Millard-Gubler syndrome?

At the base of the pons. This syndrome includes VII and VI nerve palsy and contralateral hemiplegia (**Fig. 1.34**).[43]

112. What is the function of the red nucleus?

Maintains flexor muscle tone (**Fig. 1.33**).[34]

113. What is the input of the red nucleus?

The deep cerebellar nuclei and the cerebral cortex. The dentate nuclei and the interposed nuclei of the cerebellum send fibers via the superior cerebellar peduncle that cross to the contralateral side of the midbrain to reach the red nucleus. The motor, premotor, and supplementary motor cortices send fibers to the red nucleus (**Fig. 1.35**).[34]

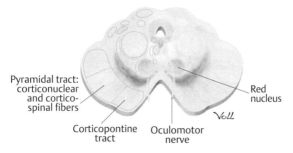

Fig. 1.33 Midbrain cross-section. (Reproduced with permission from Schuenke et al. Illustration by Markus Voll.[2])

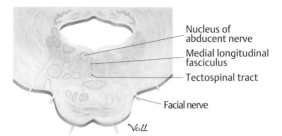

Fig. 1.34 Lower pons cross-section. (Reproduced with permission from Schuenke et al. Illustration by Markus Voll.[2])

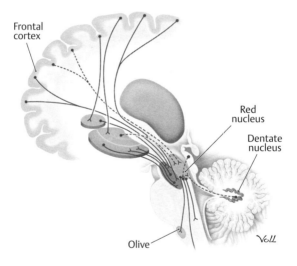

Fig. 1.35 Red nucleus afferents and efferents. (Reproduced with permission from Schuenke et al. Illustration by Markus Voll.[2])

114. What are the internal arcuate fibers?

The crossing fibers of the dorsal column fibers. The dorsal columns (gracile fasciculus and cuneate fasciculus) terminate in the medulla where they synapse in the gracile and cuneate nuclei. Axons from these nuclei then migrate ventrally around the central gray matter of the medulla and cross the midline. These crossing fibers are the internal arcuate fibers. These fibers then ascend as the medial lemniscus to reach the VPL of the thalamus (**Fig. 1.36**).

115. Where is the vertical gaze center located?

The rostral interstitial nucleus on the medial longitudinal fasciculus.

116. Crossed nasal retinal visual fibers go to which layer(s) of the LGN?

Layers I, IV, and VI. Fibers from the ipsilateral temporal hemiretina synapse in layers II, III, and V.[27]

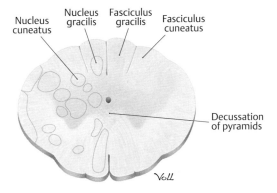

Fig. 1.36 Lower medulla oblongata cross-section. (Reproduced with permission from Schuenke et al. Illustration by Markus Voll.[2])

117. Which trigeminal nucleus receives pain and temperature sensation from the face?

The spinal trigeminal nucleus. This nucleus extends from the pons to C2 and merges caudally with the substantia gelatinosa. This nucleus also receives input from CNs VII, IX, and X (**Fig. 1.37**).[44]

118. Which trigeminal nucleus receives proprioception from the face?

The mesencephalic nucleus (**Fig. 1.37**).[44] Neurons of this nucleus are unipolar cells that receive proprioceptive information from the mandible and send projections to the trigeminal motor nucleus to mediate monosynaptic jaw jerk reflexes.

119. What does the lateral lemniscus carry?

The lateral lemniscus is the second-order neuron of the auditory pathway. It ascends in the brainstem to the inferior colliculus. A lesion of the lateral lemniscus results in partial bilateral deafness.[44]

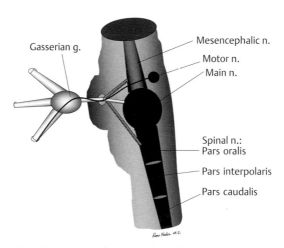

Fig. 1.37 Trigeminal nerve nuclei and functions. g, ganglion; n, nucleus. (Reproduced with permission from Nader and Sabbagh.[21])

120. Sensation from the external auditory canal that is carried by the vagus nerve arrives at which nucleus?

Sensation from the external auditory canal travels via Arnold's nerve to the superior (jugular) ganglion of CN X and then to the spinal trigeminal tract to arrive at the spinal trigeminal nucleus.[44]

121. General visceral sensation of the vagus nerve from the trachea, lungs, heart, stomach, and thoracoabdominal viscera arrives at which nucleus?

GVA (general visceral afferent) sensation as well as SVA (special visceral afferent) sensation of the vagus nerve travels to the inferior ganglion of X (nodose ganglion) and then to the solitary tract to arrive at the nucleus of the solitary tract in the medulla. The solitary nucleus also receives fibers from CNs VII and IX.[44]

■ Cranial Nerves

122. Which CN is most susceptible during carotid endarterectomy?

The hypoglossal nerve (XII). This can result in fasciculations on the tongue and paralysis of the affected side. When the patient sticks the tongue out, the tongue will deviate toward the affected side. The most common complication immediately after carotid endarterectomy surgery is hematoma in the wound bed.

123. What is the only sensory modality that reaches the cortex without being relayed from the thalamus?

Olfaction.

124. What does hypoglossal nerve palsy suggest in the setting of a skull base tumor?

Hypoglossal nerve palsy may be a manifestation of tumor infiltration into the anterior portion of the ipsilateral occipital condyle.

125. What location of the optic chiasm is the normal anatomic location? Prefixed? Postfixed?

The optic chiasm is usually located above the diaphragma sellae, but it may be prefixed and lie over the tuberculum sellae, or postfixed and lie over the dorsum sellae.[45]

126. Which CNs carry general visceral efferent fibers?

CNs III, VII, IX, and X.[44]

127. Where does the trochlear nerve decussate?

Within the superior medullary velum.[44]

128. What triggers a glossopharyngeal neuralgia "attack"?

Swallowing, talking, or chewing.

129. What is Hering's nerve?

A branch of CN IX that is the sensory limb of the carotid body. When a chemoreceptor detects changes in blood O_2 and CO_2 concentration, Hering's nerve is stimulated.[44] Heinrich Ewald Hering (1866–1948) was a German physiologist best known for his study of the reflex that initiates expiration.

130. What nerve supplies the digastric muscle?

This muscle has a dual innervation. The anterior belly of the digastric is innervated by CN V, whereas the posterior belly of the digastric muscle is innervated by CN VII.[1]

131. Which CNs pass through the foramen magnum?

The accessory nerve is the only CN that passes through the foramen magnum (**Fig. 1.13**).[44]

132. What are the symptoms of a unilateral vagal injury?

Hoarseness, dyspnea, dysphagia, ipsilateral decreased cough reflex (afferent), and uvular deviation to the normal side.

133. What does the hypoglossal nerve innervate?

All of the intrinsic and the extrinsic muscles of the tongue, except for the palatoglossus muscle, which is innervated by CN X.[44]

134. Which CN is most often involved with tumors of the upper cervical canal?

The spinal accessory nerve. Dysfunction of CN XI may manifest as torticollis and weakness of the trapezius and sternocleidomastoid muscles.

Spine and Peripheral Nerve

135. What is the largest avascular organ in the body?

The intervertebral disk.[46]

136. What is a zygapophyseal joint?

Another name for a facet joint in the spine.[46]

137. What is the most common dermatome syndrome seen with craniocervical diseases?

C2.

138. Where does the pyramidal decussation begin and where does it complete the decussation?

The pyramidal decussation begins just below the obex and is not completed until some distance below the exit of the first cervical nerve root (**Fig. 1.38**).[40]

139. Which spinal tract is compromised in a foramen magnum tumor presenting with hand weakness?

The cortical spinal tract (**Fig. 1.39**).[47]

140. What is the significance of an enlarged intervertebral foramen on radiography?

It may suggest a nerve root tumor.[48]

141. What ligament is important to divide for proper visualization of a ventral spinal tumor after dural opening in a posterior approach?

The dentate ligament.

142. At what cervical levels are the hyoid bone, the thyroid cartilage, and the cricoid?

The hyoid bone is at the level of C3, the thyroid cartilage is at C4–C5, and the cricoid is opposite C6.[49]

143. Perioral tingling and numbness in syringobulbia is due to compression of which tract?

The spinal trigeminal tract.

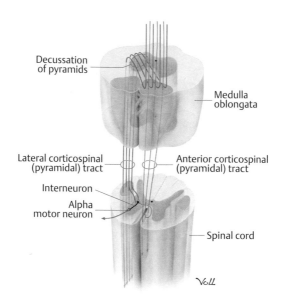

Fig. 1.38 Pyramidal tract and decussation in the medulla. (Reproduced with permission from Schuenke et al. Illustration by Markus Voll.[2])

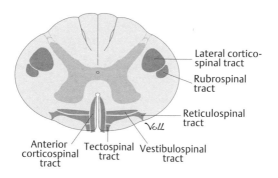

Fig. 1.39 Descending spinal cord tracts. (Reproduced with permission from Schuenke et al. Illustration by Markus Voll.[2])

144. At what level is the line drawn from one scapula tip to another when the patient is positioned prone?

T7. This is a simple technique to use because this area can be difficult to X-ray intraoperatively.[50]

145. What is a possible neuroanatomical reason why a dorsal rhizotomy may fail to relieve pain and why a dorsal root ganglionectomy may be more effective?

There may be a few nociceptive fibers that come into the cord by way of the ventral horn to terminate on the superficial layers of the dorsal horn. These aberrant fibers do not traverse the dorsal root, but do synapse in the dorsal root ganglion.[51]

146. Which ligament is the primary restraint against atlantoaxial anteroposterior translation?

The transverse ligament (**Fig. 1.40**).[49]

147. What is the caudalis portion of the spinal trigeminal tract?

It is an extension of the dorsal root entry zone and substantia gelatinosa of the trigeminal system into the lower medullary and high cervical regions.[40]

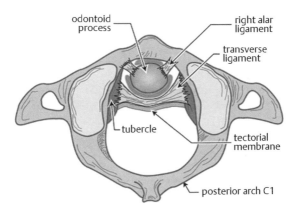

Fig. 1.40 Superior view of axis and atlas showing transverse. (Reproduced with permission from Greenberg.[16])

148. What supplies the sympathetic innervation to the arm?

The T2 and T3 ganglia.[40]

149. What is the spinal homologue of the spinal trigeminal nucleus?

The spinal dorsal horn.[46]

150. What is the other name of the dorsal ramus of the C1 nerve root?

The suboccipital nerve.[46]

151. What innervates the cervical disk?

A plexus formed by the sinuvertebral nerve dorsally and a plexus formed by the cervical sympathetic trunk ventrally.[46] Nociceptive information from cervical disks enters the trigeminothalamic tract in the upper cervical spine and may be a contributory factor in patients with cervicogenic headaches.

152. Where is the aortic bifurcation usually located?

At the midbody of L3. Anterior approaches to the lumbar spine should take into account the locations of the large vessels.

153. At what level does the spinal cord end in adults?

Between L1 and L2 (**Fig. 1.41**).[46]

154. What does a positive Babinski sign indicate?

Upper motor neuron damage.[52]

155. Loss of sensation over the webspace between the first and second toes is associated with what injury?

Injury to the deep peroneal (fibular) nerve.[52]

156. What nerve root is damaged when there is a loss of the Achilles' reflex?

S1 nerve root.[52]

157. What nerve roots are involved in the biceps reflex?

C5 and C6.[53]

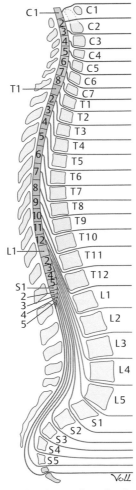

Fig. 1.41 Spinal cord in the spinal canal with segmental distribution. (Reproduced with permission from Schuenke et al. Illustration by Markus Voll.[2])

158. The L5 nerve root is associated with which reflex?

None.[52]

159. Where do the pain and temperature first-order neurons synapse in the spinal cord?

The first-order neurons have small, finely myelinated axons whose bodies are in the dorsal root ganglion. These afferents enter the cord at the dorsolateral tract (zone of Lissauer) and synapse in the substantia gelatinosa (Rexed II).

160. What are the radiographic findings in acute transverse myelitis?

Radiographic findings are usually normal, possibly with increased signal on T2-weighted magnetic resonance sequences.[54]

161. What is Pott's disease?

Tuberculous vertebral osteomyelitis. This infection, unlike most others, affects the body rather than the disks primarily.[55]

162. What are some radiographic findings that can help distinguish infection from tumor in the spine?

A characteristic radiographic finding is that destruction of the disk space is highly suggestive of infection, whereas in general the tumor will affect primarily the body and will not cross the disk space.[55]

163. What are the two most common herniated lumbar disks?

L4–L5 and L5–S1 herniated lumbar disks account for most cases (95%).[56] The reason is that the body's center of gravity is applied to the lumbar curvature.

164. What part of the intervertebral disk is an immunologically privileged site?

The nucleus pulposus is isolated from the vascular and immune systems by the anulus fibrosus and cartilaginous end plates (**Fig. 1.42**).

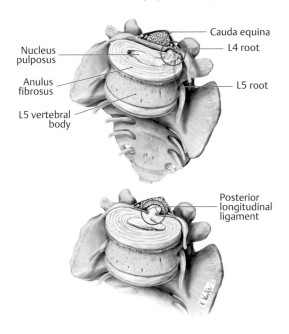

Fig. 1.42 Cross-section of intervertebral disk. (Reproduced with permission from Schuenke et al. Illustration by Karl Wesker.[2])

165. What is the unique feature of a far lateral disk herniation?

Unlike the usual disk herniation, a far lateral disk herniation impinges against the upper nerve root: an L4–L5 far lateral disk herniation will produce an L4 nerve root radiculopathy.[56]

166. What is Spurling's sign?

This is radicular pain reproduced when the examiner exerts downward pressure on the vertex while tilting the head toward the symptomatic side. This causes narrowing of the intervertebral foramen and reproduces the symptoms. This test is analogous to the straight leg raising test for lumbar disk herniation.[53] In cervical stenosis, it can be diagnostic of cervicogenic headache if it reproduces the headache.

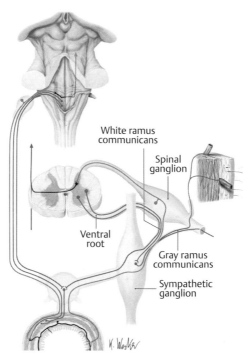

Fig. 1.43 Autonomic nervous system organization. (Reproduced with permission from Schuenke et al. Illustration by Karl Wesker.[2])

167. How do the sympathetic fibers exit the spinal cord?

Via the ventral roots by way of the white rami communicantes (**Fig. 1.43**).[46]

168. Where is the sensory loss in an axillary nerve injury?

In the lateral aspect of the shoulder.[53]

169. What are the symptoms of posterior interosseous neuropathy?

Finger extension weakness including the thumb with no wrist drop or sensory loss. The posterior interosseous nerve

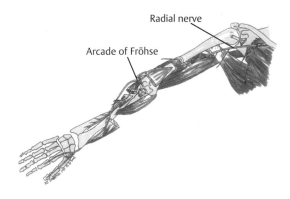

Fig. 1.44 Radial nerve anatomy and sites of entrapment.

may be entrapped at the arcade of Fröhse, which is a fibrous band that the nerve goes through when it dives into the supinator muscle (**Fig. 1.44**).[53]

170. What is meralgia paresthetica?

Also called Bernhardt-Roth syndrome, this is entrapment of the lateral femoral cutaneous nerve of the thigh. This nerve arises from L2 and L3 and enters the thigh between the inguinal ligament and the anterior superior iliac spine. This is a purely sensory nerve, and compression causes burning dysesthesia in the lateral aspect of the upper thigh.[52]

171. Which muscle of the thumb has a dual innervation?

The flexor pollicis brevis has a dual innervation by the median and ulnar nerves.[53]

172. Where is the site of entrapment of the suprascapular nerve?

Within the suprascapular notch beneath the transverse scapular ligament. Entrapment results in atrophy of the infra- and supraspinatus muscles as well as deep, poorly localized shoulder pain. This is due to the fact that this nerve carries sensation from the posterior joint capsule, but has no cutaneous representation (**Fig. 1.45**).[53]

173. Which nerve roots are usually affected in true neurogenic thoracic outlet syndrome?

The C8 and T1 nerve roots. Thoracic outlet syndrome is most commonly due to a cervical rib or an elongated C7 transverse process (**Fig. 1.45**).

174. What are the symptoms of the anterior interosseous syndrome?

Weakness of flexion of distal phalanges of the thumb (flexor pollicis longus) and index and middle fingers (flexor digitorum profundus 1 and 2). This gives the characteristic "pinch sign." In trying to pinch the tips of the index finger and thumb, the pulps touch instead of the tips. There is no sensory loss as this is a pure motor branch of the median nerve (**Fig. 1.46**).[53]

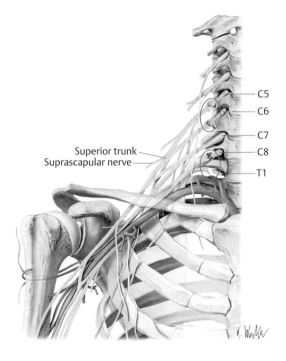

C5
C6
C7
C8
T1

Superior trunk
Suprascapular nerve

Fig. 1.45 Brachial plexus anatomy, anterior view. (Reproduced with permission from Schuenke et al. Illustration by Karl Wesker.[2])

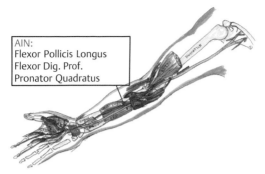

AIN:
Flexor Pollicis Longus
Flexor Dig. Prof.
Pronator Quadratus

Fig. 1.46 Median nerve anatomy and sites of entrapment. AIN, anterior interosseus nerve. (Reproduced with permission from Nader and Sabbagh.[21])

175. What toxicity must be ruled out in a patient with wrist drop?

Lead poisoning.

176. What is the difference between nociceptive pain and neuropathic pain?

Nociceptors are the nerves that sense and respond to parts of the body that suffer from damage. They signal tissue irritation, impending injury, or actual injury. When activated, they transmit pain signals (via the peripheral nerves as well as the spinal cord) to the brain. The pain is typically well localized and constant and often has an aching or throbbing quality. Visceral pain is the subtype of nociceptive pain that involves the internal organs. It tends to be episodic and poorly localized. ociceptive pain is usually time limited, meaning when the tissue damage heals, the pain typically resolves. Another characteristic of nociceptive pain is that it tends to respond well to treatment with opioids. Neuropathic pain, typically long lasting, recurrent, and lancinating in nature, is the result of an injury or malfunction in the peripheral or central nervous system. The pain is often triggered by an injury, but this injury may or may not involve actual damage to the nervous system. Nerves can be infiltrated or compressed by tumors, strangulated by scar tissue, or inflamed by infection. The pain frequently has burning, lancinating, or electric shock qualities.

177. What makes the extensor carpi radialis muscle unique?

It is innervated solely by the C6 nerve root.[53]

178. Where is the ligament of Struthers, what nerve may it compress, and what syndrome can compression of this nerve mimic?

The ligament of Struthers is present in a small percentage of the population and is found crossing the cubital fossa above the medial intermuscular septum. In this area, it may cause compression of the median nerve, which can mimic carpal tunnel syndrome. In cases of median nerve compression by the ligament of Struthers, thenar numbness is more pronounced than in carpal tunnel syndrome (where the palmar cutaneous branch is spared) (**Fig. 1.46**).[57]

179. Where is the arcade of Struthers, and what nerve may it compress?

The arcade of Struthers is located at the elbow near the medial head of the triceps. It may compress the ulnar nerve at this location. It is important in ulnar nerve transposition that the arcade of Struthers, when present, is released to prevent kinking of the ulnar nerve (**Fig. 1.47**).[57]

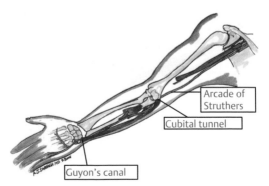

Arcade of Struthers

Cubital tunnel

Guyon's canal

Fig. 1.47 Ulnar nerve anatomy and sites of entrapment.

Cases

■ Case 1

A 70-year-old woman presents with mild intermittent headaches and double vision. Evaluation with magnetic resonance imaging (MRI) and angiogram demonstrates the lesion shown in **Fig. 1.48**. What is the diagnosis? What nerves are causing the double vision and why?

■ Case 1 Answer

This is a cavernous carotid artery aneurysm. The contents of the cavernous sinus include CNs III, IV, and V; CNs V1 and V2 are in the lateral wall of the cavernous sinus. The double vision would be related to dysfunction of CNs III, IV, and VI. These lesions have a low risk of hemorrhage, and when they do hemorrhage, it is extradural. Hemorrhage may also cause a carotid cavernous fistula.

■ Case 2

A 20-year-old man presents with the MRI in **Fig. 1.49**. He complains of difficulty looking up and blurriness in his vision. What is the likely diagnosis?

■ Case 2 Answer

A pineal region tumor. The most common tumor type in this area is a germ cell tumor, usually germinoma. Other tumor types that may present here include pineocytoma, pineoblastoma, and astrocytoma. CSF should be checked for alpha fetoprotein (AFP) found in embryonal carcinoma, endodermal sinus tumor, and teratoma. Beta human chorionic gonadotropin (HCG) can be found in choriocarcinoma and also in germinoma. Parinaud's syndrome is caused by pressure on the superior colliculus causing impaired upward gaze, lid retraction, dissociated near-light response (reaction to accommodation but not light), and pupillary dilatation. Hydrocephalus may be caused by pressure on the aqueduct. Hydrocephalus from a lesion in this area can be treated with a third ventriculostomy procedure preventing the need for shunt placement. Treatment often consists of resection; however, germinomas are quite sensitive to radiation and chemotherapy.

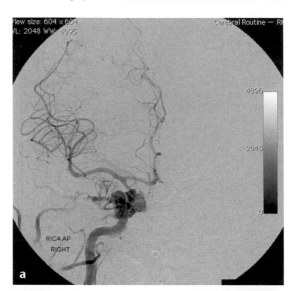

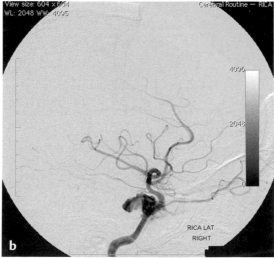

Fig. 1.48 Right carotid angiogram. AP **(a)** and lateral **(b)** views. (Courtesy of Nazih N.A. Assaad, MBBS (Hons), FRACS.)

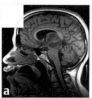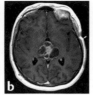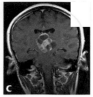

Fig. 1.49   MRI of the brain. T1-weighted images with contrast; sagittal (a), axial (b), and coronal (c) cuts.

■ Case 3

A 50-year-old left-handed patient has a lesion in the location shown in **Fig. 1.50**. What classic deficits might he present with and what would be the name of the syndrome?

■ Case 3 Answer

The patient has Gerstmann's syndrome, which is found in dominant parietal lobe lesions. Clinical findings include acalculia, agraphia without alexia, right–left confusion, and finger agnosia.

■ Case 4

A 55-year-old woman presents with severe pain extending across the buttock down toward the knee anteriorly toward the medial ankle. The MRI scan is provided in **Fig. 1.51**. What nerve root is involved? Why is the location of this disk causing symptoms in an unusual nerve root distribution?

■ Case 4 Answer

This is an extreme lateral L4–L5 disk herniation. Most disk herniations are in the paracentral region where there is a weak spot in the posterior longitudinal ligament. This tends to cause an L5 nerve root-type deficit at the L4–L5 level. Extreme lateral disk herniations impinge upon the descending nerve root either at the level of the foramen or distal to it; therefore, the L4 nerve root would be involved in this case.

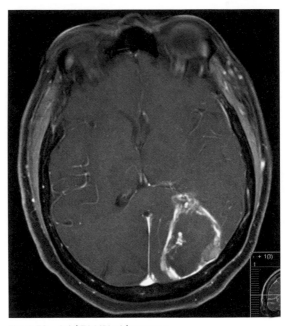

Fig. 1.50 Axial T1 MRI with contrast.

■ Case 5

A 35-year-old woman following chiropractic manipulation presents with sudden onset of severe neck pain with an ipsilateral small pupil and a drooping eyelid. An angiogram is obtained (**Fig. 1.52**). What is the differential diagnosis?

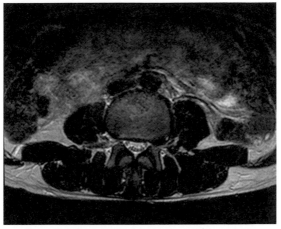

Fig. 1.51 Axial T2-weighted image revealing pathology in the left lateral recess at L4–L5.

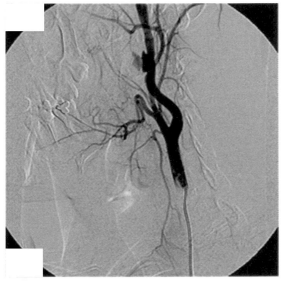

Fig. 1.52 Angiogram. Lateral view, carotid injection.

■ Case 5 Answer

An ICA dissection. This tends to cause neck pain as well as
oculosympathetic Horner's syndrome (sweat fibers travel with the ECA and usually are not affected). Horner's
syndrome causes ptosis, miosis, and anhydrosis. There will
not be anhydrosis in this case due to the location of the
dissection (third-order neuron). Anhydrosis only occurs in
first-order neuron lesions. It may also cause a CN XII deficit
and a transient ischemic attack due to embolism or occlusion, and possibly a subarachnoid hemorrhage if it enters
the dural space. The angiogram classically shows the string
sign or a double lumen. It is associated with fibromuscular
dysplasia, cystic medial necrosis, Ehlers-Danlos syndrome,
Marfan's syndrome, and syphilis. Treatment is anticoagulation therapy unless symptoms are progressing; direct surgical repair with stenting or bypass may be required. Always
caution your patients about chiropractic manipulation of
the cervical spine.

■ References

1. Standring S, Berkovitz BKB, Hacney CM. Head and neck. In: Standring S, ed. Gray's Anatomy: The Anatomical Basis of Clinical
   Practice. 39th ed. Philadelphia, PA: Elsevier; 2004:497–515
2. Schuenke M, Schulte E, Schumacher U, et al. Thieme Atlas of
   Anatomy: Head and Neuroanatomy. New York, NY: Thieme
   Medical Publishers; 2007
3. Johnson D, Shah P. Major blood vessels. In: Standring S, ed.
   Gray's Anatomy: The Anatomical Basis of Clinical Practice. 39th
   ed. Philadelphia, PA: Elsevier; 2004:1020–1025
4. Standring S, Crossman AR. Vascular supply of the brain. In:
   Standring S, ed. Gray's Anatomy: The Anatomical Basis of Clinical Practice. 39th ed. Philadelphia, PA: Elsevier; 2004:295–304
5. Rhoton AL Jr. The cavernous sinus, the cavernous venous
   plexus, and the carotid collar. Neurosurgery 2002;51(4, suppl):S375–S410
6. Rhoton AL Jr. The cerebral veins. Neurosurgery 2002;51(4, suppl):S159–S205
7. Fu EX, Kosmorsky GS, Traboulsi EI. Giant intracavernous carotid
   aneurysm presenting as isolated sixth nerve palsy in an infant.
   Br J Ophthalmol 2008;92(4):576–577
8. Rohkamm R. Brain stem syndromes. In: Color Atlas of Neurology.
   Stuttgart: Georg Thieme Verlag; 2004:70–73
9. Mumenthaler M, Mattle H. Neurology. Stuttgart: Georg Thieme
   Verlag; 2005

10. Rhoton AL Jr. The supratentorial arteries. Neurosurgery 2002;51(4, suppl):S53–S120

11. Rohkamm R. Color Atlas of Neurology. Stuttgart: Georg Thieme Verlag; 2004:186

12. Koos W, Spetzler R, Lang J. Color Atlas of Microneurosurgery: Microanatomy, Approaches and Techniques. New York, NY: Thieme Medical Publishers; 1993

13. Ropper AH, Brown RH. Hemifacial spasm. In: Adams and Victor's Principles of Neurology. 8th ed. New York, NY: McGraw-Hill; 2005:1184

14. Lister JR, Rhoton AL Jr, Matsushima T, Peace DA. Microsurgical anatomy of the posterior inferior cerebellar artery. Neurosurgery 1982;10(2):170–199

15. Rhoton AL Jr. The cerebellar arteries. Neurosurgery 2000;47(3, suppl):S29–S68

16. Greenberg MS. Handbook of Neurosurgery. 6th ed. Stuttgart: Georg Thieme Verlag; 2006:69–71

17. Rhoton AL Jr. The foramen magnum. Neurosurgery 2000;47(3, suppl):S155–S193

18. Rhoton AL Jr. Jugular foramen. Neurosurgery 2000;47(3, suppl):S267–S285

19. Rhoton AL Jr, Tedeschi H. Microsurgical anatomy of acoustic neuroma. Otolaryngol Clin North Am 1992;25(2):257–294

20. Rhoton AL Jr. The orbit. Neurosurgery 2002;51(4, suppl):S303–S334

21. Nader R, Sabbagh AJ. Neurosurgery Case Review: Questions and Answers. New York, NY: Thieme Medical Publishers; 2010

22. Rhoton AL Jr. The temporal bone and transtemporal approaches. Neurosurgery 2000;47(3, suppl):S211–S265

23. Rhoton AL Jr. The lateral and third ventricles. Neurosurgery 2002;51(4, suppl):S207–S271

24. Rhoton AL Jr. Cerebellum and fourth ventricle. Neurosurgery 2000;47(3, suppl):S7–S27

25. Lü J, Zhu XI. Microsurgical anatomy of Liliequist's membrane. Minim Invasive Neurosurg 2003;46(3):149–154

26. Jacobson S, Marcus EM. Hypothalamus, neuroendocrine system, and autonomic nervous system. In: Neuroanatomy for the Neuroscientist. New York, NY: Springer; 2008:165–188

27. Jacobson S, Marcus E. Diencephalon. In: Neuroanatomy for the Neuroscientist. New York, NY: Springer; 2008:147–164

28. Jacobson S, Marcus E. Neurotransmitters. In: Neuroanatomy for the Neuroscientist. New York, NY: Springer; 2008:39–41

29. Monkhouse S. The facial nerve. In: Cranial Nerves: Functional Anatomy. Cambridge: Cambridge University Press; 2006:66–71

30. Monkhouse S. Swallowing and speaking, bulbar palsy, pseudobulbar palsy, Broca's area. In: Cranial Nerves: Functional Anatomy. Cambridge: Cambridge University Press; 2006:77–94

31. Greenberg M. CSF. In: Handbook of Neurosurgery. 6th ed. Stuttgart: Georg Thieme Verlag; 2006:171–179

32. Greenberg M. Cortical surface anatomy. In: Handbook of Neurosurgery. 6th ed. Stuttgart: Georg Thieme Verlag; 2006:68–69

33. Jacobson S, Marcus E. Limbic system, the temporal lobe, and prefrontal cortex. In: Neuroanatomy for the Neuroscientist. New York, NY: Springer; 2008:337–374

34. Standring S, Crossman AR. Basal ganglia. In: Standring S, ed. Gray's Anatomy: The Anatomical Basis of Clinical Practice. 39th ed. Philadelphia, PA: Elsevier; 2005:419–430

35. Jacobson S, Marcus E. Subcortical white matter afferents and efferents. In: Neuroanatomy for the Neuroscientist. New York, NY: Springer; 2008:212–216

36. Yeni SN, Tanriover N, Uyanik O, et al. Visual field defects in selective amygdalohippocampectomy for hippocampal sclerosis: the fate of Meyer's loop during the transsylvian approach to the temporal horn. Neurosurgery 2008;63(3):507–513, discussion 513–515

37. Ropper A. Gerstmann syndrome. In: Adams and Victor's Principles of Neurology. 8th ed. New York, NY: McGraw-Hill; 2005:402

38. Damasio AR, Damasio H, Van Hoesen GW. Prosopagnosia: anatomic basis and behavioral mechanisms. Neurology 1982;32(4):331–341

39. Jacobson S, Marcus E. Motor systems III: cerebellum and movement. In: Neuroanatomy for the Neuroscientist. New York, NY: Springer; 2008:273–292

40. Jacobson S, Marcus E. Brain stem. In: Neuroanatomy for the Neuroscientist. New York, NY: Springer; 2008:85–120

41. Ropper A. Disorders of ocular movement and pupillary function. In: Adams and Victor's Principles of Neurology. 8th ed. New York, NY: McGraw-Hill; 2005:225

42. Ropper A. Cardinal manifestations of neurologic diseases. In: Adams and Victor's Principles of Neurology. 8th ed. New York, NY: McGraw-Hill; 2005:228

43. Ropper A. Motor paralysis. In: Adams and Victor's Principles of Neurology. 8th ed. New York, NY: McGraw-Hill; 2005:51

44. Jacobson S, Marcus E. Cranial nerves. In: Neuroanatomy for the Neuroscientist. New York, NY: Springer; 2008:121–146

45. Rhoton AL Jr. The sellar region. Neurosurgery 2002; 51(4, suppl):S335–S374

46. Waxman SG. The vertebral column and other structures surrounding the spinal cord. In: Clinical Neuroanatomy. 26th ed. New York, NY: McGraw-Hill; 2010:70–80

47. Meyer FB, Ebersold MJ, Reese DF. Benign tumors of the foramen magnum. J Neurosurg 1984;61(1):136–142

48. McCormick PC. Surgical management of dumbbell tumors of the cervical spine. Neurosurgery 1996;38(2):294–300

49. Standring S, Berkovitz B, Hacney C. Head and neck. In: Standring S, ed. Gray's Anatomy: The Anatomical Basis of Clinical Practice. 39th ed. Philadelphia, PA: Elsevier; 2005:497–515

50. Shaya MJ. Scapula tip. Neurosurgery 2007;101(1):203

51. Engsberg JR, Park TS. Selective dorsal rhizotomy. J Neurosurg Pediatr 2008;1(3):177, discussion 178–179

52. Russell SM. The lumbosacral anatomy of the lumbosacral plexus. In: Examination of Peripheral Nerve Injuries: An Anatomical Approach. New York, NY: Thieme Medical Publishers; 2006:150–163

53. Russell SM. The clinical evaluation of the brachial plexus. In: Examination of Peripheral Nerve Injuries: An Anatomical Approach. New York, NY: Thieme Medical Publishers; 2006:90–107

54. Westenfelder GO, Akey DT, Corwin SJ, Vick NA. Acute transverse myelitis due to Mycoplasma pneumoniae infection. Arch Neurol 1981;38(5):317–318

55. Ropper A. Infections of the nervous system. In: Adams and Victor's Principles of Neurology. 8th ed. New York, NY: McGraw-Hill; 2005:592–630

56. Leonardi M, Boos N. Disc herniation and radiculopathy. In: Boos N, Aebi M, eds. Spinal Disorders: Fundamentals of Diagnosis and Treatment. Berlin: Springer; 2008:481–512

57. Siqueira MG, Martins RS. The controversial arcade of Struthers. Surg Neurol 2005;64(suppl 1):S1, 17–20, discussion S1, 20–21

2 Neurophysiology

General

1. How does magnesium prevent excitotoxicity in brain injury?

Magnesium readily crosses the blood–brain barrier (BBB) and blocks various subtypes of calcium and N-methyl-d-aspartate (NMDA) channels.[1]

2. What is the most abundant excitatory neurotransmitter in the brain?

Glutamate.

3. What cellular elements compose the BBB?

Endothelial cells, astrocyte end-feet, and pericytes. The capillary endothelial cells are connected by tight junctions (**Fig. 2.1**).

4. What happens to platelet function after a subarachnoid hemorrhage?

It is enhanced, leading to an increase in platelet aggregates in the cerebral microcirculation.[3]

5. What happens to cerebral blood flow immediately after a subarachnoid hemorrhage?

Decreases.[3]

6. What is GPIIb/IIIa?

A platelet surface integrin, which is a mediator of platelet aggregation.

7. What is in the dense granules of platelets?

Serotonin, adenosine triphosphate (ATP), and platelet-derived growth factor.

8. It is thought that a disturbed balance between which peptide and molecule plays a major role in the development of vasospasm?

Endothelin-1 (vasoconstriction) and nitric oxide (vasodilatation).[3]

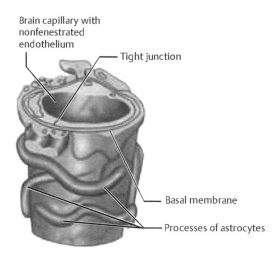

Brain capillary with nonfenestrated endothelium

Tight junction

Basal membrane

Processes of astrocytes

Blood–brain barrier (capillary)

Fig. 2.1 Blood–brain barrier showing capillary tight junction. (Reproduced with permission from Rohkamm.[2])

9. What is the name of the reaction that states that a highly reactive hydroxyl radical could be generated from an interaction between superoxide and hydrogen peroxide?

The Haber-Weiss reaction.[4]

10. What is deferoxamine?

An iron chelator. Because intracerebral hemorrhage may result in iron toxicity to the brain, iron chelation may help to reduce brain damage in these cases.[5]

11. What is the proposed mechanism of action of steroid treatment in blunt spinal cord injury?

Steroid treatment in blunt spinal cord injury is controversial. Steroids (when given within 8 hours of injury) are thought to have effects on local blood flow, inhibition of immunologic injury, and free radical–mediated lipid peroxidation and neuronal damage.[6]

12. What is S100B and how is it related to traumatic brain injury?

S100B is a protein belonging to a multigenic family of low-molecular-weight calcium-binding S100 proteins abundant in astrocytes. After traumatic brain injury, S100B protein is released by astrocytes; this protein may be neuroprotective and/or neurotrophic.[7]

13. What is factor XIII and in what diseases is it deficient?

Factor XIII is an enzyme (protransglutaminase) that stabilizes the fibrin clot and is important for cross-linking fibrin in the clotting cascade. It is deficient in leukemia, liver disease, malaria, inflammatory bowel disease, disseminated intravascular coagulopathy, and Henoch-Schönlein purpura (**Fig. 2.2**).

14. What is the (intracranial) Windkessel phenomenon?

The Windkessel phenomenon is the ability of the cerebral vasculature to expand and the ability of the cerebrospinal fluid (CSF) and venous blood to translocate to accommodate arterial pulsations and provide a smooth capillary flow in the brain.[9]

15. What is the ischemic penumbra?

The term *ischemic penumbra* has been used to define a region in which cerebral blood flow reduction has passed the threshold that leads to the failure of electrical but not membrane function. The neuron is functionally disturbed, but remains structurally intact.[10]

16. What is the role of infiltration with local anesthetic at the beginning of a case?

Infiltration with local anesthetic prevents the activation of nociceptors during surgery and substantially lessens the need for analgesic medication.[11]

17. Local anesthetic molecules are composed of a benzene ring and a quaternary amine separated by an intermediate chain. Which part of the molecule determines the metabolic pathway of the drug?

The intermediate chain.[11]

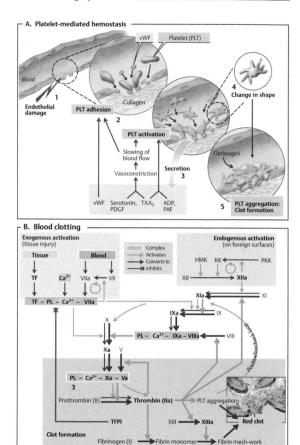

A. Platelet-mediated hemostasis

B. Blood clotting

Fig. 2.2 Outline of blood clotting cascade. (Reproduced with permission from Silbernagl and Despopoulos.[8])

18. What is the structural unit of a gap junction?

The connexon is a proteinaceous cylinder with a hydrophilic channel and is the structural unit of the gap junction. Direct electrical communication between cells occurs through gap junctions and may be important in the pathogenesis of diseases of the nervous system including epilepsy (**Fig. 2.3**).[12]

19. What are the functions of transforming growth factor β (TGF-β)?

TGF-β is a multifunctional polypeptide implicated in the regulation of various cellular processes including growth, differentiation, apoptosis, adhesion, and motility. Abnormalities in the TGF-β signaling pathway are implicated in the development and progression of brain tumors.

20. What enzyme is inhibited by acetazolamide?

Carbonic anhydrase.[13]

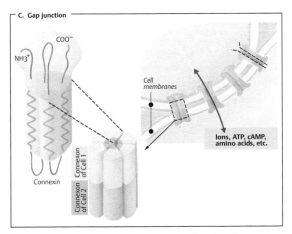

Fig. 2.3 Gap junction illustration. (Reproduced with permission from Silbernagl and Despopoulos.[8])

21. What is the difference between a bioactive Guglielmi detachable coil (GDC) and a platinum GDC?

The bioactive coil accelerates clot maturation and promotes the development of mature connective tissue and neointimal formation. The polymer used in bioactive coils is polyglycolic/poly-L-lactic acid.[14]

22. What are matrix metalloproteinases?

A family of zinc-dependent endopeptidases that mediate vascular remodeling by degrading extracellular matrix components, such as collagen and elastin.[15]

23. What is the causative mutation in Crouzon's syndrome?

Crouzon's syndrome is caused by mutations in fibroblast growth factor receptor 2 (FGFR2), leading to constitutive activation of receptors in the absence of ligand binding. This syndrome is characterized by premature fusion of the cranial sutures that leads to abnormal cranium shape, restricted brain growth, and increased intracranial pressure.

24. How does baclofen work?

Baclofen is an agonist of γ-aminobutyric acid (GABA); it reduces the release of presynaptic neurotransmitters in excitatory spinal pathways.

25. What is hypsarrhythmia?

A chaotic, high-amplitude, generalized electroencephalographic pattern characteristic of infantile spasms.[16]

26. What is "subsidence" in relation to the aging spine?

Subsidence is the loss of vertebral column height that occurs normally with aging; it may also refer to the loss of graft height after surgery. The use of dynamic plates allows normal subsidence to occur and may help bony fusion, resulting in decreased incidence of construct failures.

27. What is the genetic defect in Gorlin's syndrome?

Gorlin's syndrome is an autosomal dominant disorder resulting from mutations in the patched (PTCH) gene that predisposes to neoplasias and widespread congenital malformations.[17]

28. What is rFVIIa?

Recombinant activated factor VII can help to prevent bleeding episodes especially in hemophilic patients with inhibitors to coagulation factors VIII and IX. Administration of rFVIIa (off-label) given within 4 hours of a spontaneous intracranial hemorrhage can result in reduced hematoma growth and less intraventricular extension of the hematoma.

29. What is the name of the water channel proteins of the central nervous system (CNS), which provide a major pathway for osmotically driven water movement across plasma membranes?

Aquaporins are the water channel proteins of the brain. In normal brain, aquaporin 1 is expressed on the ventricle surface by the choroid plexus. The predominant water channel in normal brain is aquaporin 4, which is strongly expressed in the plasma membranes of astrocytes. Aquaporin proteins could be a therapeutic target for pharmacologic treatment of hydrocephalus.[18]

30. What is the most common agent used for the pharmacologic dilatation of vasospastic cerebral vessels?

Papaverine hydrochloride is a potent, nonspecific, endothelium-independent smooth muscle relaxant that produces dilatation of arteries and arterioles, as well as veins. Intra-arterial papaverine is usually administered superselectively via a microcatheter positioned proximal to the spastic vessel.

31. How do intervertebral disks receive their nutrition?

Intervertebral disks receive nutrition through passive diffusion from a network of capillary beds in the subchondral end plate region of the vertebral body.

32. What is the composition of a PEEK cage?

Polyetheretherketone (PEEK) spacers have a modulus of elasticity close to that of cortical bone. PEEK is a strong polymer that is able to withstand the compressive load of the vertebral column. Its hollow center allows for packing of autologous bone and/or demineralized bone matrix.[19]

33. What are common areas of leptomeningeal dissemination for tumors?

The most common areas of leptomeningeal dissemination of CNS tumors are the basilar cisterns, sylvian fissures, and cauda equina, most likely because of both gravity and slower rate of CSF flow in these areas.

34. What is the resting membrane potential in myelinated peripheral nerves and in the soma?

–90 mV and –65 mV, respectively. This membrane potential is largely determined by the potential of K^+, which is approximately100 times more permeable than Na^+.[20]

35. What is the mechanism of action of the botulinum toxin?

Botulinum toxin inhibits the release of acetylcholine from the presynaptic terminal and leads to loss of muscle activation (**Fig. 2.4**).

36. Where does the action potential in the neuron start?

At the axon hillock. This occurs because there are about seven times more voltage-gated Na^+ channels there, so it depolarizes much easier than the soma (**Fig. 2.5**).[20]

37. What factors determine the velocity of propagation of an action potential?

The velocity of an action potential is affected:

1. Inversely by internal resistance.
2. Inversely by membrane capacitance.
3. Proportionately by transmembrane resistance.
4. By myelin, which increases transmembrane resistance and decreases membrane capacitance.[22]

38. What is the conduction velocity of small unmyelinated nerves and large myelinated nerves?

About 0.5 and 120 m/s, respectively.[22]

39. How does hypocalcemia lead to tetany?

When there is less Ca^{2+} in the interstitial fluid, the Na^+ opens sooner (at about –80 mV), so the membrane is more excitable. In other words, hypocalcemia causes a lower threshold of membrane depolarization and action potential initiation.[23]

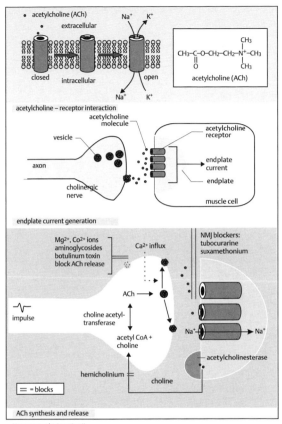

Neuromuscular junction II

Fig. 2.4 Acetylcholine receptor and modulators. (Reproduced with permission from Greenstein and Greenstein.[21])

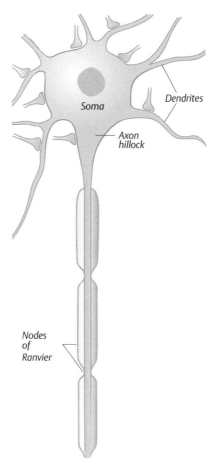

Fig. 2.5 Illustration of neuron with components. (Reproduced with permission from Silbernagl and Despopoulos.[8])

40. How can hyperventilation induce seizures?

Hyperventilation causes a respiratory alkalosis, which increases the pH. Increasing pH increases the membrane excitability and can induce seizures.

41. How big is the synaptic cleft?

20 to 30 nanometers (**Fig. 2.6**).[24]

42. What is unique about the synthesis of the neurotransmitter norepinephrine?

It is the only neurotransmitter that is synthesized within the synaptic vesicle. Dopamine α-hydroxylase is located on the membrane of the synaptic vesicle. This enzyme converts dopamine to norepinephrine (**Fig. 2.7**).[25]

43. What are the two types of acetylcholine receptors?

1. Nicotinic receptors—located in the neuromuscular junction and preganglionic endings of both sympathetic and parasympathetic fibers.
2. Muscarinic receptors—found in all postganglionic parasympathetic endings and the postganglionic sympathetic endings of sweat glands.

44. What are the two main inhibitory neurotransmitters of the CNS?

GABA and glycine.

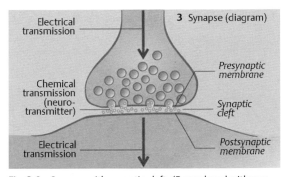

Fig. 2.6 Synapse with synaptic cleft. (Reproduced with permission from Silbernagl and Despopoulos.[8])

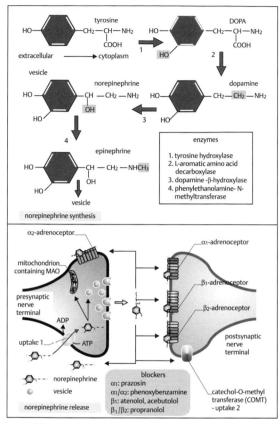

Catecholamine neurotransmitters

Fig. 2.7 Norepinephrine production from tyrosine (chemical steps). (Reproduced with permission from Greenstein and Greenstein.[21])

45. What is the mechanism of the GABA receptor?

The GABA receptor is made up of five subunits with a central Cl^- channel ($GABA_C$ receptor). This ligand-gated ion channel alters the Cl^- channel permeability and causes hyperpolarization (**Fig. 2.8**).

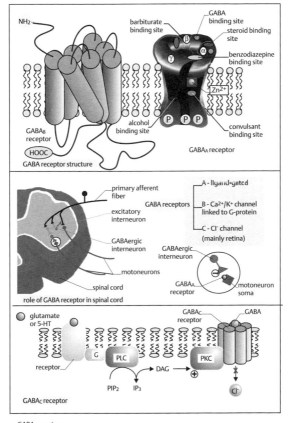

GABA receptors

Fig. 2.8 Illustration of $GABA_C$ receptor. (Reproduced with permission from Greenstein and Greenstein.[21])

46. Which body part has the largest area of representation in the primary somatosensory area (Brodmann's area 3, 1, 2)?

The lips (**Fig. 2.9**).

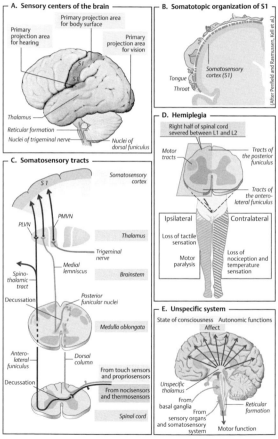

A. Sensory centers of the brain

Primary projection area for body surface

Primary projection area for hearing

Primary projection area for vision

Primary projection area for body surface

S I

S II

Thalamus

Reticular formation

Nuclei of trigeminal nerve

Nuclei of dorsal funiculus

B. Somatotopic organization of S1

Somatosensory cortex (S1)

Tongue

Throat

(After Penfield and Rasmussen, Keil et al.)

C. Somatosensory tracts

S 1

Somatosensory cortex

PLVN

PMVN

Thalamus

Trigeminal nerve

Medial lemniscus

Brainstem

Spino-thalamic tract

Decussation

Posterior funicular nuclei

Medulla oblongata

Antero-lateral funiculus

Dorsal column

Decussation

From touch sensors and propriosensors

From nocisensors and thermosensors

Spinal cord

D. Hemiplegia

Right half of spinal cord severed between L1 and L2

Motor tracts

Tracts of the posterior funiculus

Tracts of the antero-lateral funiculus

Ipsilateral

Contralateral

Loss of tactile sensation

Motor paralysis

Loss of nociception and temperature sensation

E. Unspecific system

State of consciousness   Autonomic functions

Affect

Unspecific thalamus

From basal ganglia

From sensory organs and somatosensory system

Reticular formation

Motor function

Fig. 2.9 Sensory homunculus. (Reproduced with permission from Silbernagl and Despopoulos.[8])

47. What is hyperalgia?

This is increased sensitivity to pain (decreased pain threshold). This can occur by increased sensitivity of the receptors (e.g., from sunburn of the skin which induces histamine release), facilitation in the spinal cord, or thalamic lesions.

48. What is thalamic pain syndrome?

Also known as Dejerine-Roussy syndrome, this is usually due to a posteroventral thalamic stroke and its abnormal subsequent facilitation of the medial thalamic nucleus. These patients usually have a contralateral hemianesthesia at first, with increased pain in that area in the following weeks to months.[26]

49. What causes hangover pain from excessive alcohol consumption?

Chemical irritation to the meninges.

50. What causes night blindness?

This is due to a severe deficiency in vitamin A. There is a decreased amount of photosensitive pigment present to detect decreased light. This is remedied by rapid intravenous infusion of vitamin A.[27]

51. Which area of the retina contains only cones?

The fovea, which is an area of about 0.4 mm in diameter located in the center of the macula (**Fig. 2.10**).

52. Which visual field areas do not have ocular dominance columns?

The monocular temporal crescent and the blind spot.

53. What is a scotoma?

An area of decreased vision surrounded by preserved vision in the visual field.

54. Where on the tongue is salty taste detected?

The tip of the tongue.

55. Where is the first-order neuron of the olfactory pathway located?

The first-order neurons are the olfactory cells located in the olfactory epithelium. These bipolar cells send axons through the cribriform plate to the olfactory bulb.[28]

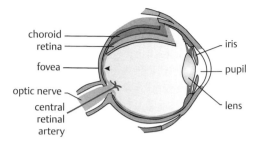

a

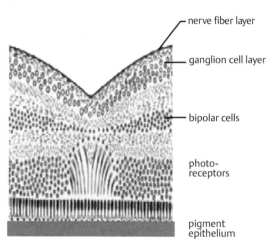

b fovea centralis

Fig. 2.10 **(a)** Cross-sectional anatomy of the human eye. **(b)** Cross-sectional anatomy of the fovea. (Reproduced with permission from Greenstein and Greenstein.[21])

56. Which proteins are involved in retrograde axonal transport and fast anterograde transport?

Kinesin and dynein, respectively. The rate of both transport modalities is approximately 400 mm/day, compared with the slow anterograde transport rate of 0.2 to 4 mm/day.[29]

57. What does a muscle spindle detect?

It detects length and velocity of change in the length of the muscle. It is in parallel with the muscle fibers and is stimulated by stretching. It increases firing with muscle stretch and decreases firing with muscle contraction (**Fig. 2.11**).[30]

58. What carries the information from the muscle spindles and the Golgi tendon organ?

The dorsal spinocerebellar tracts at 120 m/s.[30]

59. What causes decerebrate rigidity?

This is caused by a lesion between the pons and the midbrain. This results in blockage of normal stimulation input to the medullary reticular formation from the red nucleus, basal ganglia, and cortex. As a result, there is unopposed antigravity muscle tone that is stimulated by the lateral vestibular nucleus and pontine reticular nucleus.[31]

60. In the vestibular system, what is the sensory organ of the utricle and saccule?

The macula, which contains hair cells that have cilia embedded in a gelatinous layer containing calcium carbonate otoliths (**Fig. 2.12**).

61. What is the sensory organ of the semicircular canals?

The crista ampullaris, which has hair cells with cilia that project into the cupula (gel cup).[32]

62. In the vestibular system, the utricle has its macula in which plane?

The utricle has its macula on the horizontal plane, so it senses the direction of acceleration when one is upright. The saccule has its macula in the vertical plane, so it functions to detect acceleration when one is horizontal or supine (**Fig. 2.12**).[32]

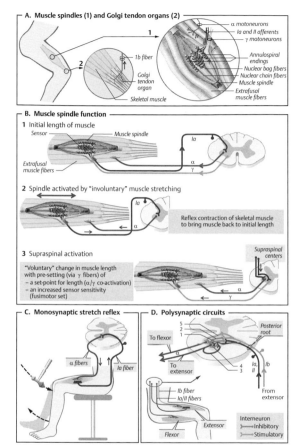

Fig. 2.11 Illustration of muscle spindle and Golgi's tendon organ. (Reproduced with permission from Silbernagl and Despopoulos.[8])

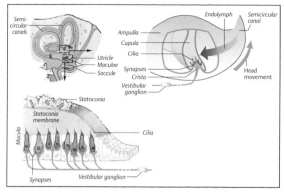

Fig. 2.12   Semicircular canal illustration with utricle, saccule, and macula. (Reproduced with permission from Silbernagl and Despopoulos.[8])

63. What is the mechanism of action of the nitrosoureas (BCNU, CCNU)?

These chemotherapy agents widely used in patients with malignant brain tumors are alkylating agents. They alkylate DNA in multiple locations causing cross-links and often produce single- or double-stranded DNA breaks, which eventually lead to tumor cell death.[33]

64. How does temozolomide work? How does Optune work?

Temozolomide works by attaching a methyl group to the DNA base guanine. This attachment prevents proper DNA replication and leads to cell death (**Fig. 2.13**).[33] Optune uses electrical tumor-treating fields to destroy mitotic spindles during cellular division.

65. What is O6-methylguanine-DNA methyltransferase (MGMT)?

MGMT is a DNA repair enzyme that can remove the methyl group placed by temozolomide, thereby negating the cytotoxic effects of temozolomide. Therefore, patients who express low levels of MGMT respond better to temozolomide (**Fig. 2.13**).[33]

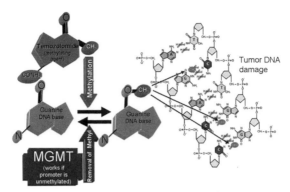

Fig. 2.13 Mechanism of action of temozolomide. (Reproduced with permission from Nader and Sabbagh.[34])

66. What kinds of waves are seen on an electroencephalogram (EEG) during REM (rapid eye movement) sleep?

Beta waves—the same as those seen when one is awake.

67. What is the effect of sleep deprivation on the autonomic system?

Sleep deprivation increases sympathetic output and decreases parasympathetic output.

68. What is the Hering–Breuer inflation reflex?

This is a reflex that is stimulated by stretch receptors in the bronchi and bronchioles. The afferent arm of the reflex is via the vagus nerve and inhibits the dorsal respiratory nucleus in the dorsal medulla to stop inspiration if the lungs are overly distended.[35]

69. What is an atonic bladder?

A flaccid bladder occurs when the bladder becomes dilated and fails to empty properly. This causes overflow incontinence. When urine accumulates in the bladder, it causes increased sensory input to the spinal cord, and this induces the micturition reflex. In atonic bladder, there is decreased sensory input to the spinal cord, so the bladder fills without proper emptying.

70. What causes vasogenic edema and cytotoxic edema?

Vasogenic edema is caused by increased BBB permeability to proteins and macromolecules. This type of edema is extracellular and is caused by vessel damage and inflammation. Cytotoxic edema is caused by an impaired Na^+/K^+ pump as occurs in ischemia. Water and electrolytes accumulate inside the cells. It is an intracellular type of edema.

71. What are the visual field findings in patients with ischemic optic neuropathy?

Ischemic optic neuropathy is the most common cause of painless monocular blindness in the elderly. This is caused by occlusion of the central retinal artery. This causes an altitudinal field deficit. One-third of cases are bilateral.

72. What is the mechanism of action of clopidogrel bisulfate (Plavix)?

Plavix is a selective inhibitor of platelet aggregation. It binds irreversibly to the adenosine diphosphate (ADP) receptor on the platelets' cell membranes. This, in turn, inhibits platelet aggregation by blocking activation of the glycoprotein IIb/ IIIa pathway.[36] Patients on Plavix who require elective surgery should stop their Plavix for at least 1 week.

73. What is the antidote for arsenic poisoning?

Dimercaprol (BAL). This is a compound that was originally developed secretly by British scientists at Oxford University during World War II. This was to be the antidote for lewisite, the arsenic-based chemical war agent. BAL stands for British anti-lewisite. Today, BAL is used to treat arsenic, mercury, lead, and other heavy metal poisoning.[37]

74. What medications increase the level of Dilantin?

Cimetidine, Coumadin, isoniazid, and sulfa drugs.[38]

75. What is the red man's syndrome?

This is a side effect of the rapid infusion of vancomycin. It is caused by histamine release producing facial flushing, pruritus, and hypotension.[39]

76. What are the effects of fentanyl and ketamine on cerebral blood flow?

Decreases and increases, respectively.

77. What are the causes of hypercortisolism (Cushing's syndrome)?

Iatrogenic, adrenocorticotropic hormone (ACTH)–secreting pituitary adenoma, adrenal tumor, and ectopic ACTH production by a pulmonary oat cell tumor or carcinoid tumor.[40]

78. What are the vitamin K–dependent factors?

Factors II, VII, IX, and X, and protein C and protein S.

79. What is the cause of febrile nonhemolytic transfusion reactions?

This occurs in approximately 3% of transfusions and is caused by antibodies to the donor white blood cells (WBCs). These patients mount a fever in 1 to 6 hours, and are treated with acetaminophen.[41]

80. What are the symptoms and signs of an acute hemolytic transfusion reaction?

Within a few minutes of the transfusion, there may be fever, dyspnea, chest pain, and hypotension. Disseminated intravascular coagulation and multiple organ failure can occur as well.[41]

81. Transfusing one unit of platelets increases the platelet count by how much?

5,000 to 10,000 and lasts for approximately 1 week.

82. What is the drug of choice in the treatment of malignant hyperthermia?

Dantrolene.

83. What is ideomotor apraxia?

This is the inability to perform a complex motor task despite the awareness of the task. These patients can perform many complex tasks automatically, but cannot perform the same acts on command. This condition is caused by a lesion of the supramarginal gyrus of the dominant parietal lobe.[42]

84. Which factors cause the oxygen–hemoglobin dissociation curve to have a right shift?

This occurs when there is decreased O_2 affinity. It is seen with increased concentrations in H^+, CO_2, temperature, and 2,3-diphosphoglycerate (2,3-DPG) (**Fig. 2.14**).

85. What are the different groups of sensory axons and what do they carry?

Sensory axons are classified into four groups, labeled I to IV:

1. Group I (Aα) fibers are the largest and fastest conducting fibers (70–120 m/s) and have two functional subgroups: Ia fibers, which are the afferents of muscle spindles, and Ib fibers, which are the afferents from the Golgi tendon organs.
2. Group II (Aβ, Aγ) fibers are slightly slower (30–70 m/s) and represent the afferents from muscle spindles as well as cutaneous touch and pressure.
3. Group III (Aδ) fibers are even smaller and slower (5–30 m/s) and carry sensations of temperature, light touch, and sharp pain.
4. Group IV (C) fibers are the slowest (0.5–2 m/s) fibers and mediate temperature and burning pain. Unlike groups I to III, group IV fibers are unmyelinated.[43]

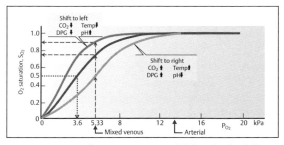

Fig. 2.14 Oxygen dissociation curve with left and right shift. (Reproduced with permission from Silbernagl and Despopoulos.[8])

86. How many basic types of striated muscle fibers are there?

There are three basic types of striated muscle fibers:

1. Type I fibers are slow-twitch or red fibers. These fibers contain large amounts of mitochondria as well as myoglobin. They contract and relax slowly and are capable of prolonged contractions without fatigue.
2. Type IIA, or fast fatigue-resistant fibers, generate rapid contractions that can be maintained for several minutes.
3. Type IIB fibers are fast fatigable fibers that contain a large amount of glycogen and have an anaerobic metabolism. They are fast-twitch fibers but cannot sustain contraction forces due to the rapid accumulation of lactic acid.[44]

87. What is the mechanism of action of tricyclic antidepressants?

They block the reuptake of serotonin and norepinephrine.

88. What are the mechanisms of cholera toxin and pertussis toxin?

Both toxins stimulate adenylyl cyclase to synthesize cyclic adenosine monophosphate (cAMP) inside the cell via two different mechanisms. Cholera toxin selectively activates the G_s (stimulatory) protein, whereas pertussis toxin inactivates the G_i (inhibitory) protein.

89. Nitrous oxide (NO) is generated from which amino acid?

Arginine. The enzyme nitric oxide synthase (NOS) generates NO from arginine.

90. In the sarcomere, which regions get shorter during contraction?

The H zone and the I band (**Fig. 2.15**).[44]

91. What is the difference between the receptive fields of bipolar cells and neurons of the primary visual cortex?

Bipolar cells have a circular receptive field, whereas neurons of the primary visual cortex have rectangular receptive fields.[43]

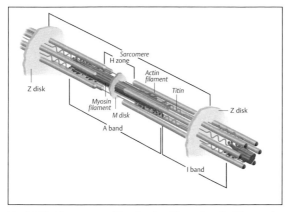

Fig. 2.15 Sarcomere with subunits. (Reproduced with permission from Silbernagl and Despopoulos.[8])

92. During which stage of sleep do night terrors occur?

Stages 3 and 4. These are the periods of deep sleep.

93. What disorder may be acquired by too rapid of a correction of hyponatremia?

Central pontine myelinolysis. The maximum safe rate of correction of hyponatremia is 0.5 mEq/L/h. Central pontine myelinolysis is a disorder characterized pathologically by dissolution of the myelin sheaths of fibers within the central aspect of the basis pontis. Clinically, the patient may suffer from spastic quadriparesis, pseudobulbar palsy, and acute changes in mental status.[45]

94. What should be prescribed to a patient with a coagulopathy associated with Coumadin?

Vitamin K and fresh frozen plasma.

95. Which is the best antiepileptic drug in the treatment of absence seizures?

Ethosuximide.[38]

96. What is the APO E gene?

Apoprotein E is produced mainly in astrocytes and is responsible for transportation of lipids within the brain. The protein mediates neuronal protection, interactions with estrogens, and modulation of synaptic proteins. Possession of the APO E4 allele has been shown to result in greater propensity to develop age-related cognitive impairment, a decrease in the synapse/neuron ratio, and increased susceptibility to exogenous neurotoxins.[46]

97. How is achondroplasia inherited? What is the specific point mutation thought to be involved?

Achondroplasia is inherited as an autosomal dominant trait, but may be caused by a sporadic mutation. A specific point mutation has been shown in the transmembrane region of FGFR3, which exerts negative control on endochondral bone formation and results in disturbed bone development.[47]

98. What is C-reactive protein (CRP)? Where is it synthesized?

CRP is an acute-phase reactant/plasma protein indicative of an acute inflammatory response. CRP expression in the peripheral blood increases in response to injury or infection. It is synthesized in the liver or adipocytes. It is normal to have a mild rise of CRP after surgery; this rise is highest on postoperative day 2 and subsides at postoperative day 5.

99. What does STIR stand for in magnetic resonance imaging (MRI)?

Short tau inversion recovery.

100. Describe the basic organization of the sleep cycle.

- Awake → Non–rapid eye movement (N-REM stage 1, 2, 3, 4) → REM → Awake.
- First third of night → N-REM > REM.
- Second third of night → N-REM ~ REM.
- Last third of night → REM > N-REM.

101. At what age do the K-complexes begin to appear in the sleep cycle?

At 6 months of age.

102. When in the sleep cycle do the K-complexes appear?

Stage 2 of N-REM.

103. What is the normal perfusion pressure breakthrough (NPPB)?

NPPB refers to the presence of possible hyperemia to the cortex surrounding an arteriovenous malformation (AVM) once this is removed. Chronic hypoperfusion around the nidus theoretically causes the vasculature to dilate to increase flow to these surrounding regions. Once the AVM is obliterated, this vasculature is unable to autoregulate.

104. Where does the facial nerve arise from? What is its course?[48]

The facial nerve is made of two roots. The motor division emerges at the pontomedullary junction, lateral to the recess between the inferior olive and the inferior cerebellar peduncle.

The sensory root, also known as the nerve of Wrisberg, emerges lateral to the motor division and just medial to the eighth cranial nerve.

Both roots enter the cerebellopontine angle cistern to reach the internal auditory canal (IAC).

The facial nerve has four segments in the temporal bone:

1. IAC from porus to fundus, running above the crista falciformis or transverse crest to pierce the dura and enter the facial canal followed by the labyrinthine artery, branch of anterior inferior cerebellar artery (AICA).
2. Labyrinthine runs anterolaterally across the axis of the petrous pyramid from the fundus to the geniculate ganglion, passing between cochlea and labyrinth, then turns posteriorly (anterior genu).
3. Tympanic or horizontal from anterior to posterior genu runs below the lateral semicircular canal in the wall of the middle ear cavity in the medial wall of the mastoid antrum.
4. Mastoid runs down vertically to the stylomastoid foramen.

105. Postcontrast enhancement of cranial nerves is considered pathologic. Is there any exception to this rule?

The labyrinthine segment of the facial nerve may enhance on postcontrast T1 due to the rich venous plexus around the nerve in this segment.[49]

106. What are the extratemporal segments of the facial nerve? Where do they arise from, where do they go, and what is their function?

Two Zebras Bit My Cat

Temporal, Zygomatic, Buccal, Marginal Mandibular, Cervical.

The temporal branch runs over the zygomatic arch in the superficial aponeurosis with branches to the posterior auricularis muscle to finally innervate the frontalis muscle and a small portion of the orbicularis oculi and corrugator supercilii mainly.

The zygomatic branches run to the lateral angle of the orbit passing over the zygomatic arch, to innervate mostly the orbicularis oculi.

The buccal branches innervate a muscle of facial expression, the buccinators, and orbicularis oris mainly.

The marginal mandibular branch supplies the muscles of the lower lip and chin, and joins with the mental branch of the inferior alveolar nerve.

The cervical branches run just below the platysma to the anterior region of the neck supplying most of its motor innervation. This muscle works with depressor labii and angular oris to move the corner of the lip.

107. What are the types of fractures of the temporal bone?

The two main types are longitudinal and transverse.

The longitudinal fracture usually runs parallel to the axis of the pyramid originating in the squamous portion of the temporal bone. It can be either anterior or posterior. If the fracture is anterior, it involves the external auditory canal with rupture of the tympanic membrane and otorrhea; if posterior, it involves the mastoid cells with the characteristic Battle's sign without involvement of the tympanic membrane.

The transverse fracture originates in the occipital bone and usually runs across the foramen magnum and posterior fossa to the contralateral petrous bone fracturing it through its short axis and therefore affecting the inner ear and the facial canal.

108. What does the cerebral perfusion pressure (CPP) represent? How is it calculated?

CPP represents the pressure at which the brain is perfused accounting for 20% of the cardiac output. It equals to the mean arterial pressure minus the intracranial pressure, having a normal value between 60 and 80 mm Hg.

109. What are the fibers of Rasmussen? What is their clinical significance?

They are anastomotic fibers between the facial and the superior vestibular nerve within the IAC, first described by Rasmussen in 1940 and subsequently described and demonstrated by others through anatomical dissections and neurophysiologic studies. They may account for vestibular disturbances in facial paralysis.[50]

110. What is the crista falciformis? What is Bill's bar? Where do the nerves run inside the IAC?

The crista falciformis or transverse crest is a bony crest that divides the internal acoustic meatus into an inferior and a superior portion.

Bill's bar further divides the meatus into a posterior and anterior component.

These four spaces are all occupied by nerves, with the posterosuperior and posteroinferior compartments occupied by the vestibular nerve and the anterosuperior and anteroinferior occupied by the facial superiorly and cochlear inferiorly (**7up/Coke down**).[51]

111. What is the most common location for hydatid cysts in the brain?

Hydatid cysts of the brain tend to occur in the distribution of the middle cerebral artery.

112. How are postoperative outcomes for epilepsy surgery measured?

The classical Engel's classification has been modified to include more information about the presence, type, and frequency of seizure activity and also the medication requirement and comparison of the present status with the preoperative.

113. What is the most common postoperative deficit in surgery for mesial temporal sclerosis? How can these be avoided?

The most common complications in resections of the amygdala and hippocampus relate to the disruption of Meyer's loop with possible contralateral homonymous superior quadrantanopsia and damage to the striatum. Several studies have demonstrated that accessing the ventricle at the inferior choroidal point and performing a resection from this point to the bifurcation of the middle cerebral artery allows for safe removal of the amygdala without injuries to the surrounding brain.[52]

114. What is defined as myokymia? What are its causes?

Myokymia is the fasciculation of the orbicularis oculi muscle, most often only on one side. This is not associated with any weakness of the eyelid. It is most commonly benign but at times is associated with hemifacial spasm, blepharospasm, or multiple sclerosis.[53]

115. What is a consequence of neurovascular compression of the left lateral medulla oblongata?

Patients affected by hemifacial spasm have been found to have arterial hypertension that resolves following microvascular decompression, especially when it was the left side that was involved.[54]

116. What is a neurovascular cause of type 2 diabetes mellitus?

As in trigeminal neuralgia, a pulsatile arterial compression has been found to be associated with the pathogenesis of diabetes mellitus. In particular, arterial compression of the right vagus nerve and medulla oblongata has been found to be associated with an increase in insulin resistance with great improvement in pancreatic function following microvascular decompression of the vagus.[55]

117. What are the distinguishing features between delirium and dementia? What are the similarities?

The two main differences between delirium and dementia are that delirium has a sudden onset and that it has a course made of resolution of symptoms and relapses. Both conditions present with attention deficits and cognitive problems including memory loss, mental decline, confusion especially at night, and problems understanding speech or talking.

118. What is Foix's syndrome? How is it different from Marie-Foix syndrome?

Foix's syndrome refers to lesions causing compression or disruption of the structures passing through the superior orbital fissure (oculomotor, trochlear, first branch of the trigeminal nerve, and abducens nerves). Clinically, it manifests with complete ophthalmoplegia, proptosis, pupillary dilation, and absent corneal reflex.

Marie-Foix syndrome is a completely different clinical entity as it is vascular in nature, being the consequence of a stroke to perforators of the basilar artery and/or the AICA causing a lateral brainstem infarct. Clinically, it manifests as hemiplegia, loss of pain and temperature sensation, limb ataxia, facial paralysis, and hearing loss or vertigo.

119. What is Balint's syndrome?

Balint's syndrome is due to bilateral superior parietal lobule lesions that manifest as optic ataxia, oculomotor apraxia, and the inability to perceive more than one object at a time.[56]

120. What is a germinal matrix hemorrhage? How are they classified? How are they treated?

It is a hemorrhage that occurs in the cellular layer between the ependyma of the lateral ventricles and the caudate where the neuronal and glial precursors migrate between the gestational ages of 5 and 28. They are graded I to IV, where I is limited to the germinal matrix and progresses all the way to include the ventricle (II), cause hydrocephalus (III), and compress deep venous structures (IV). For grade III hemorrhages, a ventricular drain is useful in relieving intracranial pressure. Grade IV has a 90% mortality rate.

121. What is referred to as otitic hydrocephalus? What is its pathophysiology?

It represents hydrocephalus following a middle ear infection that causes a thrombus to develop in the adjacent sigmoid sinus with consequent reduction of venous return and development of hydrocephalus.[57]

Cases

■ Case 1

The patient has eaten from an old dented can of beans and has developed blurred vision followed by descending quadriparesis and respiratory deterioration. What is the diagnosis?

■ Case 1 Answer

The diagnosis is likely botulism. The exotoxin causes presynaptic inhibition at the neuromuscular junction by decreasing acetylcholine release. There are no sensory changes. Symptoms progress over 2 to 4 days. Treatment is with antiserum, guanidine, and supportive respiratory care.

■ Case 2

A patient with an open leg sore develops diffuse body spasms, trismus, and aphagia. What is the diagnosis?

■ Case 2 Answer

The diagnosis is likely tetanus where the exotoxin causes presynaptic excitation of agonist and antagonist muscles (especially the masseter causing lockjaw and trismus) by inhibiting neurotransmitter release of inhibitory neurons (especially Renshaw's cells in the spinal cord). Treatment is with antitoxin, penicillin, wound débridement, diazepam, curare, and possible intubation.

■ Case 3

This patient with a brain tumor (**Fig. 2.16**) has increased signal on T2-weighted MRI around the tumor. What is causing this increased signal?

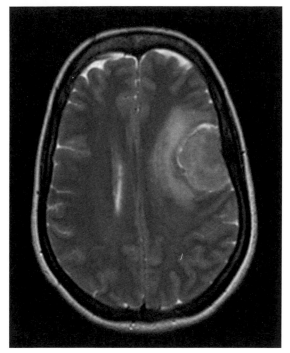

Fig. 2.16 Axial T2-weighted MRI, revealing a mass lesion in the left frontoparietal area.

■ Case 3 Answer

Tumors cause a breakdown in the BBB and release of the astrocytic foot processes and capillary endothelial tight junctions. This causes fluid to leak outside of the blood vessel between the cells. This phenomenon is vasogenic edema.

Cytotoxic edema tends to occur from swelling not between the cells but within the cells themselves due to impairment of the sodium–potassium ATP pump and retention of water within the cell. This happens as a result of hypoxia or ischemia.

■ Case 4

A patient presents with hypertension and hyperpigmentation. He has a moon face and truncal obesity with extremity wasting (**Fig. 2.17**). What is the diagnosis?

■ Case 4 Answer

Pituitary tumor secreting ACTH. This is considered Cushing's disease. Cushing's syndrome will cause similar symptoms but may also be due to the patient receiving exogenous steroids or having ectopic ACTH production. Patients will tend to present with the fatty moon face, truncal obesity, extremity wasting, easy bruising, osteoporosis, amenorrhea, peripheral neuropathy, abdominal striae, hypertension, hyperglycemia, and hyperpigmentation with increased urine and serum cortisol. In this case, the preferred treatment would be transnasal/transsphenoidal removal of the pituitary tumor. Radiosurgery would also be an acceptable

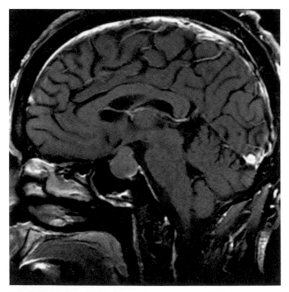

Fig. 2.17　Sagittal T1-weighted postcontrast MRI study.

treatment if ophthalmologic exam is normal, meaning that there is no mass effect to the visual apparatus.

■ References

1. Benarroch EE, Daube JR, Flemming KD, Westmoreland BF. Synaptic transmission and neurochemical systems. In: Mayo Clinic Medical Neurosciences: Organized by Neurologic Systems and Levels. 5th ed. London: Informa Healthcare; 2008:189–214
2. Rohkamm R. Color Atlas of Neurology. Stuttgart: Georg Thieme Verlag; 2004
3. Greenberg MS. Aneurysms. In: Handbook of Neurosurgery. 6th ed. Stuttgart: Georg Thieme Verlag; 2006:781–834
4. Amantea D, Marrone MC, Nisticò R, et al. Oxidative stress in stroke pathophysiology validation of hydrogen peroxide metabolism as a pharmacological target to afford neuroprotection. Int Rev Neurobiol 2009;85:363–374
5. Lullmann H, Mohr K, Ziegler A, Bieger D. Antidotes. In: Color Atlas of Pharmacology. 2nd ed. Stuttgart: Georg Thieme Verlag; 2000:172–174
6. Greenberg M. Spine injuries. In: Handbook of Neurosurgery. 6th ed. Stuttgart: Georg Thieme Verlag; 2006:698–763
7. Gonçalves CA, Leite MC, Nardin P. Biological and methodological features of the measurement of S100B, a putative marker of brain injury. Clin Biochem 2008;41(10–11):755–763
8. Silbernagl S, Despopoulos A. Color Atlas of Physiology. 6th ed. Stuttgart: Georg Thieme Verlag; 2009
9. deBoer RW, Karemaker JM, Strackee J. Hemodynamic fluctuations and baroreflex sensitivity in humans: a beat-to-beat model. Am J Physiol 1987;253(3, pt 2):H680–H689
10. Ropper A. Pathophysiology of cerebral ischemia. In: Adams and Victor's Principles of Neurology. 8th ed. New York, NY: McGraw-Hill; 2005:664–667
11. Lullmann H, Mohr K, Ziegler A, Bieger D. Local anesthetics. In: Color Atlas of Pharmacology. 2nd ed. Stuttgart: Georg Thieme Verlag; 2000:204–209
12. Kahle W. Types of synapses. In: Nervous Systems and Sensory Organs. Stuttgart: Georg Thieme Verlag; 2003:26–27
13. Lullmann H, Mohr K, Ziegler A, Bieger D. Diuretics of the sulfonamide type. In: Color Atlas of Pharmacology. 2nd ed. Stuttgart: Georg Thieme Verlag; 2000:162–163
14. Kurre W, Berkefeld J. Materials and techniques for coiling of cerebral aneurysms: how much scientific evidence do we have? Neuroradiology 2008;50(11):909–927
15. Tallant C, Marrero A, Gomis-Rüth FX. Matrix metalloproteinases: fold and function of their catalytic domains. Biochim Biophys Acta 2010;1803(1):20–28

16. Ropper A. Infantile spasms (West syndrome). In: Adams and Victor's Principles of Neurology. 8th ed. New York, NY: McGraw-Hill; 2005:280

17. Gorlin RS, Pindborg JJ, Cohen MM Jr. Syndromes of the Head and Neck. New York, NY: McGraw-Hill; 1976

18. MacAulay N, Zeuthen T. Water transport between CNS compartments: contributions of aquaporins and cotransporters. Neuroscience 2010;168(4):941–956

19. Kulkarni AG, Hee HT, Wong HK. Solis cage (PEEK) for anterior cervical fusion: preliminary radiological results with emphasis on fusion and subsidence. Spine J 2007;7(2):205–209

20. Guyton AC, Hall JE. Membrane potentials and action potentials. In: Textbook of Medical Physiology. Philadelphia, PA: Elsevier Saunders; 2006:57–71

21. Greenstein B, Greenstein A. Color Atlas of Neuroscience: Neuroanatomy and Neurophysiology. Stuttgart: Georg Thieme Verlag; 2000

22. Guyton A, Hall JE. Excitation of skeletal muscle: neuromuscular transmission and excitation-contraction coupling. In: Textbook of Medical Physiology. Philadelphia, PA: Elsevier Saunders; 2006:87–88

23. Guyton A, Hall JE. Non-bone physiologic effects of altered calcium and phosphate concentrations in the body fluids. In: Textbook of Medical Physiology. Philadelphia, PA: Elsevier Saunders; 2006:979–980

24. Guyton A, Hall JE. Physiologic anatomy of the neuromuscular junction—the motor end plate. In: Textbook of Medical Physiology. Philadelphia, PA: Elsevier Saunders; 2006:85

25. Guyton A. Humoral control of the circulation. In: Textbook of Medical Physiology. Philadelphia, PA: Elsevier Saunders; 2006:201–203

26. Ropper A. Neurogenic or neuropathic pain. In: Adams and Victor's Principles of Neurology. 8th ed. New York, NY: McGraw-Hill; 2005:120–121

27. Guyton A, Hall J. Rhodopsin-retinal visual cycle, and excitation of the rods. In: Textbook of Medical Physiology. Philadelphia, PA: Elsevier Saunders; 2006:629–630

28. Noback CR, Ruggiero DA, Demarest RJ, Strominger NL. The olfactory nerve. In: The Human Nervous System: Structure and Function. 6th ed. Totowa, NJ: Humana Press; 2005:247–248

29. Guyton A, Hall JE. Cilia and ciliary movements. In: Textbook of Medical Physiology. Philadelphia, PA: Elsevier Saunders; 2005:24–25

30. Guyton A, Hall JE. Adaptation of receptors. In: Textbook of Medical Physiology. Philadelphia, PA: Elsevier Saunders; 2005:575–577

31. Ropper A. Posturing in the comatose patient. In: Adams and Victor's Principles of Neurology. 8th ed. New York, NY: McGraw-Hill; 2005:314–315

32. Kiernan JA. Vestibular system. In: Barr's the Human Nervous System: An Anatomical Viewpoint. 8th ed. Baltimore, MD: Lippincott Williams & Wilkins; 2005:365–373

33. Flowers A, Levin VA. Chemotherapy for brain tumors. In: Kaye AH, Laws ER Jr, eds. Brain Tumors. 2nd ed. London: Churchill Livingstone; 2001:375–391

34. Nader R, Sabbagh AJ. Neurosurgery Case Review: Questions and Answers. New York, NY: Thieme Medical Publishers; 2010

35. Ropper A. The central respiratory motor mechanism. In: Adams and Victor's Principles of Neurology. 8th ed. New York, NY: McGraw-Hill; 2006:472–477

36. Lullmann H, Mohr K, Ziegler A, Bieger D. Antithrombotics. In: Color Atlas of Pharmacology. 2nd ed. Stuttgart: Georg Thieme Verlag; 2000:148–151

37. Lullmann H, Mohr K, Ziegler A, Bieger D. Antidotes and treatment of poisonings. In: Color Atlas of Pharmacology. 2nd ed. Stuttgart: Georg Thieme Verlag; 2000:302

38. Lullmann A, Mohr K, Ziegler A, Bieger D. Antiepileptic drugs. In: Color Atlas of Pharmacology. 2nd ed. Stuttgart: Georg Thieme Verlag; 2000:190–193

39. Sivagnanam S, Deleu D. Red man syndrome. Crit Care 2003;7(2):119–120

40. Greenberg M. Cushing's disease. In: Handbook of Neurosurgery. 6th ed. Stuttgart: Georg Thieme Verlag; 2006:441–442

41. Fauci AS, Braunwald E, Kasper D, et al. Transfusion and pheresis therapy. In: Harrison's Manual of Medicine. 17th ed. New York, NY: McGraw-Hill; 2009:44–46

42. Ropper A. Apraxia and other nonparalytic disorders of motor function. In: Adams and Victor's Principles of Neurology. 8th ed. New York, NY: McGraw-Hill; 2006:48–54

43. Meiss RA. Sensory physiology. In: Rhoades RA, Tanner GA, eds. Medical Physiology. 2nd ed. Baltimore, MD: Lippincott Williams & Wilkins; 2003:63–89

44. Meiss RA. Skeletal muscle and smooth muscle. In: Rhoades RA, Tanner GA, eds. Medical Physiology. 2nd ed. Baltimore, MD: Lippincott Williams & Wilkins; 2003:152–176

45. Greenberg M. Electrolyte abnormalities. In: Handbook of Neurosurgery. 6th ed. Stuttgart: Georg Thieme Verlag; 2006:12–19

46. Gee JR, Keller JN. Astrocytes: regulation of brain homeostasis via apolipoprotein E. Int J Biochem Cell Biol 2005;37(6):1145–1150

47. Richette P, Bardin T, Stheneur C. Achondroplasia: from genotype to phenotype. Joint Bone Spine 2008;75(2):125–130

48. Babakurban ST, Cakmak O, Kendir S, Elhan A, Quatela VC. Temporal branch of the facial nerve and its relationship to fascial layers. Arch Facial Plast Surg 2010;12(1):16–23

49. Osborn AG, Ric Harnsberger H, Ross J, et al. Diagnostic and Surgical Imaging Anatomy: Brain, Head and Neck, Spine. Salt Lake City, UT: Amirsys; 2006

50. Ozdoğmuş O, Sezen O, Kubilay U, et al. Connections between the facial, vestibular and cochlear nerve bundles within the internal auditory canal. J Anat 2004;205(1):65–75

51. Juliano AF, Ginat DT, Moonis G. Imaging review of the temporal bone: part I. Anatomy and inflammatory and neoplastic processes. Radiology 2013;269(1):17–33

52. Tubbs RS, Miller JH, Cohen-Gadol AA, Spencer DD. Intraoperative anatomic landmarks for resection of the amygdala during medial temporal lobe surgery. Neurosurgery 2010;66(5):974–977

53. Givner I, Jaffe NS. Myokymia of the eyelids; a suggestion as to therapy; preliminary report. Am J Ophthalmol 1949;32(1):51–55

54. Nakamura T, Osawa M, Uchiyama S, Iwata M. Arterial hypertension in patients with left primary hemifacial spasm is associated with neurovascular compression of the left rostral ventrolateral medulla. Eur Neurol 2007;57(3):150–155

55. Jannetta PJ, Fletcher LH, Grondziowski PM, Casey KF, Sekula RF Jr. Type 2 diabetes mellitus: a central nervous system etiology. Surg Neurol Int 2010;1:31

56. Amalnath SD, Kumar S, Deepanjali S, Dutta TK. Balint syndrome. Ann Indian Acad Neurol 2014;17(1):10–11

57. Gurung U, Anurag, Ullah KS, Shrivastav RP, Bhattarai H. Otitic hydrocephalus. Indian J Otol 2011;17(4):167–169

3 Neuropathology

Congenital

1. With regard to brain development, what are the primary brain vesicles? What secondary brain vesicles do they give rise to?

The neural tube gives rise to the following primary followed by secondary brain vesicles (**Fig. 3.1**)[1,2]:
- Forebrain (prosencephalon):
  - Telencephalon.
  - Diencephalon.
- Midbrain (mesencephalon):
  - Mesencephalon.
- Hindbrain (rhombencephalon):
  - Metencephalon.
  - Myelencephalon.

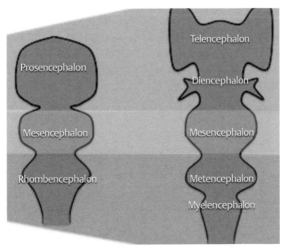

Fig. 3.1 Neural tube development: primary and secondary brain vesicles.

2. Compare primary and secondary neurulation.

A. Primary neurulation: describes the early embryologic formation of the neural plate and its subsequent closure forming the neural tube. It includes:

- Formation of the neural plate (by the neuroectoderm)—day 18 and 19.
- Development of the neural folds—day 20 to 21.
- Closure of the neural tube—starts at day 22, then the rostral neuropore closes at day 24 and the caudal neuropore at day 26.
- The resulting neural tube will eventually develop into the brain and spinal cord down to the second sacral level.

B. Secondary neurulation: describes the development of the neural tube (day 28). It is species specific; in chicks, the tube forms by canalization and multiple luminal secondary neural tubes coalesce and become the primary neurulation tube at the overlap zone.

- In mice, there is extension of the primary neural tube into the medullary rosette that is formed by recruiting cells from the caudal cell mass (CCM) beyond the second sacral level (S2).[1,3]

3. At what spinal level does the spinal cord end, during pre- and postnatal life?
- Prenatal life:
  - 12 weeks at C5.
  - 15 weeks at S3.
  - 24 weeks at S1.
- Postnatal life:
  - Newborn at L3.
  - Adult at L1–L2, end of dural and arachnoid sac at S2.[1]

4. Classify dysraphism according to embryology.
- Disorders during gastrulation (week 3, trilaminar):
  - Split cord malformation.
  - Combined spina bifida.
  - Neurenteric cysts.
  - Some myelomeningoceles.
  - Hemimyelomeningoceles.
  - Klippel-Feil syndrome.
  - Complex dysraphic malformations.
- Premature ectodermal dysjunction:
  - Lipomyelomeningocele.

- Disorders during primary neurulation (week 4):
  - Anencephaly.
  - Cranioschisis.
  - Myelomeningocele.
  - Myeloschisis.
- Disorders during secondary neurulation (week 4):
  - Dermal sinus tract.
  - Dermoid or epidermoid tumors.
  - Spina bifida occulta.
- Postneurulation disorders:
  - Encephalocele.
  - Meningocele.
  - Chiari II malformation.[3]

5. How does tissue repair differ in the fetus brain compared with the adult brain?

In early fetal life, up to the first half of the second trimester, if ischemia occurs, macrophages are attracted to the area, and phagocytosis takes place (without gliosis), producing a smooth-walled defect, which would give a pseudoprimary malformation. This is the case with hydranencephaly or a porencephalic cyst that occurs from an insult before or at early second trimester.[3]

6. In which patients do subependymal germinal matrix (GM) hemorrhages occur?

GM hemorrhage occurs in prematurely born (usually before 34 weeks of gestation) and low-birth-weight neonates (50% in neonates < 1,500 kg) mostly, within the first 3 days after delivery.[4,5]

7. What is the pathogenesis of GM hemorrhage?
- GM has the following characteristics:
  - Located in the periventricular area.
  - Contains fragile microcirculation stroma.
  - Has high levels of tissue plasminogen activator that may impair hemostasis, and receives a major percentage of the cerebral blood flow.
- The GM starts involution at 34 weeks of gestation.
- In case of hypoxic stress, autoregulation fails and excessive perfusion ruptures the GM microcirculation leading to hemorrhage.[4,5]

8. What are the grades of GM hemorrhage?

I. Confined only to GM.

II. Hemorrhage filling lateral ventricles without distension.

III. Hemorrhage filling and distending lateral ventricles.

IV. Hemorrhage extending into the neighboring parenchyma (**Fig. 3.2**).[6]

9. Where is the usual location of GM hemorrhage?

Around the GM over the head of the caudate followed by the thalamus or behind the foramen of Monro (unlike the most common site of term-baby intraventricular hemorrhage—from choroid plexus).[4,5,6]

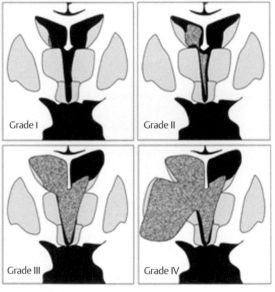

Fig. 3.2 The four grades of germinal matrix hemorrhage.

Trauma

10. Where do contusions occur most frequently?

Frontal and temporal lobes.[7]

11. What are the sources of bleeding in traumatic epidural hematoma?

The most common source of bleeding is arterial blood, mainly from the middle meningeal artery, and less commonly from a laceration of a venous sinus, such as the transverse sinus after sustaining an occipital fracture.[7]

12. What is a Duret hemorrhage?

A Duret hemorrhage is a delayed upper brainstem hemorrhage (anterior and paramedian aspects) that typically occurs in patients with rapidly evolving descending transtentorial herniation.[8]

13. What is the pathophysiology of a Duret hemorrhage?

The origin remains controversial. One theory states that it is of arterial origin, occurring due to stretching and laceration of the pontine perforating branches of the basilar artery. Another theory states a venous origin due to thrombosis and venous infarction. A multifactorial origin is more likely.[8]

14. What is a diffuse axonal injury (DAI)?

A DAI is the most severe form of traumatic axonal injury. It encompasses axonal damage throughout the hemispheric white matter and the rostral brainstem (95%). The regions involved are by definition the following: the parasagittal white matter, large fiber bundles such as the corpus callosum (92%), the internal capsule, the cerebellar peduncles, and possibly other sites where they are also known as gliding (88%), thalamic (56%), and caudate (17%) contusions.[7]

15. What is the difference between a Duret hemorrhage and brainstem small tissue-tear hemorrhages that accompany a DAI?

Both are located in the upper brainstem, but a Duret hemorrhage tends to be delayed and located in the paramedian areas, whereas DAI is typically located in the dorsolateral brainstem (**Fig. 3.3**).[7,8]

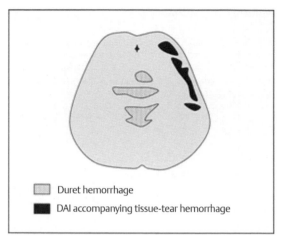

Duret hemorrhage

DAI accompanying tissue-tear hemorrhage

Fig. 3.3 Duret hemorrhages versus diffuse axonal injury (DAI) in the brainstem.

16. What is the microscopic timeline picture of a DAI?

2 to 12 hours. Axonal swellings (bulbs) develop, which can be verified by β-amyloid precursor protein (βAPP). Axonal disconnection follows; microglial clusters around degenerating axons appear at 5 to 10 days.[7]

17. Classify DAI.
- Stage I: DAI evident in frontal and temporal lobes mostly; also seen in cerebellar cortex and the internal capsule.
- Stage II: DAI also seen in corpus callosum, especially the splenium.
- Stage III: DAI also evident in brainstem and cerebellar peduncles and corticospinal tracts.

18. What are the biochemical changes in DAI?[3]
- 1 hour: neurofilament immunoreactivity.
- 4 to 5 hours: accumulation of amyloid precursor protein.
- 6 hours: ubiquitin (a marker of neural damage) is evident.
- 12 to 24 hours: axonal varicosities.
- 1 day to 2 months: axonal swelling.
- 2 months to years: wallerian degeneration and demyelination.

19. Which type of temporal bone fracture results in a conductive hearing deficit more frequently?

Longitudinal temporal bone fractures more often result in conductive hearing deficits; transverse temporal bone fractures result in disruption of the otic capsule and more often direct nerve damage with sensorineural hearing deficit. Transverse fractures are often associated with more forceful impact than longitudinal fractures; therefore, they have other associated injuries (epidural hematoma, diffuse axonal injury).[9]

Epilepsy

20. What are the layers of the neocortex, and what are the main cells that reside in these layers? What are their connections?

There are six layers in the neocortex. These are listed in **Table 3.1** with their corresponding cell types and connections.

Table 3.1 Layers of the cerebral cortex with corresponding cell types and connections[3,10]

Layer		Cell type by layer	Connections
I	Molecular	Horizontal cells (of Cajal) and Golgi cells	I & II Diffuse afferent fibers from lower brain
II	External granular	Granule cells	II & III Ipsilateral corticocortical association fibers
III	External pyramidal	Pyramidal neurons	Commissural fibers
IV	Internal granular	Stellate cells	Main sensory afferents
V	Internal pyramidal	Pyramidal neurons	Main efferent supply to brainstem/spinal cord
VI	Multiform	Fusiform or spindle cells	Efferent supply to thalamus

21. What is the most striking microscopic finding in lissencephaly type I (agyria or pachygyria)?

In lissencephaly type I, the cortex is made up of four layers[9]:

1. Molecular layer.
2. External neuronal layer—thin.
3. Sparsely cellular layer.
4. Internal neuronal layer—thick.

22. Describe the connections of the mesial temporal lobe.

These connections are illustrated in **Figs. 3.4** and **3.5**.

23. Describe the macroscopic and microscopic picture of mesial temporal lobe (hippocampal) sclerosis.

Mesial temporal sclerosis is also known as Ammon's horn sclerosis. Macroscopically, the involved hippocampus is smaller than the normal side and the temporal horn may be enlarged on the involved side. Microscopically, neuronal loss mainly occurs in the CA1 region, more so than the CA4, CA3, and CA2 regions and the dentate gyrus. This may be associated with some degree of gliosis (**Figs. 3.6 and 3.7**).[11]

24. What is Rasmussen's syndrome?

It is a rare neurologic disorder that is usually seen in children. It is characterized by a progressive unilateral neurologic deficit, which is associated with sudden onset of epilepsy that is refractory to medical treatment. Patients usually have hemiplegia, hemianopsia, and intellectual deterioration.[11]

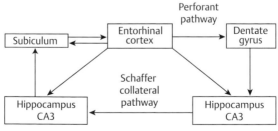

Fig. 3.4 Summary of connections of the mesial temporal lobe.

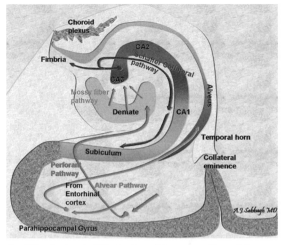

Fig. 3.5 Anatomical illustration of the connections of the mesial temporal lobe.

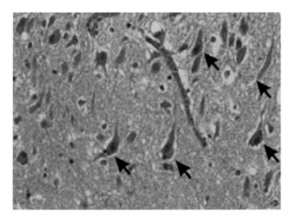

Fig. 3.6 Hippocampal sclerosis. *Arrows* show neurons; there is neuronal loss on the right-hand side of the image at the level of CA1. (Courtesy of Dr. Manuel Graeber.)

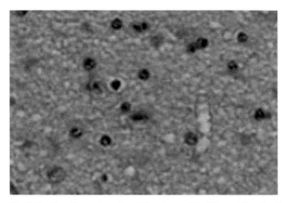

Fig. 3.7 Reactive astrocytes. (Courtesy of Dr. Manuel Graeber.)

25. What is the microscopic picture of Rasmussen's syndrome?

Rasmussen's syndrome may have features reminiscent of chronic viral encephalitis. It is characterized by the presence of[1] lymphocyte cuffs around blood vessels,[3] widespread or clustered lymphocytes and microglia (or so-called microglial nodules), and neurophagia.[4] These features are most often unilateral and located in the neocortex, hippocampus, subjacent white matter, and basal ganglia. This is seen in addition to chronic leptomeningitis.[9]

26. A 19-year-old patient had a lesion removed from the right temporal lobe after having suffered from intractable epilepsy for 15 years. What is the most likely diagnosis based on the pathology slide shown in Fig. 3.8? Describe the typical finding seen in the inset box.

Dysembryoplastic neuroepithelial tumor (DNET). The finding in the inset consists of a floating neuron. DNETs microscopically are formed of oligodendrocyte-like cells in a mucinous matrix. Microcysts are found within this matrix and suspended "floating neurons" are seen in a mucopolysaccharide-rich medium.[9]

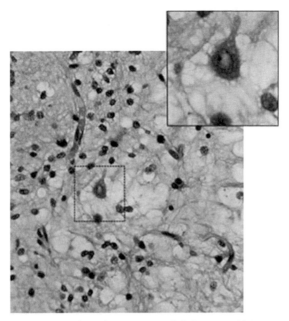

Fig. 3.8 Dysembryoplastic neuroepithelial tumor, with inset showing detail (see text). (Courtesy of Dr. Manuel Graeber.)

27. The lesion in Fig. 3.9 was removed from an epileptic patient. It was located in an epileptic focus in the pole of the right temporal lobe. What is the diagnosis? What are some other usual microscopic features of this lesion?

The diagnosis is focal cortical dysplasia. Dysplastic neurons and structural disorganization is usually seen: it depends on the type of focal cortical dysplasia, but generally this consists of disorganized hypercellular cerebral cortex with abnormal lamination (dyslamination), vacuolations, and balloon cells (cells with abundant glassy cytoplasm and an astrocyte-like morphology). Most balloon cells are vimentin positive, but others are glial (e.g., glial fibrillary acidic protein [GFAP]) or neuron-specific enolase/MAP (microtubule-associated protein)/NeuN immunoreactive (neuronal nuclei). This suggests

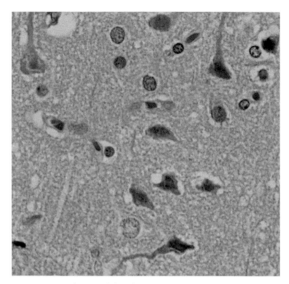

Fig. 3.9 Focal cortical dysplasia.
(Courtesy of Dr. Manuel Graeber.)

a degree of heterogeneity among the cells with partial commitment toward glial or neuronal differentiation. Thus, balloon cells may be called "noncommitted" cells. Dysplastic cortex may be positive with immature MAP2 antibody (MAP1B, MAP2C).[10,11,12]

28. How do you classify lesions caused by abnormalities of cortical development?

1. Mild malformations of cortical development:
   a. Type I: cortical ectopic neurons in or adjacent to layer 1.
   b. Type II: abnormalities outside layer 1, for example, small aggregates of white matter neurons and hippocampal dysgenesis.
2. Focal cortical dysplasia:
   a. Type I: without dysmorphic neurons or balloon cells. Type IA: dyslamination; Type IB: associated with giant or immature neurons.
   b. Type II (Taylor-type): dysmorphic neurons, architectural abnormalities ± balloon cells. Type IIA: without balloon cells; Type IIB: with balloon cells.

3. Dysplastic tumors:
   a. Dysembryoplastic neuroepithelial tumors (DNETs).
   b. Gangliogliomas.
4. Hemimegalencephaly.
5. Polymicrogyria.
6. Schizencephaly.
7. Neuronal heterotopias.[10,12]

Neoplastic

29. What are Rosenthal fibers?

They are brightly eosinophilic bodies, measuring 10 to 40 µm, with heterogeneous shapes. Their immunohistochemistry shows peripheral labeling by GFAP, ubiquitin, and αβ-crystallin; the central hyaline core does not show this labeling. They can be seen in a variety of conditions. They can be found within neoplasms, such as within juvenile pilocytic astrocytomas (JPAs), around craniopharyngiomas and multiple sclerosis plaques, and in neurologic conditions such as Alexander's disease (**Fig. 3.10**).[3]

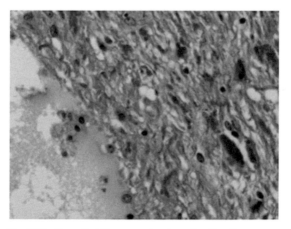

Fig. 3.10 Rosenthal fibers seen in a juvenile pilocytic astrocytoma. (Courtesy of Dr. Manuel Graeber.)

30. What are the main categories of genes that are related to tumor development? Define each.

1. Oncogenes: genes that promote growth under normal circumstances, but when mutated, promote pathologic growth.
2. Tumor-suppressor genes: genes that inhibit growth, but when mutated, lose the ability to inhibit growth.
3. Stability genes: genes that repair DNA replication errors or mutations.[13]

31. Name and describe the pathologic differences of astrocytic tumors.

There are four grades of astrocytic tumors. **Table 3.2** summarizes these grades and their respective pathologic features.[14]

32. What are the differences between primary and secondary glioblastoma (GBM)?

Primary GBM develops in older patients (55 years) and is slightly more common in men. They usually have EGFR (epidermal growth factor receptor) overexpression, PTEN (phosphatase and tensin homolog) mutations, CDKN2A (cyclin-dependent kinase inhibitor 2A) (p16) deletions, and less frequently, MDM2 (murine double minute 2) amplification. Secondary GBM develops in younger patients (39 years) and is slightly more common in women. Two-thirds of patients have TP53 mutations and no EGFR amplification.[14,15]

33. Describe the different rosettes and pseudorosettes (surrounding blood vessels) that are encountered in neurohistopathology. What tumors are they associated with?

Fig. 3.11 summarizes the different types of rosettes and their associated tumors.[16]

34. What is the most likely diagnosis based on the histopathology shown in Fig. 3.12?

Psammomatous meningioma.

Table 3.2 WHO classification of astrocytic tumors and histopathologic differentiation[13]

Grade	WHO name	Histopathology
I	Juvenile pilocytic astrocytoma	Biphasic pattern of compact bipolar cells (GFAP staining); associated with Rosenthal's fibers + loose textured multipolar cells with microcysts and eosinophilic granular bodies
I	Subependymal giant cell astrocytoma (SEGA)	Associated with tuberous sclerosis; composed of large ganglioid cells
II	Diffuse astrocytoma	Occasional nuclear atypia but no mitosis (single mitosis does not allow anaplastic diagnosis); diffusely infiltrating (fibrillary or gemistocytic) neoplastic astrocytes, moderately increased cellularity compared with normal brain
II	Pleomorphic xanthoastrocytoma	Pleomorphic lipidized cells, in a background of reticulin network and eosinophilic granular bodies
III	Anaplastic astrocytoma	Nuclear atypia, mitosis
IV	Glioblastoma multiforme	Nuclear atypia, mitosis, microvascular proliferation and necrosis
IV	Gliomatosis cerebri	Extensively diffuse (usually astrocytic) glioma at least involving three lobes, superficial and/or deep gray matter

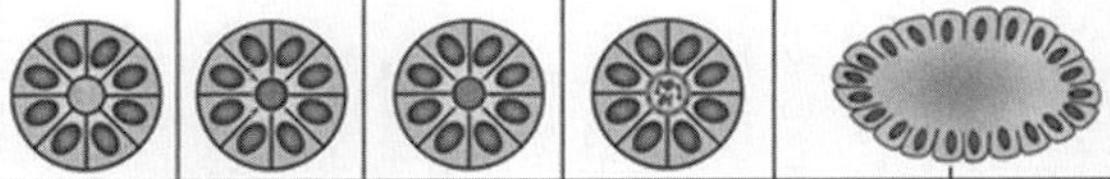

Tumors	Homer Wright rosette	Flexner-Wintersteiner rosette	True ependymal rosette	Perivascular pseudorosette	Neurocytic rosette	Pineocytomatous rosette
Medulloblastoma	☑	☑		☑		
PNET	☑			☑		
Pineoblastoma	☑	☑				
Neuroblastoma	☑					
Retinoblastoma		☑				
Ependymoma			☑	☑		
Central neurocytoma				☑	☑	
Pineocytoma						☑
GBM				☑		

Fig. 3.11 Pathologic differentiation between different types of rosettes.[14] GBM, glioblastoma; PNET, primitive neuroectodermal tumor.

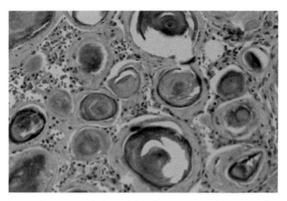

Fig. 3.12 Histopathology slide of brain tumor. (Courtesy of Dr. Manuel Graeber.)

35. A hematoxylin and eosin (H&E) histopathology slide of a metastatic lesion in the brain is presented in Fig. 3.13. What are some features of the lesion and what further immunohistochemical work-up would you perform to further define the diagnosis (origin of the metastasis seen to the left of the micrograph)?

Metastatic tumors are different from brain histology and vary according to the primary lesions that they arise from.

Immunohistochemistry is very helpful in identifying the source tumor. See **Table 3.3** for further details.

36. What is the diagnosis based on the histopathology shown in Fig. 3.14? Where is this lesion usually located? What are the typical macro- and microscopic features of this lesion?

The lesion represents a colloid cyst. These are usually located in the anterior third ventricle. Macroscopically, they are glistening cysts containing mucin (usually viscous, murky material). Microscopically, the cyst has an outer fibrous connective tissue capsule, lined by an inner well-differentiated mucin-producing or ciliated pseudostratified epithelium. The mucin is periodic acid–Schiff (PAS) positive.[17]

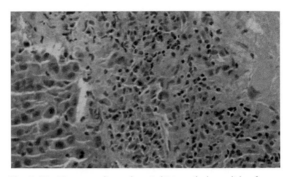

Fig. 3.13 Hematoxylin and eosin histopathology slide of a metastatic brain tumor. (Courtesy of Dr. Manuel Graeber.)

Table 3.3 Differentiation of metastatic brain tumors based on immunohistochemistry

	CK7	CK5/CK6	CK20	CAM5.2	TTF	Melan–A	Vim	CD3, CD20
Small cell lung Ca	–	–	–	+/–	+			
Non–small cell lung Ca	+	–	–	+	+			
Renal cell Ca	–	–	–	+/–	–		+	
Breast Ca	+	–	–	+	–			
Lymphoma	–	–	–	–	–			+
Melanoma	–	–	–	–	+	+		

Note: Ca, cancer; –, negative; +, positive; TTF, thyroid transcription factor; Vim, vimentin.

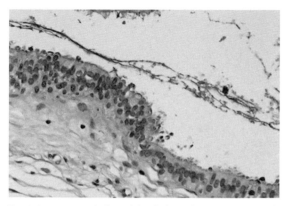

Fig. 3.14 Histopathology slide of a brain lesion. (Courtesy of Dr. Manuel Graeber.)

37. An H&E histopathology slide from a tumor resected from the suprasellar region of a 7-year-old boy is shown in Fig. 3.15. What is the diagnosis and why? Describe the two types of this tumor.

The lesion represents a craniopharyngioma (adamantinomatous type). Cords of squamous epithelium, palisaded columnar epithelium (*), wet keratin (WK), and focal keratin (K) can be seen. The types are adamantinomatous[1] (~90%) and papillary[3] (less common, very well-differentiated squamous pseudopapillary tumor of adulthood).[14,17]

38. The tumor in Fig. 3.16 was resected from the cerebellopontine angle. What is the diagnosis? What are the two distinct patterns seen in the image? What histopathologic structure would you likely see if you looked further in this tumor?

The diagnosis is schwannoma. The distinct patterns are Antoni A and Antoni B patterns seen to the left and right of the micrograph, respectively. The histopathologic structure referred to is a Verocay body.[14]

39. What are Verocay bodies?

Verocay bodies are typically densely packed whorled arrangements in palisaded cells of Antoni A areas of schwannomas.

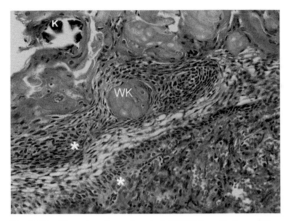

Fig. 3.15 Hematoxylin and eosin (H&E) histopathology slide of a brain tumor. *, palisaded columnar epithelium; K, focal keratin; WK, wet keratin. (Courtesy of Dr. Manuel Graeber.)

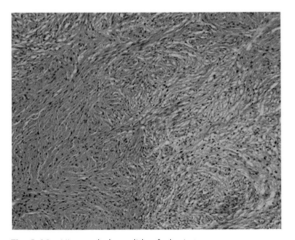

Fig. 3.16 Histopathology slide of a brain tumor. (Courtesy of Dr. Manuel Graeber.)

40. What are Antoni A and Antoni B areas?

Antoni A is an area of dense histologic patterns and Antoni B is an area of loose histologic patterns in schwannomas.

41. Other than schwannomas, which other tumor may show a dual histologic pattern?

Pilocytic astrocytoma.

42. Which staining is positive in schwannoma?

S-100, Leu 7, laminin, vimentin, and collagen IV.

43. The image in Fig. 3.17 is from an intraventricular tumor removed from a 29-year-old woman. What is the most likely diagnosis? What are the microscopic features of this tumor?

The diagnosis is central neurocytoma. This lesion is a neuroepithelial tumor formed of uniform round cells with nucleus-free areas of neuropil. They typically present a low proliferation rate. This tumor is synaptophysin positive.[14]

44. Reticulin stain is positive in which tumors?

- Ganglioglioma.
- Hemangiopericytoma.
- Pituitary tumor.
- Lymphoma.
- Glomus tumor.
- Hemangioblastoma.

45. Which bone tumors have giant cells?

Aneurysmal bone cyst and giant cell tumor.

46. S-100 staining is positive in which tumors?

- Schwannoma.
- Eosinophilic granuloma.
- Paraganglioma.
- Hemangioblastoma.
- Chordoma.
- Esthesioneuroblastoma.
- Meningioma (20% of the time).[14]

47. Which are the specific immunohistochemical markers for melanoma?

MART-1 and HMB-45.

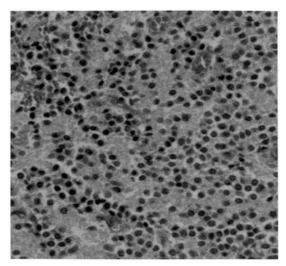

Fig. 3.17 Histopathology slide of an intraventricular brain tumor. (Courtesy of Dr. Manuel Graeber.)

48. Which subtype of meningioma shows PAS positivity?

Secretory meningioma.

49. Which other stains are positive in secretory meningiomas that are not positive in any other kind of meningioma?

Cytokeratin and carcinoembryonic antigen (CEA).

50. Which are the two common positive immunohistochemical stains in meningiomas?

Ethidium monoazide (EMA) and vimentin.

51. Which immunohistochemical stains are positive in hemangiopericytoma?

Reticulin, vimentin, and von Willebrand factor (perivascular spaces).

52. How does EMA staining help in differentiating meningioma from hemangiopericytoma?

EMA staining is positive in meningioma and negative in hemangiopericytoma.[14]

53. Name immunohistochemical markers used in the diagnosis of germinoma.

Placental alkaline phosphatase (PLAP) and c-Kit.

54. What are blepharoplasts?

Blepharoplasts are the intracytoplasmic basal bodies of cilia present in apical portions of the cells in ependymomas that stain with phosphotungstic acid hematoxylin (PTAH).

55. Which tumors have blepharoplasts: ependymomas or choroid plexus papilloma?

Ependymomas.

56. Can a monosomy of chromosome 22 differentiate between WHO grade I and grade II meningioma?

No, chromosome 22 monosomy cannot differentiate between grade I and grade II meningiomas, although trisomy and tetrasomy of chromosome 22 are seen in higher-grade meningiomas [14]

57. Which other chromosomes are associated with meningioma progression?

An alteration of chromosome 1 is also needed in addition to chromosome 22 deletion for progression of meningioma.

58. Other than chromosome 1, are there other chromosomes associated with higher-grade meningiomas?

Chromosome 14 deletion along with chromosome 22 monosomy is also seen in higher-grade meningiomas.

59. What are Schwann's cells derived from?

Neural crest cells.

60. What is the mode of inheritance of von Recklinghausen's neurofibromatosis (neurofibromatosis type 1 [NF1])?

Autosomal dominant on chromosome 17, although as much as 50% occur by spontaneous mutation.[18]

61. Histologically, what is the name given to the cells that are seen in chordomas?

Physaliphorous or "bubble-bearing" cells.[19]

62. The presence of uniform cell density and nuclei surrounded by a rim of clear cytoplasm giving a "fried egg" appearance on H&E stain is consistent with which tumor?

Oligodendroglioma. These perinuclear halos are the result of artifact from the delay in formalin fixation in a surgical specimen.[20]

63. Which neoplasm is characterized by the Reed-Sternberg binucleated cells?

Hodgkin's lymphoma. About 20% of these patients develop neurologic complications involving the skull or meninges.[21]

64. What is the classic histologic finding in retinoblastomas?

Flexner-Wintersteiner rosettes.[22]

65. What are the small, round, blue cell tumors of childhood?

1. Neuroblastomas.
2. Chondrosarcoma.
3. Rhabdomyosarcoma.
4. Lymphoma.
5. Ewing's sarcoma.

Degenerative

66. How do you classify human prion disease?[22]

1. Idiopathic: sporadic Creutzfeldt–Jakob disease (CJD) and sporadic fatal insomnia.
2. Familial: familial CJD, Gerstmann-Sträussler-Scheinker disease, prion disease associated with octapeptide repeat region insertional mutations, fatal familial insomnia.
3. Acquired:
   a. From human: kuru, iatrogenic CJD.
   b. From bovine: variant CJD.

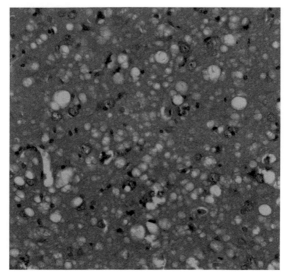

Fig. 3.18 Histopathology slide of a brain lesion. (Courtesy of Dr. Manuel Graeber.)

67. Fig. 3.18 shows an H&E slide from a biopsy of a brain lesion taken from the cortex of a patient suspected to have CJD. Are the findings on the slide representative of what you would expect to see in CJD? Why or why not?

Yes, this represents CJD. There are multiple vacuoles giving a spongiform appearance. Unlike edema, the vacuoles are not empty.[23]

68. Fig. 3.19 shows a silver stain of a brain lesion taken at autopsy of a patient with dementia. What is the likely diagnosis? On what factors do you base your diagnosis?

The most likely diagnosis is Alzheimer's disease based on the presence of senile plaques and neurofibrillary tangles, as well as neuronal loss.[24]

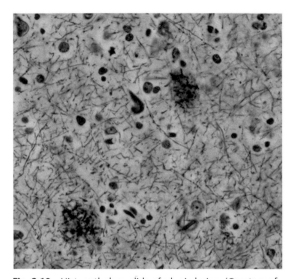

Fig. 3.19 Histopathology slide of a brain lesion. (Courtesy of Dr. Manuel Graeber.)

69. What are senile plaques?

They are deposits of neuropil. They contain an Aβ peptide that is derived from a fragment of amyloid precursor protein (APP; a neuronal protein that is encoded on chromosome 21).[24]

70. What are neurofibrillary tangles?

Intracellular inclusion bodies, mainly containing tau protein.[23]

71. How does Alzheimer's disease appear macroscopically?

Cerebral atrophy most strikingly in the mesial temporal structures, followed by atrophy in the parietal and frontal lobes. The occipital lobe is usually unaffected. Temporal horns are usually widened due to the atrophy.[24]

72. What are the most useful sequences to detect foci of cortical dysplasia and other epileptogenic lesions on magnetic resonance imaging (MRI)?

For a long time, the standard sequence to detect epileptogenic lesion has been the rapid acquired gradient echoes (MPRAGE), able to create a highly contrasted image of different anatomical structures. Recently a double inversion recovery (DIR) has been developed that yields even better results in detecting this type of abnormality with a higher specificity and that is also very useful in detecting plaques in multiple sclerosis (MS).[25]

73. What is referred to as "pancake brain"? What are the pathologic features of this condition?

This is a radiological sign of alobar holoprosencephaly (HPE). In this condition, the cerebral hemispheres are fused with the presence of a single ventricle. The fusion of the cerebral hemispheres and different deep gray matter structures can be present in different degrees. This condition is associated with other midline abnormalities outside the brain in the facial structures.[26]

74. What is vacuolar myelopathy? What reversible cause can it mimic?

Vacuolar myelopathy is a form of myelopathy that affects the posterior columns of the spinal cord, especially in the thoracic spine, and is associated with late stages of human immunodeficiency virus (HIV) infection with very low CD4 count. It resembles the neurologic symptoms of B_{12} deficiency and should be differentiated from that with laboratory work-up and replacement. It is thought to be caused by a cytokine activation.[27]

75. What are optic pathway gliomas (OPGs)? What are they associated with? What is their clinical course?

OPGs are tumors of the optic pathways that can involve the optic nerve, chiasm, optic tract, and optic radiations. They can be associated with NF1 or be sporadic. Their clinical course depends on the tumor type. NF1-associated OPGs are usually pilocytic astrocytoma and have a benign course with 50% of the patients not presenting any symptoms and with long-term indolent course. The sporadic form of OPG is more aggressive with higher-grade glial lesions with visual compromise in up to 75% of cases.[28]

76. What is MELAS? What are the most relevant pathologic features?

MELAS syndrome (mitochondrial myopathy, encephalopathy, lactic acidosis, and strokes) is a mitochondrial cytopathy. Muscle biopsy demonstrates ragged red fibers on modified Gomori's trichrome and succinate dehydrogenase stains. Molecular analysis commonly demonstrates A3243G mutation on mitochondrial DNA.[29]

77. What are the differences in adult onset versus pediatric onset of Lhermitte-Duclos disease (LDD)?

LDD is a pathologic entity that is either hamartomatous or WHO grade I (dysplastic gangliocytoma). All cases of adult onset LDD present a PTEN mutation and are now thought to be a manifestation of Cowden's disease. On microscopy, there is a diffuse enlargement of the granular layers of the cerebellum that are filled with ganglionic cells. The cerebellar architecture is preserved.[30]

78. What is the site of origin of juvenile angiofibroma? How does this possibly correlate with its pathogenesis?

Juvenile angiofibroma tends to originate around the sphenopalatine foramen in young men.

If there is an incomplete regression of the first branchial arch artery around the sphenopalatine foramen during puberty, this is thought to be susceptible to growth hormones and to cause the "birth" of juvenile angiofibroma as a true vascular malformation. This is further supported by overexpression of VEGFR and tenascin in these lesions as well as lack of pericytes and disruption of the basement membrane and muscular layer of the vessels.[31]

79. What are the pathologic features of Sturge-Weber syndrome?

Sturge-Weber syndrome is a neurocutaneous disorder. It manifests with angiomas that involve the meninges and the skin of the face in the distribution of V1 and V2 that look dark like port-wine due to venous dilation. The pathologic features are related to its pathogenesis as Sturge-Weber syndrome is due to the formation of a vascular plexus under the ectoderm of the cephalic portion of the neural tube that fails to regress around the sixth week.[32]

80. What is a thyroglossal duct cyst? What is their treatment?

Thyroglossal duct cysts are the second most common neck mass after lymphadenopathy. They develop from remnants of the thyroid gland. In 1 to 2% of cases they can have malignant transformation, which is one of the reasons to remove them even if asymptomatic.[33]

81. Esthesioneuroblastoma is one of the small blue cell tumors. How can it be differentiated from the others?

The demonstration of human achaete-scute 1 gene expression (HASH1) is diagnostic in cases of undifferentiated tumors arising from the sinonasal tract as it is expressed in immature olfactory cells.[34]

82. What is the IDH wild-type glioblastoma?

It is a subtype of glioblastoma that does not demonstrate any mutation in the IDH1 and IDH2 genes. This is almost exclusively seen in primary glioblastomas. Diffuse astrocytomas, oligodendrogliomas, and oligoastrocytomas that have progressed to glioblastoma present a mutation in IDH1/IDH2 in >70% of cases and all cases that have progressed from astrocytoma.[35]

83. What is a RELA-positive ependymoma?

It refers to a subgroup of supratentorial ependymomas that demonstrates a fusion gene—the C11orf95-RELA, which causes activation of the NF-kappaB pathway. The presence of this mutation is important as these patients have poor outcome compared with the other subtypes of ependymoma in the supratentorial compartment.[35]

84. What are WNT-activated medulloblastomas? How does their prognosis differ from SHH-activated medulloblastomas?

Medulloblastomas are neuroectodermal tumors of the cerebellum (PNET) that are very common in the pediatric population and that account for 10 to 20% of all primary brain tumors in this age group. They are labeled as grade IV neoplasm. If they demonstrate WNT activation either by accumulation of β-catenin or detection of monosomy of chromosome 6 or mutation in CTNNB1, they demonstrate an excellent prognosis with overall survival of almost all patients that are treated. SHH-activated medulloblastomas have a far worse prognosis.[35]

■ References

1. Moore KL, Persaud TVN. The Developing Human: Clinically Oriented Embryology. Philadelphia, PA: WB Saunders; 1993

2. Parent A. Carpenter's Human Neuroanatomy. Baltimore, MD: Williams & Wilkins; 1996

3. Ellison D, Love S, Chimelli L, Harding B, Lowe JS, Vinters HV. Neuropathology—A Reference Text to CNS Pathology. St. Louis, MO: Mosby; 2004

4. Morioka T, Hashiguchi K, Nagata S, et al. Fetal germinal matrix and intraventricular hemorrhage. Pediatr Neurosurg 2006;42(6):354–361

5. Takashima S, Itoh M, Oka A. A history of our understanding of cerebral vascular development and pathogenesis of perinatal brain damage over the past 30 years. Semin Pediatr Neurol 2009;16(4):226–236

6. Papile LA, Burstein J, Burstein R, Koffler H. Incidence and evolution of subependymal and intraventricular hemorrhage: a study of infants with birth weights less than 1,500 gm. J Pediatr 1978;92(4):529–534

7. Geddes JF, Graham DI. Central nervous system trauma. In: De Girolami U, Poirier J, Gray F, eds. Escourolle & Poirier's Manual of Basic Neuropathology. 4th ed. Philadelphia, PA: Butterworth-Heinmann; 2004:57–74

8. Parizel PM, Makkat S, Jorens PG, et al. Brainstem hemorrhage in descending transtentorial herniation (Duret hemorrhage). Intensive Care Med 2002;28(1):85–88

9. Saraiya PV, Aygun N. Temporal bone fractures. Emerg Radiol 2009;16(4):255–265

10. Palmini A, Lüders HO. Classification issues in malformations caused by abnormalities of cortical development. Neurosurg Clin N Am 2002;13(1):1–16, vii.

11. Thom M, Scaravilli F. Neuropathology of epilepsy. In: De Girolami U, Poirier J, Gray F, eds. Escourolle & Poirier's Manual of Basic Neuropathology. 4th ed. Philadelphia, PA: Butterworth-Heinmann; 2004:269–280

12. Palmini A, Najm I, Avanzini G, et al. Terminology and classification of the cortical dysplasias. Neurology 2004;62(6, suppl 3):S2–S8

13. Vogelstein B, Kinzler KW. Cancer genes and the pathways they control. Nat Med 2004;10(8):789–799

14. Louis DN, Ohgaki H, Wiestler OD, Cavenee WK. WHO Classification of Tumours of the Central Nervous System. 4th ed. Lyon: International Agency for Research and Cancer (IARC); 2007

15. Kleihues P, Ohgaki H. Primary and secondary glioblastomas: from concept to clinical diagnosis. Neuro Oncol 1999;1(1):44–51

16. Wippold FJ II, Perry A. Neuropathology for the neuroradiologist: rosettes and pseudorosettes. AJNR Am J Neuroradiol 2006;27(3):488–492

17. Berger PC, Scheithauer BW, Vogel FS. Surgical Pathology of the Nervous System and Its Coverings. 4th ed. New York, NY: Churchill Livingstone; 2002

18. Kleihues P, Cavanee WK. Pathology and Genetics of Tumors of the Nervous System. Lyon: World Health Organization; 2000

19. Riopel C, Michot C. Chordomas [in French]. Ann Pathol 2007;27(1):6–15

20. Takeuchi Y, Kanamori M, Kumabe T, et al. Collision tumor of anaplastic oligodendroglioma and gangliocytoma: a case report. Brain Tumor Pathol 2009;26(2):89–93

21. Chang KC, Chang Y, Jones D, Su IJ. Aberrant expression of cyclin A correlates with morphogenesis of Reed-Sternberg cells in Hodgkin lymphoma. Am J Clin Pathol 2009;132(1):50–59

22. Ts'o MO, Fine BS, Zimmerman LE. The Flexner-Wintersteiner rosettes in retinoblastoma. Arch Pathol 1969;88(6):664–671

23. Ironside JW, Frosch MP, Ghetti B. Human prion disease. In: De Girolami U, Poirier J, Gray F, eds. Escourolle and Poirier's Manual of Basic Neuropathology. 4th ed. Philadelphia, PA: Butterworth-Heinmann; 2004

24. Low J, Duyckaerts C, Frosch MP. Pathology of degenerative disease of the nervous system. In: De Girolami U, Poirier J, Gray F, eds. Escourolle and Poirier's Manual of Basic Neuropathology. 4th ed. Philadelphia, PA: Butterworth-Heinmann; 2004

25. Ryan ME. Utility of double inversion recovery sequences in MRI. Pediatr Neurol Briefs 2016;30(4):26

26. Chavhan GB, Shroff MM. Twenty classic signs in neuroradiology: a pictorial essay. Indian J Radiol Imaging 2009;19(2):135–145

27. Di Rocco A, Simpson DM. AIDS-associated vacuolar myelopathy. AIDS Patient Care STDS 1998;12(6):457–461

28. Rasool N, Odel JG, Kazim M. Optic pathway glioma of childhood. Curr Opin Ophthalmol 2017;28(3):289–295

29. Lorenzoni PJ, Scola RH, Kay CS, et al. MELAS: clinical features, muscle biopsy and molecular genetics. Arq Neuropsiquiatr 2009;67(3A):668–676

30. Louis DN, Ohgaki H, Wiestler OD, et al. The 2007 WHO classification of tumours of the central nervous system. Acta Neuropathol 2007;114(2):97–109 Erratum in Acta Neuropathol 2007 Nov;114(5):547

31. López F, Triantafyllou A, Snyderman CH, et al. Nasal juvenile angiofibroma: current perspectives with emphasis on management. Head Neck 2017;39(5):1033–1045

32. Roach ES. Neurocutaneous syndromes. Pediatr Clin North Am 1992;39(4):591–620

33. Gioacchini FM, Alicandri-Ciufelli M, Kaleci S, Magliulo G, Presutti L, Re M. Clinical presentation and treatment outcomes of thyroglossal duct cysts: a systematic review. Int J Oral Maxillofac Surg 2015;44(1):119–126

34. Carney ME, O'Reilly RC, Sholevar B, et al. Expression of the human Achaete-scute 1 gene in olfactory neuroblastoma (esthesioneuroblastoma). J Neurooncol 1995;26(1):35–43

35. Louis DN, Perry A, Reifenberger G, et al. WHO classification of tumours of the central nervous system. Acta Neuropathol 2016;131(6):803–820

4 Neuropharmacology

Neurotransmitters

1. What are the most important central nervous system (CNS) transmitters?

Glutamic acid, γ-aminobutyric acid (GABA), acetylcholine, dopamine, norepinephrine, serotonin (5HT), and opioid peptides.[1]

2. What is the mechanism of action of glutamic acid?

Excitatory by increasing the influx of cations by direct coupling and G-protein linked on the NMDA (N-methyl-d-aspartate) receptor. This receptor is a potential target for ketamine and phencyclidine (PCP).[1]

3. What is the mechanism of action of acetylcholine?

Excitatory and inhibitory on muscarinic receptors by decreasing and increasing potassium efflux by coupling diacylglycerol (DAG) and cyclic adenosine monophosphate (cAMP) receptors, respectively—excitatory on nicotinic receptor.[1]

4. What is the mechanism of action of GABA?

Inhibitory by increasing the influx of potassium by direct coupling—potential target for anticonvulsants, sedatives, hypnotics, and some muscle relaxants.[1]

5. Name the different GABA receptor agonists.

- Barbiturates—increase the duration of Cl^- ion channel opening.
- Benzodiazepines—increase frequency of Cl^- ion channel opening.
- Propofol acts on $GABA_A$.
- Baclofen acts on $GABA_B$.
- Valproic acid at high concentrations acts on GABA.[2]

6. What is the mechanism of action of flumazenil?

Flumazenil is a benzodiazepine receptor antagonist and decreases the frequency of Cl^- ion channel opening.[2]

7. What is the nonbenzodiazepine drug that binds to a benzodiazepine receptor?

Zolpidem. Used in sleep disorders. It is not effective for chronic anxiety, seizure disorders, or muscle relaxation. It has less tolerance and dependence.[2]

8. Name a nonbenzodiazepine anxiolytic.

Buspirone: a partial $5HT_{1A}$ receptor. It has no dependence effects and no symptoms of withdrawal.[2]

9. What are the important effects/side effects to remember when prescribing benzodiazepines?

They have sedative, amnestic, anxiolytic, antidepressant, and muscle relaxant properties. All are contraindicated in the first semester of pregnancy. If combined with opioids, this may result in hypotension and ventilatory depression. Those with long-duration action can result in cumulative sedation and impairment of intellectual and psychomotor function, and those with short half-life are less likely to sedate, but are more prone to cause withdrawal or rebound depression.[2,3]

10. What are the clinical findings of benzodiazepine withdrawal syndrome?

They include hypertension, tachycardia, muscle twitching, tremulousness, diaphoresis, confusion, dysphoria, and seizures.[2,3]

11. Summarize the effect of the main benzodiazepines, including onset of action, duration, and dosage.

Benzodiazepines are summarized in **Table 4.1**.[4]

12. What is the pharmacologic strategy in Parkinson treatment?

To restore normal neurotransmitter balance by:

- Increasing dopamine activity.
- Decreasing acetylcholine activity at muscarinic (M) receptors in the striatum.

Drugs may improve symptoms, but do not alter the natural course of the disease.

Table 4.1 Commonly used benzodiazepines[4]

Drug	Dose	Onset	Duration	Comments
Midazolam	1–2 mg IV	Rapid	Short (the shortest)	Four times more potent than diazepam; excellent anticonvulsant; always monitor patient
Clorazepate	15–60 mg/d, divided	Rapid	Long	
Diazepam	2–10 mg BID-QID	Rapid	Long (the longest)	
Flurazepam	30 mg	Rapid/intermediate	Long	
Alprazolam	0.25–0.5 mg TID	Intermediate	Intermediate	Antidepressant effects
Chlordiazepoxide	5–10 mg TID	Intermediate	Long	
Lorazepam	1 mg TID	Intermediate	Intermediate	Not metabolized in liver
Halazepam	20–40 mg TID	Intermediate	Long	
Oxazepam	10–15 mg TID	Intermediate/slow	Intermediate/short	Not metabolized in liver
Temazepam	15–30 mg	Intermediate/slow	Intermediate	Not metabolized in liver
Prazepam	20–60 mg/d, divided	Slow	Long	

Abbreviations: BID, twice daily; IV, intravenously; QID, four times daily; TID, three times daily.

13. What are the drugs that increase dopamine function?

Levodopa is converted to dopamine by a dopa-decarboxylase. *Carbidopa* inhibits the peripheral decarboxylation and increases CNS availability of L-dopa. The former drug does not cross the blood–brain barrier (BBB).[3]

14. What are the actions of tolcapone and entacapone?

They inhibit peripheral catechol-*O*-methyltransferase (COMT), enhancing the CNS uptake of L-dopa and possibly reducing its on–off effects.[3]

15. What are the two dopamine receptor agonists?

Bromocriptine had been used as an adjuvant to levodopa. Because of its secondary effects such as hallucinations, confusion, and psychosis, it has been replaced by *pramipexole* and *ropinirole. Selegiline* is a selective monoamine oxidase (MAO) type B inhibitor that increases dopamine in the CNS.[3]

16. What are the drugs that decrease acetylcholine function?

Benztropine and trihexyphenidyl. These drugs are M receptor blockers. They reduce tremor and rigidity, reduce extrapyramidal symptoms, exacerbate tardive dyskinesias, and cause atropinelike effects.[3]

17. Why do antipsychotic drugs cause atropinelike effects, postural hypotension, and sexual dysfunction?

They block dopamine D_2 receptors, but they also block muscarinic and α receptors, causing atropinelike effects and postural hypotension and sexual dysfunction, respectively.[3]

18. What are the other side effects of a dopamine receptor antagonist?

Akathisia, acute dystonic reaction, extrapyramidal dysfunction, and endocrine dysfunction such as prolactinemia.[3]

19. Extrapyramidal dysfunction can be reduced by using the new dopamine receptor antagonists. Provide examples of these drugs and their effects.

Clozapine blocks D_2c and $5HT_2$ receptors, but it may cause severe agranulocytosis and a weekly blood test is required. Olanzapine blocks $5HT_2$ receptors and improves negative symptoms.[3]

20. What are the side effects after chronic dopaminergic receptor blockage?

After the use of older antipsychotic drugs, akathisia and tardive dyskinesia present months later (e.g., Haldol); both are reversible when the medication is stopped and when anticholinergic medications are initiated such as benztropine mesylate and trihexyphenidyl.[3]

21. What is neuroleptic malignant syndrome?

The neuroleptic malignant syndrome is an idiosyncratic life-threatening reaction to a neuroleptic medication. Patients present with hyperthermia, cardiovascular instability, muscle rigidity, and altered mental status due to enhanced sensitivity of dopamine receptors to blocking agents. This life-threatening condition can be treated with bromocriptine and dantrolene.[3]

22. What are the mechanisms of action of a tricyclic antidepressant?

They block the reuptake of norepinephrine and serotonin. They block muscarinic and a receptors, cause sedation, decrease seizure threshold, and have cardiotoxicity.[3]

23. What is the mechanism of action of the selective serotonin reuptake inhibitors (SSRIs) and what are their common side effects?

These include fluoxetine, paroxetine, and sertraline; they block the reuptake of serotonin (5HT). Their side effects are anxiety, agitation, bruxism, sexual dysfunction, seizures, and transitory weight loss.[3]

24. What is serotonin syndrome?

Serotonin syndrome is a potentially life-threatening adverse drug reaction that may occur as a consequence of excess serotonergic activity in the CNS. It includes diaphoresis, rigidity, myoclonus, hyperthermia, instability of the autonomic nervous system, and seizures.

Epilepsy

25. Name the drugs of choice for generalized tonic-clonic seizures and their mechanism of action.

Valproic acid, phenytoin, and carbamazepine. They decrease axonal conduction by preventing Na^+ influx through fast Na channels.[4]

26. What is the first-line drug for complex partial seizures?

Carbamazepine.[4]

27. What is the mechanism of action of the first-line drug for absence seizures?

Ethosuximide. It decreases presynaptic Ca^{2+} influx through type-T channels in thalamic neurons.[4]

28. What are the most common side effects of phenytoin?

Sedation, ataxia, diplopia, acne, gingival overgrowth in children, hirsutism, osteomalacia, and hepatotoxicity.[4]

29. What are the side effects of valproic acid?

Pancreatitis, hepatotoxicity, and thrombocytopenia.[2]

30. List some of the medications frequently used in neurosurgery that can lower seizure threshold.[2,3]

- Antidepressants: baclofen, phenytoin at supratherapeutic levels.
- Analgesics: meperidine, fentanyl, and tramadol.
- Anesthetics: methohexital and enflurane.
- Benzodiazepines.
- Barbiturates and withdrawal of antiepileptic drugs.
- Antibiotics: cefazolin, imipenem, and metronidazole.
- Radiographic contrast materials.

31. What are the pharmacologic choices to treat seizures including status epilepticus?

- *Lorazepam* has several advantages: it can be given quickly with an antiseizure duration of 12 to 24 hours. It controls seizures in up to 90% of cases when compared with diazepam (76%). It has become the drug of choice. Dosage is as follows: 0.1 mg/kg (IV); usually 2 to 4 mg intravenously (IV) over 2 minutes and may administer again in 5 minutes.
- *Diazepam* or *midazolam* (10 mg) intranasally, buccally, or intramuscularly (IM) if no IV access available.
- *Fosphenytoin* 20 mg/kg IV at 150 mg/min with continuous monitoring; may cause hypotension and cardiac depression.
- *Continuous IV midazolam* (load 0.2 mg/kg followed by 0.2–2 mg/kg).
- *Continuous IV propofol* (load 1–2 mg/kg to 10 mg/kg followed by 1–15 mg/kg/h titrated to electroencephalographic [EEG] seizure control or burst suppression); be careful to guard against propofol infusion syndrome.
- *IV valproate* 30 to 40 mg/kg over 10 minutes followed by another 20 mg/kg if necessary. Levels may decrease if given concomitantly with meropenem or amikacin. Recent data have shown that it is a very good alternative; it does not cause sedation or hypotension. It may be associated with platelet dysfunction.
- *Continuous IV pentobarbital* (load 5 mg/kg at up to 50 mg/min, repeat 5 mg/kg boluses, followed by 0.5–10 mg/kg/h titrated to EEG seizure control or burst suppression).
- *Thiamine* 100 mg IV and 50 mL of D50 (50% dextrose in water) IV.[4]

32. What is the mechanism of action of levetiracetam?

It is not well understood, but it involves binding to the synaptic vesicle protein SV2A. It has rapid titration, no drug interaction, and a good safety profile. Not metabolized by the liver, although dosage should be reduced in the presence of renal failure and extra doses should be given after dialysis. Doses are 500 to 1,500 mg orally (PO) or IV. No need to check levels.[4]

Anesthetics, Analgesics, and Anti-inflammatories

33. What is propofol infusion syndrome?

Propofol infusion syndrome is a rare and potentially fatal condition associated with high doses and long-term use of propofol. The syndrome produces metabolic acidosis, cardiac failure, rhabdomyolysis, hypotension, and death. Propofol should not be administered for more than 4 to 5 days. Extreme caution must be taken when using doses greater than 5 mg/kg/h or when usage of any dose exceeds 48 hours in critically ill adults.[5]

34. Who are most likely to suffer from propofol infusion syndrome?

Although propofol infusion syndrome was initially described in the pediatric population, occurrence in the adult population has been reported with increased frequency. The syndrome occurs in critically ill patients receiving high-dose propofol (> 5 mg/kg/h), steroids, and elevated catecholamine levels (endogenous or exogenous).[5]

35. What are the findings in an intrathecal baclofen pump overdose?

Hallucinations, seizures, confusion, psychotic behavior, respiratory depression, hypotension, and coma.[6,7]

36. What is the time course for intrathecal baclofen withdrawal syndrome?

Intrathecal baclofen withdrawal syndrome usually manifests over 1 to 3 days, but can be fulminant in presentation. Treatment is restoration of baclofen, but IV benzodiazepine may be required.[6,7]

37. What are the toxic doses of acetaminophen?

Rare at doses of < 4,000 mg/d, usually > 1 0 g/d, but may occur at lower doses in patients with previous liver disease such as alcoholism, viral hepatitis, and autoimmune hepatitis, as well as in patients taking cytochrome P-450 enzyme-inducing drugs.[3]

38. What are the concepts that need to be kept in mind when prescribing nonsteroidal anti-inflammatory drugs (NSAIDs)?

They do not create dependence. After a maximum dose, they do not have further analgesia effects (ceiling effect). Taking them with meals/antacids and via IV route does not reduce gastrointestinal (GI) side effects; misoprostol (synthetic prostaglandin) may be effective in the reduction of such effects. All of them have a reversible inhibitory platelet function. Acetylsalicylic acid (aspirin) has an irreversible effect and inhibits platelet function for the 8- to 10-day life of the platelet. All of them cause water and sodium retention and potential nephrotoxicity.[2,3]

39. Discuss individual features of specific NSAIDs.

See **Table 4.2**.

40. What are the most common antispasmodics used in spine surgery?

Although very commonly used after spine surgery, there is very little evidence of beneficial effect and their use in acute low back pain is dubious. Some of them are cyclobenzaprine, methocarbamol, and carisoprodol. Diazepam is a very efficient benzodiazepine (see above) to treat muscle spasms.[2,3]

Table 4.2   Individual features of specific nonsteroidal anti-inflammatory drugs

Aspirin	Unique effectiveness in pain from bone metastasis (spine)
Ibuprofen	Associated with Reye's syndrome in children
Ketorolac	Only parenteral NSAID. Very useful in neurosurgery patients who are very sensitive to narcotics. Usual safe doses in a healthy adult: 30 mg IV or IM every 6 hours, with a maximum of 120 mg/d
Celecoxib	COX-2 inhibitor; 200 mg twice daily is a good dose[2,3]

Abbreviations: IM, intramuscularly; IV, intravenously; NSAIDs, nonsteroidal anti-inflammatory drugs

41. What are the mechanisms of action of anti-inflammatory steroids?

They include decreased leucocyte migration, increased lysosomal membrane stability decreasing phagocytosis, decreased capillary permeability, and decreased platelet activation, COX-2 expression, and interleukins.[2,3]

42. What is the half-life of cortisone?

90 minutes.[3]

43. What is a normal physiologic replacement of steroids (under no stress)?

Prednisone 5 mg every morning and 2.5 mg every night PO *or* hydrocortisone 10 mg every morning and 5 mg every night.[8]

44. Which dose of steroids is unlikely to cause hypothalamic–pituitary–adrenal axis suppression?

Less than 40 mg of prednisone (or its equivalent) given in the morning for less than 1 week. Axis suppression will certainly occur after 40 to 60 mg daily of hydrocortisone (or its equivalent) after 2 weeks. After a month or more of steroids, the axis may be depressed for almost 1 year.

45. What are the equivalent corticosteroid doses?

Dexamethasone 0.75 mg, methylprednisolone 4 mg, prednisone 5 mg, hydrocortisone 20 mg, and cortisone 25 mg.[2,3]

46. What are other common side effects of steroids?

Hypertension, sodium and water retention, growth suppression in children, GI bleeding, pancreatitis, impaired wound healing, hyperglycemia, glaucoma, osteoporosis, avascular necrosis of the hip or other bones, infections, hypercoagulopathy (inhibits tissue plasminogen activator), leukocytosis (even in the absence of infection), and hiccups (usually responds to chlorpromazine 25 to 50 mg three times daily PO).[2,3]

47. What are the neurologic side effects of steroids?

Mental agitation, "steroid psychosis," spinal epidural lipomatosis, multifocal leukoencephalopathy, and pseudotumor cerebri.[2,3]

48. What is the mechanism of action of opioid analgesics?

Opioid receptors are of multiple subtypes, all G-protein linked. Activation of presynaptic opioid receptors causes inhibition of Ca^{2+} influx through voltage-regulated ion channels, decreasing neurotransmitter release. Activation of postsynaptic opioid receptors results in increased K^- efflux causing inhibition.[1,2]

49. What are important characteristics of opioid analgesics?

Overdose is possible with potential seizure and respiratory depression. Physical and psychologic tolerances may develop. They have no ceiling effects.[2,3]

50. List examples of weak opioids, their dosage, and delivery times.

- Codeine 30 to 60 mg IM/PO every 3 hours as needed (PRN).
- Propoxyphene 1 to 2 tablets PO every 4 to 6 hours PRN.
- Tramadol 50 to 100 mg PO every 4 to 6 hours PRN. This opioid binds to μ-opioid receptors inhibiting the reuptake of serotonin and norepinephrine.[2,3]

51. Discuss dosages, onset, and duration of the most common opioids used in neurosurgery and spine surgery.

See **Table 4.3** for details.[2,3]

52. What is the antidote for morphine overdose?

Naloxone.[2]

53. What is the primary indication for dexmedetomidine (Precedex; Hospira, Inc., Lake Forest, IL), its mechanism of action, and most common side effect?

Dexmedetomidine (Precedex) is indicated to treat anxiety; it provides opioid-sparing analgesia and sedation without respiratory depression. It is approved for use in intubated and nonintubated patients. It is a highly selective α-2 agonist with a common side effect of bradycardia.[9,10]

Table 4.3 Most common opioids used in neurosurgery (the doses are equianalgesic for severe pain)[2,3]

Drug name	Dose and route	Duration	Comments
Hydrocodone	10 mg + 325 mg APAP 1–2 tab every 4–6 hours; 5 mg + 500 mg APAP 1–2 tab every 4–6 hours	4–6 hours	Do not exceed 4,000 mg of APAP in 24 hours
Codeine	130 mg IM; 200 mg PO	3.5 hours	
Morphine	20–60 mg PO or 10 mg IM or 2–3 mg IV	4–7 hours	Respiratory depression. Morphine oral is a long-acting PO form.
Hydromorphone	7.5 mg PO; 1.5 mg IM	3 hours	
Meperidine	75 mg IM; 300–400 mg PO	4–6 hours	Long-term or high doses not recommended because its metabolites can cause agitation and CNS hyperactivity (delirium and seizures); severe encephalopathy if given with MAOIs
Oxycodone	15 mg IM; 30 mg PO	2–3 hours for acetaminophen and 12 hours for oxycodone	
Fentanyl patch	1 patch	72 hours	Not for postop analgesic due to risk of respiratory depression

Abbreviations: APAP, acetaminophen; CNS, central nervous system; IM, intramuscularly; IV, intravenously; MAOI, monoamine oxidase inhibitor; PO, orally.

54. Why is dexmedetomidine useful in functional neuro-surgery?

It provides successful sedation without interfering with electrophysiologic monitoring, thus allowing brain mapping during awake craniotomy and microelectrode recording during implantation of deep-brain stimulators.[9,10]

55. What are the effects of dexmedetomidine in traumatic spinal cord injury?

It decreases inflammation. Serum levels of TNF-α and IL-6 were significantly reduced in Wistar rats after spinal cord injury after treatment with dexmedetomidine.[9,10]

56. Is the innate immune response potentiated by dexmedetomidine?

Yes, in the presence of inflammation, a sedative such as dexmedetomidine may act in an anti-inflammatory rather than proinflammatory manner.[9]

57. What are the two types of antiemetics and their characteristics?

Phenothiazine and nonphenothiazine. Phenothiazine antiemetics, promethazine and prochlorperazine, lower the threshold for seizures and should be used with caution following craniotomy and head injury. Other alternatives are trimethobenzamide, which is very effective for nausea related to posterior fossa surgery, dimenhydrinate, and diphenhydramine. Metoclopramide may cause extrapyramidal symptoms that respond to diphenhydramine. Ondansetron is the most common drug used to treat nausea and vomiting related to chemotherapy and surgery.[2,3]

58. Why is the use of acid inhibitors in neurosurgery patients important?

The risk of stress ulcers is high in patients with CNS pathology. These pathologies include brain and spinal cord injury, brain tumors, intracerebral hemorrhage, syndrome of inappropriate antidiuretic hormone secretion (SIADH), CNS infection, and ischemic stroke. Other nonneurologic factors that contribute are the use of steroids, burns, hypotension, respiratory failure, coagulopathies, renal/hepatic failure, and sepsis. Diencephalon and brainstem pathologies may reduce the vagal output that leads to hypersecretion of gastric acid and pepsin.[3,8]

59. What are the acid inhibitors commonly used in neurosurgery patients?

Ranitidine 150 mg PO twice daily or 50 mg IV every 8 hours. *Famotidine* 40 mg PO daily—this drug may cause thrombocytopenia. *Omeprazole* inhibits the final step in acid secretion by gastric parietal cells. It should not be used long term as the trophic effects may lead to gastric carcinoid tumors; it decreases the effectiveness of prednisone and the clearance of warfarin and phenytoin. Doses are 20 to 40 mg twice daily. *Sucralfate* appears to be superior to H2 antagonists with a lower incidence of pneumonia; doses are 1 g PO four times daily on an empty stomach. Cimetidine is not recommended because of its interactions with multiple other medications.[3,8]

60. What is the mechanism of action of ondansetron?

It inhibits $5HT_3$ receptors found in the area postrema and the peripheral sensory and enteric nerves. Its activation opens ion channels. It decreases emesis in chemotherapy and postoperatively.[2,3]

Antimicrobials

61. What are the main physiochemical properties influencing antimicrobial penetration into the CNS?
- *Ionization*: Ionized (polar) compounds are less likely to cross the BBB.
- *Lipophilicity*: Highly lipophilic drugs penetrate the CNS more (unequal distribution, highly lipophilic drugs will accumulate in lipid-rich brain structures and minimally in cerebrospinal fluid [CSF] and extracellular spaces).
- *Molecular weight*: Substances > 500 to 800 daltons penetrate with difficulty the BBB (e.g., vancomycin or amphotericin B), especially an intact barrier.
- *Protein binding*: Highly protein-bound drugs have reduced CNS penetration.
- *Active transport*: Active transport cells in the choroid plexus may excrete drugs.[11]

62. What are the factors to be considered when starting empiric antimicrobial therapy?

The most likely infectious agent, which in turn depends on patient age, immune status, and setting (community or nosocomial).[11]

63. Is antibiotic prophylaxis for ventilated patients necessary to prevent pneumonia?

Studies have demonstrated the use of cefuroxime 1,500 mg for 2 doses or ampicillin-sulbactam 3 g for 3 days after intubation reduces the incidence of subsequent pneumonia.[11]

64. What is the pharmacologic approach in the case of suspected ventriculitis/meningitis associated with a neurosurgical procedure including an external ventricular drain (EVD), head trauma, or shunt infection?

EVD and/or shunt infections frequently involve grampositive organisms (*Staphylococcus epidermidis* and *Staphylococcus aureus*, including methicillin-resistant *S. aureus*). Around 25% of these infections are secondary to gramnegative organisms, such as *Escherichia coli*, *Klebsiella*, *Acinetobacter*, and *Pseudomonas* species. Vancomycin plus cefepime or meropenem is recommended. Any infected hardware should be replaced, removed, or externalized. Intraventricular and intrathecal administration of antibiotics may be necessary.[11]

65. What is important to remember when treating a brain abscess?

Always obtain a specimen. The type of pathogen depends on patient-specific risk factors. A brain abscess is often polymicrobial (around 60%), with anaerobic bacteria in up to 49% of cases. Organisms frequently isolated are *Streptococcus milleri*, *Bacteroides* species, *Enterobacteriaceae*, and *S. aureus*. Initial coverage for immunocompetent patients is vancomycin, ceftriaxone or cefotaxime, and metronidazole. Keep metronidazole even if an anaerobic source is not identified on culture. Patients who had recent neurosurgery or head injury with a possible nosocomial source should be treated with a third- or fourth-generation cephalosporin with antipseudomonal activity (ceftazidime or cefepime) along with vancomycin and metronidazole. Treatment should continue for 6 to 8 weeks.[11]

66. What is the rationale for the use of steroids in bacterial meningitis?

Experimental data have shown that an inflammatory response in the subarachnoid space contributes significantly to morbidity and mortality. Dexamethasone given before or with the first dose of antibiotics and then every 6 hours for 4 days improves outcome. There are no data to support steroids in patients who have meningitis related to CSF shunts and after neurosurgical procedures.[11]

67. Name some of the antibiotics for intrathecal and intraventricular use.

They include *vancomycin* with doses of 10 to 20 mg/d for a few days until the cultures become negative, *gentamicin* and *tobramycin* with doses of 5 to 10 mg/d, and *amikacin* 10 to 20 mg/d. Preservative-free formulations should be used for intraventricular administration. No antimicrobial agent has been approved by the Food and Drug Administration for intraventricular use.[11]

68. What are the side effects of intraventricular vancomycin?

Ototoxicity, CSF eosinophilia, seizures, altered mental status, and local tissue irritation.[11]

69. What are the alternatives in the case of multidrug-resistant *Acinetobacter* and *Pseudomonas* ventriculitis?

Polymyxin B and colistimethate with doses of 5 to 20 mg/d— the optimal duration is unknown.[11]

70. Which vitamin should be coadministered with isoniazid for tuberculosis treatment?

Pyridoxine, vitamin B_6, should be administered to prevent peripheral neuropathy.[11]

71. What is the main side effect of ethambutol?

Optic neuritis that can lead to blindness.[11]

Intensive Care: Vasogenic and Hematologic

72. What are the best options to treat hypertension when high intracranial pressure is present (e.g., traumatic brain injury [TBI])?

Sympathomimetic-blocking agent drugs such as β-blocking drugs (propranolol, esmolol, labetalol) or centrally acting α receptor agonists (clonidine or α-methyldopa).[12]

73. Why is nicardipine a good alternative to manage hypertension in neurovascular pathologies (e.g., TBI, subarachnoid hemorrhage, intraparenchymal hemorrhages)?

It is a short-acting continuous-infusion agent with a reliable dose–response relationship and favorable safety profile. It has been shown to reverse vasospasm.[12]

74. Which of the following vasodilating antihypertensive agents cross the BBB: nitroprusside, calcium channel blockers, hydralazine, adenosine, nitroglycerin?

They all do. As vasodilating antihypertensive agents, these drugs have the potential to increase cerebral blood flow, impair autoregulation, and increase intracranial pressure.[12,13]

75. Besides nimodipine, what are other effective options for vasospasm prophylaxis?

In addition to the standard course for vasospasm prophylaxis, that is, nimodipine 60 mg every 4 hours or 30 mg every 2 hours, the following can also be used: *HMG Co A* (3-hydroxy-3-methyl-glutaryl-CoA) *reductase inhibitors* (statins) have been shown to reduce inflammation, increase production of *nitric oxide* through upregulation of nitric oxide synthase, and prevent thrombogenesis. Animal as well as human research studies have reported decreased vasospasm-related ischemic deficits after subjects received statins either before or after subarachnoid hemorrhage. *Pravastatin* or *simvastatin* in 40-mg or 80-mg daily doses, respectively, is commonly used. Continuous *infusions of magnesium* have been effective in reducing cerebral vasospasm—specific doses and serum target levels are still under investigation.[12,14]

76. What is the specific mechanism of action of nimodipine?

Nimodipine blocks L-type calcium channels. The L-type channel is the major influx route for calcium ions in smooth muscle.

77. In addition to nimodipine and the triple-H therapy, are there any more options to treat vasospasm?

Intraventricular nicardipine, intra-arterial milrinone, nitric oxide, and clazosentan are new alternatives for the treatment of refractory vasospasm.

78. How is intraventricular nicardipine used in the treatment of vasospasm?

Intraventricular nicardipine can be used to treat severe vasospasm in doses of 4 mg every 12 hours for 5 to 17 days.[15]

79. What is the clinical use of milrinone?

Intra-arterial followed by systemic milrinone for 14 days demonstrated a significant enlargement in diameter of vasospastic intracranial arteries. The systemic dose started at 50 µg/kg/min and was titrated to 1.5 µg/kg/min.[16]

80. What is the mechanism of action of clazosentan?

Clazosentan, an endothelin receptor antagonist, has been shown to decrease moderate and severe vasospasm and is currently being evaluated in phase III trials.[17]

81. What is the treatment for SIADH?

Fluid restriction (800–1,000 mL/d). An alternative is demeclocycline, which is an antibiotic that inhibits ADH's action on the collecting duct of the kidney, producing water diuresis.[12]

82. What is the treatment for cerebral salt wasting (CSW)?

Replacement of intravascular volume with normal saline.[12]

83. What is the treatment for diabetes insipidus (DI)?

Most of the time, DI is transient and does not require management other than to monitor inputs and outputs. If necessary, desmopressin at 2 to 4 µg every 8 to 12 hours IM or IV can be given.

84. What is another clinical use of desmopressin?

Desmopressin (0.3 µg/kg) can be used in thrombocytopenia or platelet dysfunction including platelet dysfunction related to acetylsalicylic acid (aspirin) or clopidogrel. Desmopressin releases von Willebrand factor from the endothelium.[12]

85. What is the mechanism of action of warfarin?

It inhibits the hepatic synthesis of vitamin K–dependent clotting factors: I, VII, IX, and X. It has no effect on factors already synthesized.[18]

86. What are the options to reverse the effects of warfarin?

Vitamin K (10 mg IV or IM for a few days), factor VII, and protein C activation peptide (PCP; factor IX).[18]

87. For emergent reversal of anticoagulation in warfarin-consuming patients, will factor VIIa correct the international normalized ratio (INR) and the underlying coagulopathy?

No, factor VIIa will reverse the INR but will not replace the vitamin K–dependent factors (II, VII, IX, X). Factor VIIa is thought to act by binding to the surface of activated platelets, forming a stable clot. The optimal dose for the reversal of warfarin is not known, and ranges from 10 to 20 µg/kg. Vitamin K and fresh frozen plasma are required to replace inactivated factors.[18]

88. Which medications and foods can increase the levels of warfarin?

Cimetidine, metronidazole, trimethoprim-sulfamethoxazole, fluconazole, amiodarone, and grapefruit—they have in common the liver enzyme CYP3A4.[18]

89. What is the mechanism of action of heparin?

It inhibits the activity of several clotting factors (IIa, IXa, Xa, XIa, XIIa) via activation of antithrombin III.[3]

90. What are the side effects of heparin?

Bleeding, osteoporosis, heparin-induced thrombocytopenia, and hypersensitivity. Low-molecular-weight heparins can be used in case of hypersensitivity, but the risk of thrombocytopenia is still present.

91. What is the mechanism of action of acetylsalicylic acid (aspirin) and for how long will the effects last?

Acetylsalicylic acid (aspirin) blocks irreversibly the enzymatic conversion (by inhibiting cyclooxygenase 1 [COX-1]) of arachidonic acid to prostaglandins and thromboxanes, lasting 7 to 10 days, the life span of platelets.

92. What is the mechanism of action of clopidogrel (Plavix)?

It blocks adenosine diphosphate (ADP) receptors on platelets decreasing its activation. Its effects can be reversed by the administration of platelets and desmopressin (DDAVP).[3]

93. What are the treatment options for von Willebrand's disease?

Cryoprecipitate—which is rich in factors VII and XIII, fibrinogen, VW factor, and desmopressin (DDAVP)—facilitates the release of von Willebrand factor from epithelial cells.

Toxicology

94. Name the antidote for organophosphates, lead, iron, and arsenic.

Atropine/pralidoxime, ethylenediaminetetraacetic acid (EDTA), deferoxamine, and dimercaprol, respectively.[2,3]

95. What is the antidote for copper, iron, lead, and mercury intoxication?

Penicillamine.[2,3]

96. What is the antidote for carbon monoxide intoxication?

Oxygen.

97. What are the mechanisms of action of cocaine?

It blocks dopamine, norepinephrine, and serotonin reuptake in the CNS causing tachycardia, hypertension, mydriasis, hyperactivity, psychotic episodes, hallucinations, dyskinesias, and decreased appetite. Complications resulting from toxicity are arrhythmias, myocardial infarction, stroke, subarachnoid hemorrhage, and convulsions, which can lead to death.[19]

98. What is the common presentation and time course of stroke associated with cocaine?

Seventy percent of strokes after intranasal and IV cocaine use are hemorrhagic. Most strokes tend to occur within an hour of use, especially for "crack" (freebase form, smokable) and IV injection. Others occur within 3 hours. Infarction of the brain, spinal cord (usually anterior spinal artery), or retinal artery occurs less frequently than hemorrhage, but is more common with smoking "crack" cocaine. Patients tend to develop their infarct within a few hours of use or wake up with a deficit the morning after.[19]

99. What are the mechanisms of action of amphetamines?

They block the reuptake of norepinephrine and dopamine, and release amines into the circulation. Amphetamines have effects and toxicity similar to those of cocaine.[19]

100. What is a thromboelastogram (TEG) and what does it measure?

TEG is a laboratory technique that allows monitoring of all components of the coagulation cascade from platelet activation to clot formation and lysis.[20]

101. What are the components of the TEG and how can this information be used?

The r-time measures the time it takes for the formation of the fibrin clot.

The k-time measures the time it takes for the clot to achieve a certain level of clot strength.

Alpha-angle measures how effective the cross-linking is between fibrin clots.

Maximum amplitude measures the strength of the clot and therefore the interaction between platelets and fibrin via GPII/IIIb.

LY30 measures fibrinolysis.[20]

102. Is the use of anticonvulsants recommended following subarachnoid hemorrhage (SAH)?

Prophylactic anticonvulsants may be used in the postictal period but short term unless the patient has risk factors for the development of seizures or the SAH was accompanied by intracerebral hematoma.[21]

103. Following SAH, is prophylactic hypervolemia recommended to prevent delayed cerebral ischemia?

Hypervolemia is not indicated for the prevention of delayed cerebral ischemia, but only for its treatment in the setting of vasospasm.[21]

104. When is tranexamic acid or aminocaproic acid indicated in patients with SAH?

When the aneurysm cannot be repaired within 72 hours from the ictus or there is a significant risk for rebleeding.[21]

105. In patients with spontaneous intracranial hypertension (ICH), how should blood pressure be managed? What about long term?

In patients that present with elevated blood pressure (150–220 systolic), it is safe to lower SBP to 140 mm Hg if there are no associated contraindications, as it can improve outcomes. After the acute management of ICH, it is important to maintain good control of BP with a systolic no more than 130 and a diastolic of 80 mm Hg.[22]

106. In anticoagulant-related ICH, when should anticoagulation be restarted? What type?

The exact timing to restart anticoagulation following an anticoagulant-related ICH is uncertain. If the patient does not have a mechanical valve, anticoagulation needs to be withheld at least for 4 weeks to avoid a possible rebleed. If aspirin is warranted it may be restarted a few days following the hemorrhagic event as a single agent, but there are no certainties in regard to the best time to do so.[22]

107. What is to be considered when treating anemia in patients with SAH? When should a patient be transfused?

The first of the most important two things to consider in approaching the SAH patient with anemia is that increasing the oxygen-carrying capacity of the blood by transfusing red cells will allow more oxygen to be carried to the brain, to the potential areas of vasospasm. The second is that these red cells will not necessarily get where they are needed, as with an increase in hemoglobin, the viscosity of the blood also increases, potentially exacerbating the potential ischemia of the regions downstream from the spastic vessels. There is no magic level of hemoglobin that should trigger a transfusion, but it seems that SAH patients tend to do better with an HB around 9 g/dL.[23]

108. What is the main characteristic of normal saline that makes it suitable for fluid resuscitation? What is the most common possible electrolyte abnormality when using normal saline in fluid resuscitation?

The fact that it has the same osmolality as plasma (286 mOsm/kg H_2O). Normal saline is different in its electrolyte composition and pH. In fact it has a higher concentration of chloride (154 mEq/L vs 90–106 in plasma) that in cases of large volume supplementation may place the patient at risk of hyperchloremic metabolic acidosis.[24]

109. How is vancomycin dosed? What are the things that need to be considered when dosing vancomycin?

Vancomycin has a long half-life and therefore a loading dose may help in reaching target concentration quickly, especially in those patients with sepsis, meningitis, or endocarditis.

Subsequent doses are based upon the patient's creatinine clearance and body weight.

Vancomycin levels and renal function are monitored in patients that will undergo therapy for more than 3 days. Vancomycin troughs are drawn 30 minutes before the fourth dose.[25]

110. When giving normal saline, what is the net effect on the extracellular volume and why?

25% of the normal saline given will remain in the intravascular space, and the sodium will rise slightly according to the amount of normal saline given and the volume of the extracellular fluid in the patient. In normovolemic patients, there are 14 L of ECF, so if 1 L of normal saline is given, this will only add 150 mmol of Na in total.[24] The fact that the sodium is higher in the normal saline will also attract an extra 100 mL from the intracellular compartment to the extracellular one.

111. How is the volume deficit best estimated in a critically ill patient? How is it defined?

The volume deficit in a critically ill patient is monitored by serially measuring the weight of the patient, with mild deficit represented by an acute loss in 4% of the initial weight, moderate in 6 to 8% and severe in 15%. Severe volume deficit can cause cardiovascular compromise.

112. In fluid resuscitation of a neurosurgical patient with traumatic brain injury, what fluid needs to be avoided and why?

Ringer's lactate. For two main reasons: First, it is a hypotonic solution and therefore can exacerbate cerebral edema. Second, it can bind to the citrated anticoagulants in blood products.[26]

113. 3L of D5W provides 500 kcal/d, which is enough to avoid catabolism of proteins. What is the reason for which D5W is not routinely used in critically ill patients?

In noncritically ill patients only 5% of the infused dextrose will be converted to lactate, while it has been shown that in the critically ill patients up to 85% of the dextrose gets converted to lactate.[27]

114. What is the main reason why dextrans have limited use in trauma patients as plasma expanders?

Dextran is a colloid that expands the intravascular space with less volume than crystalloids, and more specifically 1 L of dextran increases the intravascular space by 800 mL while 1 L of NS only adds 180 mL. They find limited use in trauma patients due to their side effects that include anaphylactic reactions and potential inhibition of the coagulation cascade.[28]

115. What is the effect of urea in hyponatremia? When is it appropriate to give?

Urea is an osmotic agent; it gets excreted pulling water out of the extracellular space and allowing for passive reabsorption of sodium in the impermeable segment of the loop of Henle. It is a good treatment when the mechanism of the hyponatremia is uncertain and CSW versus SIADH is still being worked up.[29]

116. How is hypernatremia corrected?

Free water deficit is calculated with the equation 140 mEq/L × 0.6 × usual body weight/$[Na]_{current}$

Half the water deficit is given over the first 24 hours and the remainder over the following 24 to 48 hours.

117. How is SIADH differentiated from CSW?

The only reliable method to differentiate SIADH and CSW is to measure the fractional excretion of urate (FE urate), correct the hyponatremia with hypertonic saline, and then remeasure the FE urate. If the FE urate normalizes (range 4–11%), it was SIADH; if FE urate remains elevated (> 11%), it was CSW.[30]

118. Phenylephrine is very useful to reach BP goals in critically ill patients. When is it not indicated in neurosurgery and why?

Phenylephrine has selective α-1 adrenergic effect and for this reason has good hypertensive effect that at times may cause reflex vagal tone with subsequent bradycardia due to increase in vagal tone.[31]

119. Dopamine is used with caution as a pressor in neurosurgical patients given that it may worsen cerebral edema. What is the first-line pressor in patients with traumatic brain injury? In what type of neurosurgical patients has dopamine been widely used as first choice?

Norepinephrine has been demonstrated to improve brain oxygenation compared with dopamine without worsening in cerebral edema. Furthermore, the use of dopamine may affect the release of some pituitary hormones. Dopamine has been the first-line choice of pressor in patients with spinal cord injury, although recent evidence did not demonstrate significant difference in neurologic improvement.

120. What nonbarbiturate agent is used in aneurysm surgery to achieve burst suppression and is thought to be neuroprotective?[32]

Propofol has been used as a neuroprotective agent when used to achieve burst suppression in aneurysm surgery, especially when the use of temporary clips is warranted. This is linked to its properties of reducing cerebral metabolic rate, reducing blood flow and intracranial pressure. Unfortunately, this seemed to work only in experimental animal models and failed to lead to improvement in postoperative outcomes in the clinical setting, probably as it provokes persistent pial vessel constriction.[33]

■ References

1. Kandel E, Schwartz J, Jessell T. Principles of Neural Science. New York, NY: McGraw-Hill Medical; 2000
2. Katzung BG. Basic & Clinical Pharmacology. Stamford, CT: Appleton & Lange; 2000
3. Brunton L, Blumenthal D, Buxton I. Goodman and Gilman's Manual of Pharmacology and Therapeutics. New York, NY: McGraw-Hill Professional; 2007
4. Abou Khaled KJ, Hirsch LJ. Updates in the management of seizures and status epilepticus in critically ill patients. Neurol Clin 2008;26(2):385–408, viii
5. Vasile B, Rasulo F, Candiani A, Latronico N. The pathophysiology of propofol infusion syndrome: a simple name for a complex syndrome. Intensive Care Med 2003;29(9):1417–1425
6. Coffey RJ, Edgar TS, Francisco GE, et al. Abrupt withdrawal from intrathecal baclofen: recognition and management of a potentially life-threatening syndrome. Arch Phys Med Rehabil 2002;83(6):735–741
7. Deer TR, Raso LJ, Coffey RJ, Allen JW. Intrathecal baclofen and catheter tip inflammatory mass lesions (granulomas): a reevaluation of case reports and imaging findings in light of experimental, clinicopathological, and radiological evidence. Pain Med 2008;9(4):391–395
8. Greenberg MS. Handbook of Neurosurgery. 6th ed. New York, NY: Thieme Medical Publishers; 2006
9. Gertler R, Brown HC, Mitchell DH, Silvius EN. Dexmedetomidine: a novel sedative-analgesic agent. Proc Bayl Univ Med Cent 2001;14(1):13–21
10. Rozet I. Anesthesia for functional neurosurgery: the role of dexmedetomidine. Curr Opin Anaesthesiol 2008;21(5):537–543

11. Ziai WC, Lewin JJ III. Update in the diagnosis and management of central nervous system infections. Neurol Clin 2008;26(2): 427–468, viii

12. Rangel-Castilla L, Gopinath S, Robertson CS. Management of intracranial hypertension. Neurol Clin 2008;26(2):521–541, x

13. Urrutia VC, Wityk RJ. Blood pressure management in acute stroke. Neurol Clin 2008;26(2):565–583, x–xi

14. Sillberg VA, Wells GA, Perry JJ. Do statins improve outcomes and reduce the incidence of vasospasm after aneurysmal subarachnoid hemorrhage: a meta-analysis. Stroke 2008;39(9):2622–2626

15. Goodson K, Lapointe M, Monroe T, Chalela JA. Intraventricular nicardipine for refractory cerebral vasospasm after subarachnoid hemorrhage. Neurocrit Care 2008;8(?):247–252

16. Fraticelli AT, Cholley BP, Losser MR, Saint Maurice JP, Payen D. Milrinone for the treatment of cerebral vasospasm after aneurysmal subarachnoid hemorrhage. Stroke 2008;39(3):893–898

17. Macdonald RL, Kassell NF, Mayer S, et al; CONSCIOUS-1 Investigators. Clazosentan to overcome neurological ischemia and infarction occurring after subarachnoid hemorrhage (CONSCIOUS-1): randomized, double-blind, placebo-controlled phase 2 dose-finding trial. Stroke 2008;39(11):3015–3021

18. Aiyagari V, Testai FD. Correction of coagulopathy in warfarin associated cerebral hemorrhage. Curr Opin Crit Care 2009;15(2):87–92

19. Enevoldson TP. Recreational drugs and their neurological consequences. J Neurol Neurosurg Psychiatry 2004;75(suppl 3):iii9–iii15

20. Thakur M, Ahmed AB. A review of thromboelastography. Int J Periop Ultrasound Appl Technol 2012;1(1):25–29

21. Sander Connolly E, Rabinstein AA, Carhuapoma JR, et al., on behalf of the American Heart Association Stroke Council, Council on Cardiovascular Radiology and Intervention, Council on Cardiovascular Nursing, Council on Cardiovascular Surgery and Anesthesia, and Council on Clinical Cardiology. Guidelines for the management of aneurysmal subarachnoid hemorrhage. Stroke 2012. https://doi.org/10.1161/STR.0b013e3182587839

22. Hemphill JC, Greenberg SM, Anderson CS, et al. Guidelines for the Management of Spontaneous Intracerebral Hemorrhage. Stroke 2015;STR.0000000000000069, originally published May 28, 2015

23. Oddo M, Milby A, Chen I, et al. Hemoglobin concentration and cerebral metabolism in patients with aneurysmal subarachnoid hemorrhage. Stroke 2009;40(4):1275–1281

24. Lobo DN, Dube MG, Neal KR, Simpson J, Rowlands BJ, Allison SP. Problems with solutions: drowning in the brine of an inadequate knowledge base. Br J Surg 2000;87(S1):53

25. Ye ZK, Chen K, Chen YL, Zhai SD. A protocol for developing a clinical practice guideline for therapeutic drug monitoring of vancomycin. J Huazhong Univ Sci Technolog Med Sci 2016;36(3):469–472 [Medical Sciences]

26. Haddad SH, Arabi YM. Critical care management of severe traumatic brain injury in adults. Scand J Trauma Resusc Emerg Med 2012;20:12

27. Günther B, Jauch KW, Hartl W, Wicklmayr M, Dietze G, Heberer G. Low-dose glucose infusion in patients who have undergone surgery. Possible cause of a muscular energy deficit. Arch Surg 1987;122(7):765–771

28. Coats TJ, Heron M. The effect of hypertonic saline dextran on whole blood coagulation. Resuscitation 2004;60(1):101–104

29. Pierrakos C, Taccone FS, Decaux G, Vincent J-L, Brimioulle S. Urea for treatment of acute SIADH in patients with subarachnoid hemorrhage: a single-center experience. Ann Intensive Care 2012;2(1):13

30. Maesaka JK, Imbriano L, Mattana J, Gallagher D, Bade N, Sharif S. Differentiating SIADH from cerebral/renal salt wasting: failure of the volume approach and need for a new approach to hyponatremia. J Clin Med 2014;3(4):1373–1385

31. Kroppenstedt SN, Sakowitz OW, Thomale UW, Unterberg AW, Stover JF. Norepinephrine is superior to dopamine in increasing cortical perfusion following controlled cortical impact injury in rats. In: Czosnyka M, Pickard JD, Kirkpatrick PJ, Smielewski P, Hutchinson P, eds. Intracranial Pressure and Brain Biochemical Monitoring. Acta Neurochirurgica Supplements. Vol 81. Vienna: Springer; 2002

32. Pfister D, Strebel SP, Steiner LA. Effects of catecholamines on cerebral blood vessels in patients with traumatic brain injury. Eur J Anaesthesiol Suppl 2008;42:98–103

33. Mahajan C, Chouhan RS, Rath GP, et al. Effect of intraoperative brain protection with propofol on postoperative cognition in patients undergoing temporary clipping during intracranial aneurysm surgery. Neurol India 2014;62(3):262–268

5 Cranial Neurosurgery

General

■ History and Physical Examination

1. What is the most common type of headache?

Tension headache is the most common. Other types of headaches are migraine headaches and cervicogenic headaches.

2. What lesions can produce a head tilt?

Trochlear (fourth) nerve palsy, anterior vermis lesion, and tonsillar herniation. In myasthenia gravis, the head tilts back.[1]

3. What is the term for the vermicular movement of the face in a patient with pontine demyelination?

Myokymia.[2]

4. What disorders can benefit from deep brain stimulation (DBS) of the ventral intermediate (VIM) thalamic nucleus?

Essential tremor and parkinsonian tremor.[3,4]

5. What region of the internal capsule may be affected in a patient with dysarthria and clumsy-hand syndrome?[5]

The genu.

6. Dilute pilocarpine (0.1–0.125%) may constrict what type of pupil?

An Adie pupil. This is possibly because of denervation supersensitivity as the normal pupil reacts only to 1% pilocarpine. A pharmacologic pupil (dilated for the purpose of examination by an ophthalmologist) will not constrict with 1% pilocarpine; however, a pupil that is dilated from a compressive third cranial nerve (CN) palsy may constrict with 1% pilocarpine.[6]

7. What is the term given when the consensual light reflex is stronger than the direct light reflex?

Afferent pupillary defect. The lesion is ipsilateral to the side of the impaired direct reflex.[7]

8. What is the most common cause of spontaneous diplopia in middle-aged people?

Orbital Graves' disease is the most common cause of spontaneous diplopia in this age group. It can present with normal thyroid function tests. The inferior and medial rectus muscles are involved first. The patient may present with marked lid edema, lid retraction, and ophthalmoplegia. Dysthyroid disease may occur unilaterally and with normal thyroid function tests, which makes this diagnosis difficult. Steroids are helpful in the acute setting.[8]

9. Which Parkinson-like disease manifests with vertical gaze palsy?

Progressive supranuclear palsy (also known as Steele-Richardson-Olszewski syndrome).[7]

10. In one-and-a-half syndrome, which eye movement is preserved?

Abduction of the unaffected eye.[9]

11. How can one differentiate an oculomotor palsy from an aneurysm versus an oculomotor palsy from diabetic neuropathy?

An oculomotor palsy in diabetes usually occurs with pain and may occur with pupillary sparing, which helps to distinguish it from an aneurysmal cause. Anatomically, the parasympathetic fibers on the oculomotor nerve are at the periphery; therefore, a compressive lesion such as an aneurysm will compromise these fibers first.[10]

12. What disease is characterized by ataxia, myoclonus, positive immunoassay for 14–3–3 protein, and bilateral sharp waves on electroencephalogram (EEG)?

Creutzfeldt-Jakob disease (CJD).[11]

13. What tests can be performed to differentiate an actual seizure from a pseudoseizure?

EEG, serum prolactin level, and muscle enzyme studies.[11]

14. What type of electrical activity occurs with an absence seizure?

3 Hz per second spike and wave.[12]

15. How does the diplopia of myasthenia gravis differ from the diplopia of a compressive lesion?

The diplopia of myasthenia is intermittent, whereas the diplopia of a compressive lesion is constant or worsening.[7] A useful bedside test to distinguish myasthenia gravis from other causes of ptosis is the ice pack test explained by Liu and Chen.[13] A decrease in ptosis (> 5 mm) can be seen with 2 minutes of ice pack over the affected eye.

16. What extraocular muscle may be involved if a horizontal object appears slanted?

Superior oblique muscle.[14]

17. How does one differentiate the hypertension caused by a pheochromocytoma from essential hypertension?

Clonidine suppression test (reduces only essential hypertension). If no decrease in plasma catecholamine levels is detected after giving a 0.3-μg/kg oral test dose, the study is considered positive (pheochromocytoma).[15]

18. What do lesions of the bilateral hippocampi produce?

Recent memory impairment.[16]

19. In what percentage of left-handed subjects is the left hemisphere dominant?

Over 75%.[17]

20. What are the clinical symptoms of normal pressure hydrocephalus (NPH)?

The chief feature is gait disturbance; the other two major components are memory loss, usually for recent events, and urinary incontinence. These features are similar to Alzheimer's disease, but in Alzheimer's disease the memory loss is out of proportion to the gait disorder. A good clue to NPH is that gait disturbance is usually the first symptom to appear and may precede the other symptoms by months to years. If rigidity and tremor occur, these patients can be diagnosed incorrectly with Parkinson's disease. Other diseases in the differential diagnosis are depression and multi-infarct dementia. A computed tomography (CT) scan of the brain in NPH shows large ventricles out of proportion to atrophy. The cerebrospinal fluid (CSF) pressure measured by lumbar puncture is not high for unknown reasons. A good test to show that an NPH patient may improve with a ventriculo-peritoneal shunt is to place a lumbar drain for a few days and watch for any improvement (especially of gait, which is very predictive).[18] It is also beneficial to discharge the patient home and have the symptoms reappear as a reconfirmation of NPH. The patient can then be scheduled electively with assurance that symptoms should improve with a shunt.

21. What is the name of the area involved with cortical inhibition of bladder and bowel voiding that is damaged in NPH?

The paracentral lobule.[18]

22. What other diseases must first be ruled out to be confident about the diagnosis of NPH?

Vascular dementia, Parkinson's disease, dementia with Lewy's bodies, cervical spondylotic myelopathy, and peripheral neuropathy.[18]

23. What are the synapses that occur in the pupillary reflex?[19]

- An afferent impulse through the optic nerve to the superior colliculus.
- The superior colliculus to the Edinger-Westphal nuclei bilaterally.
- From the Edinger-Westphal nucleus through the third CN to the ciliary ganglion.
- From the ciliary ganglion via the short ciliary nerves.

24. If there is a problem with pupillary response, where is the lesion in relation to the lateral geniculate body?

Anterior to the lateral geniculate body.[20]

25. What are some causes of circumoral paresthesia?

Hypocalcemia, hyperventilation, syringobulbia, and neurotoxin fish poisoning.[21]

26. What is significant about the pitch of tinnitus?

Low-pitch tinnitus is seen in conductive deafness and Ménière's disease; high-pitch tinnitus is seen with sensori-neural deafness.[22]

27. What is the significance of a "transverse smile" in a patient with myasthenia gravis?

A myasthenic snarl (or transverse smile) may be seen with bulbar muscle involvement in myasthenia gravis.[23]

28. What diseases may manifest as facial myokymia?

Intrinsic brainstem glioma or multiple sclerosis (MS).[2]

29. What maneuver can elicit nystagmus characteristic of benign positional vertigo?

The Dix-Hallpike maneuver. The examiner turns the head of the seated patient to one side and pulls the patient back-ward into a supine position with the head hanging over the edge of the examining table; the patient then looks straight ahead and the examiner observes for positional nystagmus, which is indicative of benign positional vertigo.[24]

30. What are some characteristics of benign positional vertigo?

Fatigability is often seen and nystagmus is characteristic with rotatory movement in one eye and vertical movement in the other eye. Patients describe a "critical position" that either elicits the vertigo or alleviates the vertigo.[24]

31. What are some characteristics of Ménière's disease?

Spontaneous bouts of prolonged vertigo, fluctuating hearing loss (poor speech perception), tinnitus, and excessive endolymph within the scala media. It may mimic an acoustic neuroma.[22]

32. What are the major signs and symptoms of lateral medullary infarction?

Vertigo, nausea, vomiting, intractable hiccups, diplopia, dysphagia, dysphonia, ipsilateral sensory loss of facial pain and temperature, ipsilateral Horner's syndrome, contralateral pain, and temperature loss of the limbs and trunk. This is also known as Wallenberg's syndrome.[25]

33. What differentiates ptosis due to third CN palsy from ptosis in Horner's syndrome?

Horner's syndrome ptosis is partial and disappears on looking up.[26]

34. What localizing value is the presence of anhidrosis in Horner's syndrome?

If the lesion is proximal to the internal carotid artery (ICA) origin or involves the external carotid artery circulation, then the anhidrosis is present along the face due to dysfunction of cervical sympathetic output. If the lesion is more proximal (along the first- or second-order neuron level), then the anhidrosis may involve a greater portion of the hemibody.[26]

35. What are some causes of partial ptosis from a first-order Horner syndrome?

A first-order Horner syndrome involves the nerves from the posterolateral hypothalamus to the intermediolateral cell column (at C8–T2). Its causes include an Arnold-Chiari malformation, basal meningitis, basal skull fracture, lateral medullary syndrome, demyelinating disease, an intrapontine hemorrhage, neck trauma, pituitary tumor, and syringomyelia.[26]

36. What pharmacologic test can be used to determine if Horner's syndrome is second order or third order?

Hydroxyamphetamine drops placed in the eye of a patient with Horner's syndrome with intact postganglionic fibers (i.e., first- or second-order neuron lesions) dilate the pupil to an equal or greater extent than a normal pupil, whereas in an eye with damaged postganglionic fibers (third-order neuron lesions) and in a normal pupil the pupil does not dilate after hydroxyamphetamine drops.[26]

37. What is Bell's phenomenon?

On attempting to close the eyes and show the teeth, one eye does not close and the eyeball rotates upward and outward.[27]

38. What are some nutritional causes of dementia?

Wernicke-Korsakoff syndrome (thiamine deficiency), vitamin B12 deficiency, and folate deficiency.

39. What is the name of the inherited disorder that presents with migraine (often hemiplegic) in early adult life, progressing through transient ischemic attacks (TIAs) and subcortical strokes to early dementia?

CADASIL. The disease CADASIL (cerebral autosomal dominant arteriopathy with subcortical infarcts and leukoencephalopathy) is a recently identified cause of stroke and vascular dementia. CADASIL is identified by finding mutations in a gene called NOTCH3, which influences how cells in blood vessels grow and develop.[28]

40. What tests or procedures can one perform to determine if a patient with NPH will benefit from a shunt?[19]

- The presence of β waves can be noted with intracranial pressure (ICP) monitoring for more than 4 hours over a 24-hour period.
- After lumbar CSF drainage for a few days, there is clinical improvement.

41. What is the most common cause of cardioembolic stroke?

Atrial fibrillation.[29]

42. What arteries supply macular vision?

Posterior cerebral artery (PCA) and middle cerebral artery (MCA).[30]

43. What are symptoms of color desaturation in MS?

Patients complain about their perception of color, for example, the perception of red color as different shades of orange or gray.[31]

44. In acoustic schwannomas, when tumors are greater than 2 cm the trigeminal nerve may be involved, causing facial pain, numbness, and paresthesias. What sign on CN examination may be an early manifestation of this phenomenon?

Depression of the corneal reflex on the side of the tumor is an early sign. Facial weakness is surprisingly uncommon despite marked CN VII compression.

45. At what diameter of the carotid vessel lumen does a carotid bruit manifest on auscultation?

Carotid artery bruits, often atherosclerotic in nature, become audible when the residual vessel lumen diameter approaches 2.5 to 3 mm; they later disappear as the lumen is thinned to 0.5 mm.[32,33]

46. What are some features of Cushing's syndrome?

Moon face, acne, hirsutism and baldness, buffalo-type obesity, purple striae over flank and abdomen, bruising, muscle weakness and wasting, osteoporosis, hypertension, susceptibility to infection, and diabetes mellitus.

47. What are conditions that may result in upgaze palsy?

Tumor on the quadrigeminal plate or pineal region (Parinaud's syndrome), hydrocephalus or other causes of elevated ICP, Guillain-Barré syndrome, myasthenia gravis, botulism, and hypothyroidism.

48. In what percentage of patients will phenytoin result in a skin rash?

About 5 to 10%.[34,35]

49. What is the diagnosis (until proven otherwise) of an adult patient who presents with recurrent meningitis without any other predisposing conditions?

CSF fistula. Recurrent meningitis in an infant may be a manifestation of basal encephalocele.

50. What is the other name of the disease known as cupulolithiasis?

Benign positional vertigo.[36]

51. What causes horizontal diplopia?

Paresis of one or both of the sixth CNs. This may occur, for example, with pseudotumor cerebri as a false localizing sign. The firm attachment of the abducens nerve at the pontomedullary junction and its attachment to the dural elements as it passes into the Dorello canal make it susceptible to stretch forces in cases of high ICP.[37]

52. A cherry red spot in the retina is seen in which conditions?

- Tay-Sachs disease.
- Niemann-Pick disease.
- Pseudo-Hurler's syndrome (GM1 ganglioside).

53. Retinitis pigmentosa is seen in which conditions?

- Friedreich's ataxia.
- Refsum's disease.
- Cockayne's syndrome.
- Kearns-Sayre syndrome.

54. What is cerebellar mutism?

Mutism seen in children usually 1 to 4 days after a vermian lesion resection that may take weeks to months to resolve.

55. What is the House-Brackmann classification of a seventh CN injury?

- Grade I: normal.
- Grade II: mild deformity and mild synkinesis.
- Grade III: moderate damage, good eye closure, forehead function is preserved.
- Grade IV: no forehead function, partial eye closure.
- Grade V: no eye closure.
- Grade VI: total paralysis, no tone.[38,39]

56. Which questions should be asked regarding seventh CN palsy?

- Ask about history of diabetes mellitus, pregnancy, autoimmune disorders, and ear/parotid surgery.
- Also inquire about otalgia, otorrhea, vertigo, and blurred vision as well as taste.

57. What is Melkersson-Rosenthal syndrome?

Triad of recurrent orofacial edema, recurrent seventh CN palsy, and lingua plicata.[40]

58. What is Ramsay Hunt syndrome?

- Herpes zoster oticus.
- Third most common cause of seventh CN palsy.

59. What is Heerfordt's syndrome?

- Uveoparotid fever.
- Seventh CN palsy in sarcoidosis.[41]

60. Bilateral seventh CN palsy is indicative of which infectious disease?

Lyme disease.

61. What is Millard-Gubler syndrome?

Ipsilateral sixth and seventh CN palsy and contralateral hemiparesis.[42]

62. What is Brissaud-Sicard syndrome?

Ipsilateral CN VII hemispasm and contralateral hemiparesis.[42]

63. What is Foville's syndrome?

Ipsilateral CN VI and VII involvement and horizontal gaze paralysis with contralateral hemiparesis.[42]

64. What is Panayiotopoulos' syndrome?

Benign occipital lobe epilepsy in children (40% idiopathic). Presents between 1 and 14 years of age and includes eye deviation and myoclonic jerks. It is sleep induced and has a good prognosis.[43]

■ Techniques

65. What is the diameter in millimeters of a 12-French suction tip used in neurosurgery?

Three French units equal 1 mm. A 12-French suction catheter has an outer diameter of 4 mm at the tip. The French gauge was devised by Joseph-Frédéric-Benoît Charrière, a 19th-century Parisian maker of surgical instruments, who defined the "diameter times 3" relationship.

66. What is exposed from a properly placed burr hole at the keyhole area?

The frontal dura in the upper half and the periorbita in the lower half.

67. Where is the keyhole in relation to the frontozygomatic point?

Directly above the frontozygomatic point.[44]

68. What is the significance of the frontozygomatic point?

It is the location on the lateral orbital bone (~2.5 cm from the zygoma attachment) which, if connected with the 75% point (three-fourths of the distance from the nasion to the inion), approximates the location of the sylvian fissure.[44]

69. An incision reaching the zygoma that is more than 1.5 cm anterior to the ear may interrupt what nerve?

The branch of the facial nerve that passes across the zygoma to reach the frontalis muscle.[44]

70. Where are the skull landmarks for upper and lower rolandic points?

Upper point is 2 cm behind the "50% point" and the lower point is midway on the zygoma. Connecting these two points approximates the location of the central sulcus.[39]

71. How can the internal auditory canal be identified below the floor of the middle fossa?

By drilling along a line approximately 60 degrees medial to the axis of the arcuate eminence, near the middle portion of the angle between the axis of the greater superficial petrosal nerve (GSPN) and the axis of the arcuate eminence (**Fig. 5.1**).[38]

72. What types of variations on the subfrontal operative route are used to access a suprasellar craniopharyngioma or other lesions of the third ventricle?

Lamina terminalis approach, opticocarotid approach through the opticocarotid triangle, subchiasmatic approach below the optic chiasm, and transfrontal–transsphenoidal approach through the planum sphenoidale and sphenoid sinus (**Fig. 5.2**).[46]

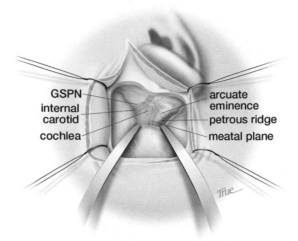

Fig. 5.1 Middle fossa approach for resection of vestibular schwannoma with labeled landmarks. GSPN, greater superficial petrosal nerve. (Reproduced with permission from Badie.[45])

73. What operative approach can be used for a tumor of the tegmentum of the midbrain?

Subtemporal transtentorial approach.

74. What length of temporal tip may be safely removed from the nondominant side?

6 to 7 cm.[48]

75. What are the initial steps in performing a superficial temporal artery biopsy?

Trace out the artery's course with Doppler ultrasound, determine branching pattern, sample the frontal branch by dissecting the artery under microscope, and obtain a segment 3 to 5 cm long.[49]

76. What is the inferior frontal gyrus on the dominant hemisphere called?

Broca area.

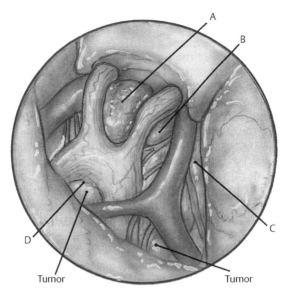

Fig. 5.2 Variation routes of the subfrontal approach to access suprasellar mass: A, between optic nerves; B, opticocarotid triangle; C, carotid–oculomotor triangle; D, lamina terminalis. (Reproduced with permission from Sekhar and Fessler.[47])

77. Through which triangle may one access the posterior fossa dura anterior to the sigmoid sinus?

The Trautmann triangle.[50]

78. Following the GSPN will lead to which ganglion?

The geniculate ganglion.

79. What part of the internal capsule lies very close to the foramen of Monro?

The genu of the internal capsule.[51]

80. After a callosal opening, how can one determine if one has opened the left or right lateral ventricle?

By observing the relationship of the thalamostriate vein and choroid plexus; the thalamostriate vein is located lateral to the choroid plexus (**Fig. 5.3**).[52]

81. After a callosal opening, if a surgeon determines that there are no intraventricular structures present, what most likely is the cause assuming the surgeon has proceeded correctly up to this point?

The surgeon has entered a cavum septum pellucidum.[52]

82. How can one enlarge the foramen of Monro in an operation for a large colloid cyst?

The ipsilateral column of the fornix can be incised at the anterosuperior margin of the foramen of Monro of the nondominant side. There is a risk of memory loss anytime the fornix is manipulated. If access is needed to the midportion of the third ventricle, opening the tela choroidea medial to the choroid plexus is a safe pathway.[52]

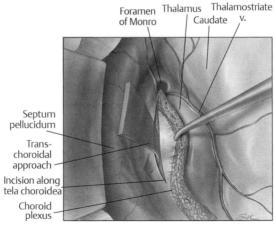

Fig. 5.3 Transcallosal approach to the lateral and third ventricles. (Reproduced with permission from Badie.[45])

83. What nucleus of the thalamus may be damaged while opening the body of the choroidal fissure?

The dorsomedial nucleus.[52]

84. What areas of bone may need to be removed to successfully clip a low-lying basilar artery aneurysm?

The posterior clinoids, or a portion of the dorsum sellae. An anterior petrosectomy may also be performed to clip the aneurysm.[53]

85. What are the boundaries in performing an anterior petrosectomy?

Behind the petrous ICA, in front of the internal acoustic meatus, and medial to the cochlea.[54]

86. What are the pterional routes to a basilar aneurysm?

Opticocarotid triangle, between carotid bifurcation and optic tract, carotid–oculomotor triangle above the posterior communicating (PComm) artery, and carotid–oculomotor triangle below the PComm artery.[53]

87. In what cases would one approach an anterior communicating (AComm) artery aneurysm from the left?

In a dominant left A1, dome pointing to the right, another left-sided aneurysm, possibly a left-sided blood clot.[55]

88. For a craniotomy, what are reasons to use a linear incision, a "lazy S" incision, a flap incision, and a zigzag incision?

A linear incision increases blood supply to the wound. A "lazy S" incision is used to prevent the incision line in the dura from lying directly underneath the incision in the skin. A flap incision is used so that scalp blood flow is not compromised (the base cannot be too short, and remember that blood flow is coming from inferior to superior). A pedicle that is narrower than the width of the flap may result in the flap edges becoming gangrenous. A zigzag coronal incision (sometimes called a stealth incision) is used in craniosynostosis surgery to minimize the visibility of incisional scalp alopecia in children. A zigzag coronal incision also provides greater access to the anterior and posterior skull in craniosynostosis surgery.

89. What is the technique for placing a ventriculoatrial (ventriculovenous) shunt?

An incision is made across the anterior border of the sternomastoid muscle, and the jugular vein is identified. The vein is tied off distally and a small opening made into the jugular vein to pass the shunt down the jugular vein into the right atrium of the heart. Using electrocardiographic monitoring, the atrium is indicated by the P wave configuration becoming more and more upright, and when it becomes a bi-phasic P wave, the tip has just entered the atrium, which is the optimal placement. Intraoperative fluoroscopy is used to confirm that the catheter is at the T6 level. Shunt nephritis is a complication of vascular shunts.[56]

90. Where is the distal entry point of a ventriculopleural shunt?

An incision is made between the second and third ribs lateral to the midclavicular plane, and the tubing is inserted after puncture of the parietal pleura.

91. During posterior fossa surgery, brisk venous bleeding occurs on midline dural opening. What is the source of the bleeding and what can be done to stop it?

The circular sinus can bleed during posterior fossa decompression. This bleeding is best controlled with hemostatic clips.

92. What are the landmarks and trajectory for frontal ventriculostomy or shunt placement and occipital ventriculostomy or shunt placement?

A frontal burr hole is best placed 10 cm from the nasion and 3 cm right of midline (unless there is a reason not to cannu-late the right lateral ventricle). It is best to aim the catheter midway between the lateral orbital rim and the tragus, in the direction of the medial canthus. Aiming directly at the tragus places the end of the catheter at the third ventricle. For frontal cannulation, 6 cm of catheter is inserted below the dura. For an occipital approach, select the point 7 cm above the inion and 3 cm to the right of the midline (unless there is a reason not to cannulate from the right). With this trajectory, the catheter is aimed 1 cm above the nasion. For the occipital approach, 10 cm of catheter is used; however, it is best to measure the exact distance needed on the preoperative CT scan. Occipital catheter placement may have a lesser chance of seizure disorder and better cosmesis than a frontal catheter.[57]

■ Operative Anatomy

93. What bones form the hard palate?

The anterior part is formed by the maxilla and the palatine bones form the posterior part.

94. What veins are connected at the torcula?

The superior sagittal sinus, transverse sinus, straight sinus, and occipital sinus.

95. What bones form the zygomatic arch?

The anterior part is formed by the zygoma and the posterior part is formed by the squamosal part of the temporal bone.

96. What bones form the nasal septum?

The perpendicular plate of the ethmoid and the vomer.

97. What bones form the clivus?

The sphenoid bone and occipital bone.

98. What nerve carries parasympathetic innervation of the parotid gland?

The auriculotemporal nerve.

99. Which cerebellar peduncle carries only afferent fibers?

The middle cerebellar peduncle.

100. Which thalamic veins join the thalamostriate vein?

None of them—despite its name.

101. The superior orbital fissure provides a communication between what two areas?

The orbit and the middle fossa.

102. The lamina terminalis extends upward from the optic chiasm and blends into what structure?

The rostrum of the corpus callosum.[58]

103. What cistern is contained in the posterior incisural space?

The quadrigeminal cistern.

104. The lateral and medial posterior choroidal arteries are branches of which circle of Willis artery?

The PCA.

105. How does CSF secreted from the choroid plexus enter the subarachnoid space?

Via the fourth ventricular foramina of Magendie and Luschka.

106. What is the rate of CSF formation?

About 500 mL per day (or 0.33 mL per minute) under normal conditions.[59]

107. What is the normal diameter of the supraclinoid ICA?

4 to 5 mm.[60]

108. What ligament does the abducens nerve pass under?

The petrosphenoid ligament.

109. Where does the basal vein originate and through which cisterns does it pass?

The basal vein originates on the surface of the anterior perforated substance and it courses through the crural and ambient cisterns to reach the quadrigeminal cistern and join with the internal cerebral vein.

110. What is the most medial structure in the cavernous sinus?

The ICA.[61]

111. What are the 10 anatomical triangles identified near the cavernous sinus?

The 10 triangles in the cavernous sinus area can be grouped into three regions with the triangles grouped as follows (**Fig. 5.4**)[61]:

1. The parasellar region:
   - The anteromedial triangles.
   - The paramedian triangles.
   - The oculomotor triangles.
   - The Parkinson triangles.

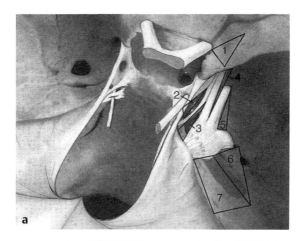

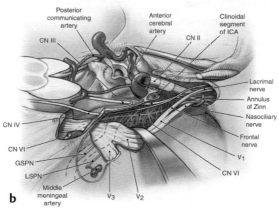

Fig. 5.4 **(a)** Triangles of the cavernous sinus. 1, anteromedial; 2, paramedian; 3, Parkinson; 4, anterolateral; 5, lateral; 6, Glasscock (posterolateral); 7, Kawase (posteromedial). (Reproduced with permission from Tamme et al.[41]) **(b)** Surgical anatomy of the cavernous sinus and basal region. GSPN, greater superficial petrosal nerve; ICA, internal carotid artery; LSPN, lesser superficial petrosal nerve. (Reproduced with permission from Sekhar and Fessler.[47])

2. The middle cranial fossa area:
    - The anterolateral triangles.
    - The lateral triangles.
    - The posterolateral (Glasscock) triangles.
    - The posteromedial (Kawase) triangles.
3. The paraclival region:
    - The inferomedial triangles.
    - The inferolateral (trigeminal) triangles.

■ Preoperative Assessment

112. What is the most common side effect of mannitol?

Renal failure.

113. When do the majority of perioperative myocardial infarctions (MIs) occur?

Between postoperative days 3 and 5.

114. What is the best method in current use to assess cerebral metabolism quantitatively?

Positron emission tomography (PET).

115. Why are inhalational anesthetics referred to as "uncoupling" agents with respect to cerebral hemodynamics and metabolism?

They decrease cerebral metabolism, but increase cerebral blood flow through vasodilatation. If an inhalational agent is to be given to a patient with poor intracranial compliance, hyperventilation should be initiated prior to induction. Isoflurane has less of an effect on cerebral blood flow than other agents.[39,62]

116. When should the use of nimodipine in vasospasm be reconsidered?

In the face of diminished cardiac contractility, use of nimodipine (which is a negative inotrope) may exacerbate the cardiac complications.

117. What should be considered in the evaluation of a patient who is scheduled for an elective craniotomy for meningioma who is hyponatremic and hypotensive, but otherwise healthy?

Adrenal insufficiency.

118. What types of coagulopathies are not detected by prothrombin time/partial thromboplastin time/international normalized ratio (PT/PTT/INR) and platelet counts?

Dysfibrinogenemia, von Willebrand's disease, factor XIII deficiency, and aspirin/Plavix use.

119. What disorders can lead to platelet sequestration?

Hypersplenism associated with cirrhosis, Gaucher's disease, and sarcoidosis.

120. In what patient population does steroid use increase the risk of gastrointestinal hemorrhage?

Patients with preexisting ulcer disease.

121. Oxygen transport is maximal when hematocrit is in what range?

30 to 32%.

122. What finding on a CT scan of the head would be predictive of the success of a third ventriculostomy for hydrocephalus?

Triventricular hydrocephalus (or obstructive hydrocephalus) from aqueductal stenosis or blockage of third ventricular outflow.[63]

123. What are the basic types of morphology of cerebral aneurysms?

Saccular, dissecting, and fusiform. The morphology of the aneurysm influences surgical and/or endovascular treatment.

Trauma and Emergencies

■ Trauma

124. What is the most common cause of subarachnoid hemorrhage (SAH)?

Head trauma.[64]

125. What is the most common cause of CSF leakage?

Head trauma; having a skull fracture doubles the patient's risk of a CSF leak. CSF leaks may occur from the nose (rhinorrhea), ear (otorrhea), or orbit (mimicking tears).[64]

126. How can one differentiate if nasal drainage is CSF or nasal secretion?

The primary distinction between CSF and nasal drainage is the glucose level. Glucose is present in CSF (at 50% of the serum level) but not in nasal drainage. A protein level of less than 1 g per liter is suggestive of CSF. The double-ring sign ("halo sign") seen on the bed sheets or clothing of patients with nasal drainage is only suggestive of a CSF leak; the β2-transferrin test can confirm the presence of CSF.[65]

127. What is the best initial treatment for a CSF leak?

Bed rest and head elevation. Most leaks stop within 3 days. If after 3 days the leak persists, lumbar drainage may be used. Rarely is surgery needed to repair the source of the leak. The use of prophylactic antibiotics is controversial and may select for more virulent bacteria should infection occur.[65]

128. What is the major cause of spontaneous intracranial hypotension?

Spontaneous CSF leaks. Diffuse pachymeningeal enhancement on magnetic resonance imaging (MRI) is the most common imaging finding. Patients often complain of headache that is alleviated by lying flat. A CT myelogram or radionucleotide cisternogram may be used to find the leak site.[65]

129. What are the areas most prone to diffuse axonal injury after head trauma?

Corpus callosum and superior cerebellar peduncle.[66]

130. What is the microscopic hallmark of diffuse axonal injury?

Axonal retraction balls, which are eosinophilic globular swellings at the proximal and distal sites of disrupted axons. They are formed by axoplasm and driven by altered axoplasmic transport.[66]

131. Regarding bullet wounds to the skull, which site is typically smaller, the entrance or exit wound?

In through-and-through missile wounds to the skull, the entrance wound is typically smaller.

132. What radiologic view is necessary to fully appreciate an occipital bone fracture and a maxillary sinus fracture on plain X-ray films?

The Towne view[67] and Water's view, respectively.

133. Which allele predisposes one to greater risk of Alzheimer's disease after a head injury?

Apolipoprotein E4 (APOE4).

134. What area of the intracranial facial nerve is most commonly damaged by blunt trauma?

The area of the facial nerve around the geniculate ganglion.[68]

135. What is the Schirmer test?

This test distinguishes facial nerve injuries proximal and distal to the geniculate ganglion. The test involves placing a narrow strip of thin paper on the conjunctiva to assess for lacrimation. Injuries proximal to the geniculate ganglion tend to produce a dry eye, whereas injuries distal to the ganglion do not interfere with lacrimation. Whether the location of the facial nerve injury is proximal or distal to the geniculate ganglion is important because the choice of surgical approach differs with different sites of injury.[68]

136. What types of temporal bone fractures more frequently result in external manifestations such as otorrhea of CSF and tympanic membrane perforation?

Longitudinal fractures more frequently result in external signs of injury, whereas transverse fractures generally spare the middle ear, tympanic membrane, and external auditory canal. For this reason, transverse fractures manifest fewer external signs of injury. Transverse fractures most commonly pass through the otic capsule; longitudinal fractures typically spare the otic capsule.[68]

137. Why is an EEG sometimes ordered in cases of lowered level of consciousness after trauma?

To rule out subclinical status epilepticus.[69]

138. What range of cerebral perfusion pressures are accommodated by cerebral autoregulation?

60 to 160 mm Hg.[70]

139. How does one calculate cerebral perfusion pressure?

Cerebral perfusion pressure equals the mean arterial pressure (MAP) minus the ICP (CPP = MAP - ICP).[71]

140. Cerebral perfusion pressure should be maintained above what number after a severe head injury?

70 mm Hg.[71]

141. How does one calculate MAP?

Twice the diastolic pressure is added to the systolic pressure; then all are divided by 3. MAP = (2D + S)/3. It is two times the diastolic because the majority of the cardiac cycle is in diastole.[71]

142. At what blood flow rate does electrical activity of the cerebral cortex fail?

About 20 mL/100 g/min.[71]

143. What brainstem reflexes are mandatory to test in performing brain death evaluation?

Pupil reflex, corneal reflex, oculovestibular reflex, oculocephalic reflex, and gag reflex. Additional tests that should be performed are checking for a response to deep central pain and the apnea test. The patient should be checked for normothermia and normal blood pressure, and show no evidence of drug or metabolic intoxication.[72] Sodium level should be near normal.

144. In using auditory evoked potentials in the evaluation of brain death, what wave is necessary for the test to be valid?

Wave I, at least on one side.[72]

145. What are some medications that are neuroprotective?

Corticosteroids, free radical scavengers, calcium channel blockers, glutamate antagonists, mannitol, and barbiturates.

146. A trauma patient with a broken leg is neurologically stable, but deteriorates after manipulation of his broken leg by the orthopaedic service on hospital day 5. What is the most likely cause of the deterioration in this patient?

Fat emboli syndrome.

147. Why is a bifrontal exposure often needed in trauma cases for persistent rhinorrhea?

Fractures of the anterior fossa often extend across the midline.

148. What does the literature state about prophylactic antibiotics for CSF leaks after traumatic head injury?

An article in *Lancet* states that the use of prophylactic antibiotics only encourages the resistance and late attacks of meningitis; therefore, they are *not* recommended.[73]

Prophylactic antibiotics, in the setting of no fever or symptoms, are abused by the medical community. Gut flora dramatically changes even with a single dose of antibiotics, and this can hamper the normal immune system that would have otherwise prevented a potential infection.

149. What does the literature state about hyperventilation in the setting of traumatic brain injury?

Hyperventilation of head-injured patients may do more harm than good by decreasing cerebral perfusion pressure and delivery of O_2 and glucose. There are no good prospective, randomized studies to date to support the use of hyperventilation in head injury.[74]

150. What is a possible diagnosis of a young adult with a family history of migraines who presents to the emergency room after head trauma and complains of blindness?

Trauma-triggered migraine with transient cortical blindness.[74]

151. How can an acute subdural hematoma appear isointense to brain in a multitrauma patient?

When the hematocrit is less than approximately 23%, this may cause an acute subdural to appear isointense to brain. Another possibility is in the setting of coagulopathy.[75]

152. Why are epidural hematomas more frequently seen in younger adults than in the elderly?

The dura is thinner and more adherent to the skull in the elderly. This decreases the ease with which the dura tears in relation to an overlying skull fracture. Epidural hematomas are much more common in children and young adults than in the elderly, probably because of the flexibility of the skull and the readiness with which the dura strips off the bone (**Fig. 5.5**).

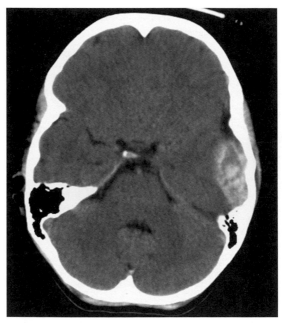

Fig. 5.5 CT scan without contrast showing epidural hematoma in a pediatric patient. Note the early uncal herniation.

153. How are epidural hematomas different in children and adults?

In children, epidural hematomas are caused by venous bleeding more often than in adults (where the usual culprit is the middle meningeal artery). In retrospective studies, it is therefore not surprising that 60% of children and 85% of infants with epidural hematomas had no disturbance of consciousness at the time of injury.[76]

154. Barbiturates are the most common class of drugs used to suppress cerebral metabolism in the setting of major cerebral trauma. What is the typical dosage of pentobarbital and what tests can be used to make sure the right amount is given?

A loading dose of 10 mg/kg is administered over 30 minutes and then 5 mg/kg per hour is administered over 3 hours. If systolic blood pressure drops by more than 10 mm Hg or the perfusion pressure falls below 60 mm Hg, the loading dose infusion should be slowed. A maintenance infusion of 1 to 3 mg/kg per hour is begun after loading is completed. The infusion is titrated to burst suppression on the EEG and a serum level of 3 to 4 mg/dL. When checking for brain death, remember that the level of pentobarbital must be less than 10 μg/mL.[74]

155. Where on the carotid artery is the most common location for a traumatic aneurysm?

Most traumatic aneurysms of the carotid artery are located on the segment between the proximal and distal dural rings. They are pseudoaneurysms that may project medially into the sphenoid sinus. They may present with the classic triad of head injury with basal skull fracture, unilateral visual loss, and epistaxis.[77]

156. What are some shortcomings of the Glasgow Coma Scale (GCS)?

It does not allow the assessment of eye opening in periorbital trauma, verbal response in intubated patients, and brainstem function or reflexes. The GCS also works poorly for patients in the first 2 years of life. The GCS, however, remains the standard for defining the level of consciousness after head injury and is a reliable and independent predictor of long-term outcome. The GCS is also used for patients who have not sustained trauma, such as postoperative patients.

157. Finding a linear skull fracture on radiologic exams in a conscious patient increases the risk of intracranial hematoma by how much?

400-fold according to a study by Mendelow et al.[78]

158. What is the definition of an "early" posttraumatic seizure? What is a "late" posttraumatic seizure?

An early posttraumatic seizure is one that occurs within the first 7 days of an injury; those that come after 7 days are called late posttraumatic seizures. About 10% of adults with early seizures will develop status epilepticus. Prophylactic phenytoin therapy may be stopped in about 1 to 2 weeks to prevent early posttraumatic seizures; however, there is no proof that phenytoin or other anticonvulsants prevent late posttraumatic seizures.

159. What is the preferred method of intubation in a patient with a basal skull fracture?

Orotracheal intubation. There is a possibility of entering the cranium through the cribriform plate with a nasotracheal intubation.

160. What are the prerequisites for a growing skull fracture?[74]

- The skull fracture occurs in infancy or early childhood.
- There is a dural tear at the time of the fracture.
- There is brain injury at the time of the fracture with displacement of leptomeninges and possibly brain through the dural defect.
- There is subsequent enlargement of the fracture to form a cranial defect.

■ Emergencies

161. A fall in end-tidal CO_2 could be the only clue to what emergency?

Air embolus.

162. How is air embolism treated?

Packing the wound with wet sponges, lowering the patient's head, using jugular venous compression, rotating the patient's left side downward, aspirating from the venous line that is in the right atrium, and ventilating the patient while maintaining adequate blood pressure and heart rate.

163. What are some cases where hyperemia of the brain can occur?

Head trauma, after carotid endarterectomy or stenting, and after excision of an arteriovenous malformation (AVM).

164. How is the diagnosis of disseminated intravascular coagulation confirmed?

Low platelet count, prolonged PT, elevated fibrin degradation products, and reduced fibrinogen levels.

165. What is the treatment of a cluster headache in a patient who is in excruciating pain?

Oxygen, sumatriptan, analgesics, or a combination of these. Restlessness and agitated behavior are reported symptoms in 93% of cluster headache patients. Steroids may be helpful in some patients.

166. Which drug is best in the immediate control of seizures in status epilepticus?

Lorazepam is better than diazepam or phenytoin.[69]

167. What is the treatment algorithm for status epilepticus?

Lorazepam 4 mg (or 0.1 mg/kg) intravenously (IV) over 2 minutes, may repeat after 5 minutes. Simultaneously load with phenytoin 1,200 mg (or 20 mg/kg), or 500 mg if already on phenytoin. Phenobarbital may be given up to 1,400 mg at a rate of less than 100 mg/min. If seizures continue, consider general anesthesia. It is also important in the initial stages of status to send laboratories for electrolyte levels and antiepileptic drug levels if the patient is already on an agent. A normal saline IV drip may be started and 50 mL of 50% glucose given, as well as 100 mg of thiamine. Other agents that may be used if the above measures are not effective include pentobarbital (while watching for circulatory depression and being prepared to use a pressor), midazolam, or propofol.[69]

168. What are the signs and symptoms of myxedema coma and how is it properly treated?

Myxedema coma is an emergency of hypothyroidism. The signs are hypotension, bradycardia, hyponatremia, hypoglycemia, hypothermia, and hypoventilation. Treatment consists of IV fluids, intubation if necessary, IV glucose, 400 mg hydrocortisone IV over 24 hours, and 0.5 mg levothyroxine IV followed by 0.05 mg levothyroxine per day.[79]

169. What are the three places that a shunt may be occluded?

The entry point (proximal occlusion), the valve system (valve obstruction), and the distal end (distal catheter occlusion). A CT scan of the head, a shunt series, and palpation of the valve are important in determining the site of the occlusion.

170. A patient with a prior history of pituitary tumor presents with a sudden onset of headache and rapid visual failure with extraocular nerve palsies. What is the most likely diagnosis and how is it treated acutely?

This is pituitary apoplexy, which can clinically mimic an SAH. Death may follow unless urgent steroid treatment is started.

171. How should life-threatening cerebellar swelling from infarction be managed (Fig. 5.6)?

Resection of cerebellar infarction has been advocated in patients in whom life-threatening deterioration is occurring from focal cerebellar swelling, herniation, and brainstem compression or secondary fourth ventricular obstruction and hydrocephalus. A ventriculostomy may be needed as a temporizing measure in anticipation of surgery; however, one must be cognizant of the risk of upward herniation.

172. What are the drugs used in neuroleptic malignant syndrome?

Bromocriptine (dopamine receptor agonist) and dantrolene (muscle relaxant). Neuroleptic malignant syndrome is a rare condition seen with dopamine antagonist and long-acting depot neuroleptic preparations. Drowsiness, fever, tremor, and rigidity occur suddenly.

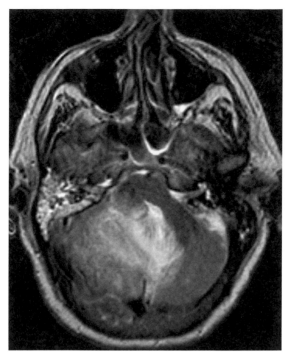

Fig. 5.6 Life-threatening cerebellar swelling from right cerebellar hemisphere infarction.

173. What is the most common cerebral vascular complication encountered during pregnancy?

SAH is the most common cerebral vascular complication encountered during pregnancy. The risk of rupture parallels the hemodynamic changes, reaching an apex in the third trimester, in concert with blood volume changes. Aneurysms are most prone to rupture during the seventh and eighth months of pregnancy and at delivery.[80]

174. What is the most common site in the brain of hypertensive cerebral hemorrhage?

The putamen.

175. What are the signs and symptoms of addisonian crisis and how is it properly treated?

Addisonian crisis is an adrenal insufficiency emergency with symptoms of mental status changes and muscle weakness. Signs of postural hypotension, shock, hyponatremia, hyperkalemia, hypoglycemia, and hyperthermia may be seen. For a glucocorticoid emergency, administer 100 mg IV hydrocortisone (Solu-Cortef; Pfizer Pharmaceuticals) immediately (STAT) and then 50 mg IV every 6 hours. Concurrently, one should also give cortisone acetate 75 to 100 mg intramuscularly (IM) STAT, and then 50 mg IM every 6 hours. For a mineralocorticoid emergency, it is best to give desoxycorticosterone acetate 5 mg IM twice daily.[81]

176. What is central pontine myelinolysis?

A rare disorder of pontine white matter producing insidious flaccid quadriplegia and mental status changes. This disorder results from correcting hyponatremia too rapidly; Na^+ should be corrected no faster than 10 mEq/L in 24 hours.

177. What is neurogenic pulmonary edema?

Neurogenic pulmonary edema is associated with SAH, head trauma, and seizure disorder. It is caused by an increased capillary permeability in the lungs associated with an increase in sympathetic discharge. Treatment is aimed at reducing ICP, maintaining positive pressure ventilation, and supportive care.

178. How is an acute attack of migraine headache best treated?

Prochlorperazine (Compazine; Brentford, Middlesex) 10 mg IV.

179. What potential emergency can occur intracranially if nitrous oxide anesthesia is not discontinued prior to closure of the dura during surgery?

Tension pneumocephalus.

180. What are the most common complications of the transoral operative route?

CSF leakage and infection.

Neoplasms

181. What is the name of a cystic tumor of the suprasellar region that arises from neuroectodermal remnants of Rathke's pouch?

Craniopharyngioma (**Fig. 5.7**).[82]

182. What preoperative medication can lessen general and cardiac risks in patients with a growth hormone (GH)–secreting tumor?

Somatostatin analogue.[83]

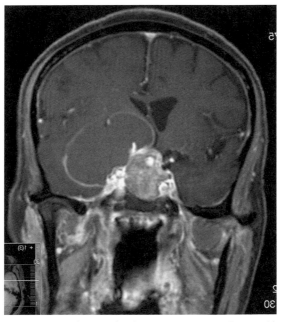

Fig. 5.7 Coronal T1-weighted magnetic resonance image with contrast demonstrating a craniopharyngioma with suprasellar cystic extension.

183. Which type of embryonic lesion can present with calcification in the sella area and erode through the posterior clinoids?

Craniopharyngioma. Erosion of the posterior clinoids may also occur from chronic increases in ICP for a variety of reasons.[82]

184. What type of tumor can erode the internal acoustic meatus, the petrous apex, the clivus, the sellar floor, the orbital foramen, and the jugular foramen?

- Internal acoustic meatus: an acoustic schwannoma.
- Petrous apex: a trigeminal schwannoma.
- Clivus: a chordoma.
- Sellar floor: large pituitary tumors.
- Orbital foramen: an optic nerve glioma.
- Jugular foramen (the bone): a glomus jugulare tumor.

Also, note that an aneurysm may erode through bone, such as an aneurysm eroding through the sphenoid sinus presenting with epistaxis.[84]

185. What diseases may produce generalized bone erosion and generalized hyperostosis?

Multiple myeloma produces generalized bone erosion. Paget's disease usually results in generalized hyperostosis. Recall that a meningioma results in focal hyperostosis.[84]

186. What is the most common extradural neoplasm involving the clivus?

A chordoma (**Fig. 5.8**). The two subgroups of chordoma are the typical and the chondroid; it is suggested in the literature that chondroid features portend a better prognosis.[84]

187. What is the immunohistochemical staining profile of a chordoma versus a chondrosarcoma?

Chordomas virtually always stain positive for keratin with variable S-100 expressivity. Chondrosarcomas lack epithelial markers, but are nearly always positive for S-100.[85]

188. If chordomas are histologically benign, what features make this lesion clinically malignant?

The malignant potential of a chordoma arises from the critical location at which these tumors arise as well as from their locally aggressive nature, high rate of recurrence, and occasional tendency to metastasize.[86]

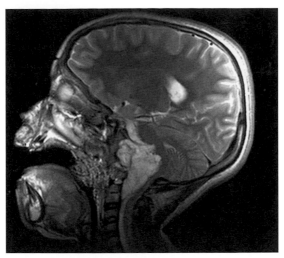

Fig. 5.8 Sagittal T2-weighted magnetic resonance image demonstrating a clival chordoma with severe brainstem compression.

189. What are the most common and the second most common sites of origin for chordoma?

The sacrum and the clivus, respectively.

190. What is the classic triad for cervicogenic headaches?

Suboccipital headache, eye pressure, and tinnitus.

191. Prophylactic cranial irradiation may be considered part of the standard treatment of patients with what disease?

Small cell lung carcinoma.[87]

192. Which neurosurgical lesion is currently most commonly removed by endoscopic methods?

A colloid cyst (**Fig. 5.9**).

193. Where are colloid cysts found?

The anterior roof of the third ventricle.[88]

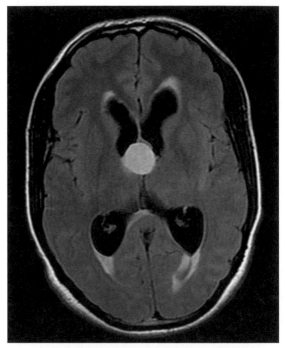

Fig. 5.9 Axial fluid-attenuated inversion recovery (FLAIR) magnetic resonance image demonstrating a colloid cyst of the third ventricle.

194. How do colloid cysts cause death?

They cause obstructive hydrocephalus that if left untreated may lead to death.[89]

195. What is the most common intraorbital tumor found in adults?

A cavernous hemangioma. These are benign, slow-growing vascular lesions. They can manifest as a painless, progressively proptotic eye. They are mostly unilateral, but bilateral cases have been reported. No predilection exists for race or ethnicity.[90]

196. What is the second most common type of intracranial schwannoma?

A trigeminal schwannoma (the vestibular type is the most common).

197. What is the most common presentation of a choroid plexus tumor?

Intracranial hypertension.[91]

198. What are the differences in location of a choroid plexus papilloma between an adult and a child?

Choroid plexus papillomas are rare benign tumors of the central nervous system (CNS) that occur mostly in children and have a slight male predominance. These tumors are usually found in the left lateral ventricle in children (**Fig. 5.10**) and the fourth ventricle in adults. They account for less than 1% of all intracranial tumors.[84]

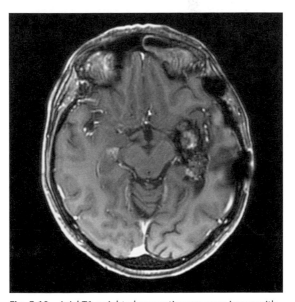

Fig. 5.10 Axial T1-weighted magnetic resonance image with contrast demonstrating a choroid plexus papilloma of the left temporal horn.

199. How can a surgeon differentiate tumor from radiation necrosis?

PET, single-photon emission computed tomography (SPECT), and/or biopsy.[84]

200. What type of histochemical stain do pathologists use to differentiate collagen from glial tissue?

Trichrome.[92]

201. What is the median survival time for malignant glioma?

9 months.

202. What is the significance of elevated choline peaks and reduced *N*-acetyl-aspartate (NAA) levels in spectroscopic evaluation of brain tumors?

Increased choline levels indicate increased membrane turnover. NAA (which reflects neuronal integrity) is reduced in tumors. The combination of both of these findings indicates tumor infiltration (**Fig. 5.11**).[93]

203. What are the prognoses for midbrain, medullary, and pontine gliomas?

Survival rates are best for midbrain and worst for pontine gliomas. Medullary gliomas are intermediate.

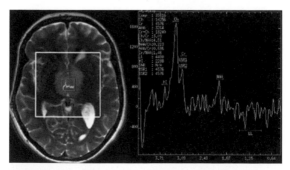

Fig. 5.11 Magnetic resonance spectroscopy of thalamic infiltrating glioma showing elevated choline peak and reduced NAA peak.

204. What CSF tumor marker is positive in germinomas?

Placental alkaline phosphatase.[94]

205. Which pineal region tumor is most sensitive to radiation?

A germinoma.[95]

206. What serum marker should you look for in a patient with a pineal region tumor?

β-Human chorionic gonadotropin (HCG) and α-fetal protein (AFP), because these neoplasms are of germ cell origin. β-HCG is elevated in choriocarcinomas. AFP is elevated in embryonal carcinomas and yolk sac tumors.

207. What tests can one perform to distinguish a primary tumor from an MS plaque when there is an enhancing lesion on MRI?

Visual evoked potentials, oligoclonal bands, and immunoglobulin G (IgG). The patient's history is also important.[31]

208. What are the three most common focal brain lesions in human immunodeficiency virus (HIV)?

Toxoplasmosis, primary lymphoma, and progressive multifocal leukoencephalopathy (PML).

209. What cancer is sensitive to chemotherapy and radiation, is usually never operated on, and exhibits paraneoplastic syndromes such as syndrome of inappropriate antidiuretic hormone secretion (SIADH) or syndrome of ectopic adrenocorticotropic hormone (ACTH) production?

Small cell lung cancer.

210. What modality can distinguish primary lymphoma of HIV from other focal mass lesions associated with HIV?

A fluorine-18 fluorodeoxyglucose (18-FDG) PET scan. Lymphomas have a higher uptake than toxoplasmosis or PML.[96]

211. What is the median survival of a child with a pontine tumor?

9 to 12 months.

212. When is radiation therapy indicated in oligodendroglioma?

For anaplastic transformation. Chemotherapy is recommended for all cases of oligodendroglioma. Loss of 1p/19q predicts an almost 100% response rate to procarbazine, lomustine (CCNU), and vincristine (PCV) chemotherapy in oligodendroglial tumors.[97]

213. What is the preferred approach for a lesion situated entirely within the atrium of the ventricle?

Posterior transcortical approach directed through the superior parietal lobule.[98]

214. What approaches are best suited for pineal region tumors?

Occipital transtentorial or infratentorial supracerebellar.

215. What diagnostic test is recommended for a pediatric patient with a posterior fossa tumor?

MRI of the spine to rule out drop metastases.

216. What are the survival rates of the four grades of gliomas?[99]

Grade I: 8 to 10 years; grade II: 7 to 8 years; grade III: ~2 years; grade IV: < 1 year.

217. What is the role of surgery in PCNSL?

No role for debulking; only biopsy if there is a question as to the lesion. Primary central nervous system lymphoma (PCNSL) may mimic a glioblastoma multiforme (GBM) radiographically.

218. What is Collins' law?

Collins' law (or rule) states that a congenital tumor may be considered cured if it does not recur within a period equal to the person's age plus 9 months after surgery. This rule does have some exceptions and may be applicable ~80% of the time.[100]

219. What is the recurrence rate for benign meningiomas?

2 to 3% in 5 years.[101] It is important to take periodic MRIs with contrast to assess any recurrence and to treat recurrence after open surgery with radiosurgery.

220. Where do meningiomas arise from?

Arachnoid cap cells present in the arachnoid granulations (convexity meningiomas) and in the arachnoid layers of the meninges (for nonconvexity meningiomas).[102]

221. What is the rate of malignant change of meningiomas?

1 to 2%.[101]

222. How do meningiomas of the foramen magnum present?

Pyramidal weakness initially affecting the ipsilateral arm, followed by the ipsilateral leg, spreading to the contralateral limbs when the tumor enlarges.[103]

223. What is the chromosomal abnormality found in meningiomas?

Over 70% of these tumors have monosomy 22.[104]

224. What are the most common CNS locations of meningiomas?

90% are cranial, 9% are spinal. The most common intracranial locations in order of highest occurrence are parasagittal, convexity, sphenoid tuberculum, olfactory groove, foramen magnum, optic sheath, tentorial, and intraventricular.[105]

225. From where do convexity meningiomas derive their blood supply?

The external carotid artery branches.

226. What bony skull abnormality is most often seen with meningiomas?

Hyperostoses. This is thought to occur because meningiomas secrete osteoblastic factors promoting bone growth.[105]

227. Which hormone receptors do meningiomas exhibit?

Progesterone and estrogen. This may explain why meningiomas are more common in women and why they tend to grow with pregnancy and breast cancer.

228. What is Foster-Kennedy syndrome?

Optic atrophy in one eye and papilledema in the other eye with anosmia. This syndrome is sometimes seen with olfactory groove meningiomas.[106]

229. What is the median survival for an oligodendroglioma that enhances with gadolinium? What is the median survival for an oligodendroglioma that does not enhance?

The median survival from the initial diagnosis of all low-grade oligodendrogliomas is 4 to 10 years, but only 3 to 4 years for anaplastic oligodendrogliomas (those that enhance). Oligodendrogliomas are chemosensitive. Patients with anaplastic oligodendrogliomas who have a loss of heterozygosity on chromosome 1p or combined loss of heterozygosity on 1p and 19q survive substantially longer (~10 years) than patients who lack these genetic changes.[107]

230. When is the facial nerve encountered in the cerebellopontine (CP) angle during the resection of an acoustic neuroma and during the resection of a CP angle meningioma?

In acoustic neuromas, the facial nerve lies anterosuperior to the tumor and is typically encountered late in surgery. In CP angle meningiomas, the facial nerve may lie at the posterior tumor edge and may be injured early in surgery unless it is identified.

231. Any patient younger than 40 years with a unilateral acoustic neuroma should also be evaluated for what condition?

Neurofibromatosis type 2 (NF2).[108]

232. What do brainstem auditory evoked potentials show in a patient with acoustic schwannoma?

A delay of wave V latency on the affected side.

233. What medication may shrink a neurosarcoid mass at the skull base?

A corticosteroid.[109]

234. What laboratory tests can support the diagnosis of sarcoid?

Elevated serum and CSF angiotensin-converting enzyme, elevated serum immunoglobulins, elevated serum calcium, elevated CSF cell count (monocytes), IgG, Ig index, and presence of oligoclonal bands. Nervous system involvement occurs in ~8% of sarcoid patients. Sarcoid usually involves the meninges, skull base, CNs, and pituitary stalk. Immunosuppression with corticosteroids is usually indicated and long-term therapy is required.[109]

235. What are some slow-growing, painless calvarial masses?

Osteoma, ossifying fibroma, chondroma, hemangioma, epidermoid, dermoid, meningioma, fibrous dysplasia, and nonossifying fibroma.[84]

236. What is the most common primary skull neoplasm?

Osteoma.[110]

237. Which malignancies are associated with neurofibromatosis type 1 (NF1)?

Malignant peripheral nerve sheath tumors, pheochromocytoma, and leukemia.[111]

238. What osseous lesion and condition are usually seen with NF1?

Sphenoid dysplasia and thinning of long bones.[112]

239. What is the mode of inheritance of NF2?

Autosomal dominant on chromosome 22.[113]

240. Where are chordomas found?

Almost all chordomas occur near the clivus or sacrum.[114,115]

241. What is the difference between an osteoid osteoma and an osteoblastoma?

Size. These are benign bone tumors. When the lesion is 2 cm or less, it is called an osteoid osteoma; if it is larger than 2 cm in size, it is referred to as an osteoblastoma.[116]

242. What is Gardner's syndrome?

Gardner's syndrome is characterized by intestinal polyposis with frequent malignant degeneration, benign soft tissue neoplasms, and multiple osteomas of the skull and mandible.[110]

243. What is the most common location for epidermoid tumors?

The CP angle.

244. What are some cerebral metastases in pediatric patients?

Neuroblastoma, rhabdomyosarcoma, and Wilms' tumor.

245. What are the radiosensitive cerebral metastases?

Small cell lung cancer, multiple myeloma, germinoma, lymphoma, and leukemia.

246. Where do metastatic brain tumors appear?

At the gray–white junction.

247. What are the most common hemorrhagic metastatic brain tumors?

In order of highest occurrence: lung, breast, renal cell carcinoma, choriocarcinoma, and melanoma.

248. Which metastatic brain tumor is associated with the shortest life expectancy?

Melanoma.[117]

249. Which brain lesion is associated with gelastic seizures?

Hypothalamic hamartomas.[118]

250. Besides a brain MRI, which other diagnostic procedures are needed in a patient with an ependymoma?

A spinal MRI and a lumbar puncture (if not contraindicated).

251. What are the most common tumors of the jugular foramen?

Also called glomus jugulare tumors, paragangliomas are most common, followed by schwannomas and meningiomas. Paralysis of the lower CNs is often the initial symptom of tumors arising in the jugular foramen. In the case of a paraganglioma, patients may present with hearing loss, pulsatile tinnitus, and facial paralysis if the tumor is very large.[119]

252. What is the most common presenting sign of a glomus tumor?

Unilateral hearing loss due to invasion of the middle ear.[120]

253. What is the most common vessel supplying a glomus jugulare tumor?

The ascending pharyngeal artery.[121] It is the smallest branch of the external carotid artery.

254. What laboratory studies should be done preoperatively in the work-up of a glomus tumor? How would that affect perioperative management?

A 24-hour urine sample should be analyzed for vanillylmandelic acid, metanephrines, and catecholamines to determine the secretory status of the tumor. A secreting tumor would need to be managed with α-blockers 2 weeks before surgery and with a β-blocker the day before surgery to prevent a hypertension crisis.

255. What CNs are most commonly affected by the growth of a glomus jugulare tumor?

CNs IX, X, and XI (those nerves that pass directly through the jugular foramen), CN VII (the facial nerve, usually along the mastoid segment), and CN XII (the hypoglossal nerve).[122]

256. What is the differential diagnosis for a cerebral ring–enhancing lesion?

Glioma, lymphoma, infection, demyelinating plaque, radiation necrosis, resolving hematoma, cysticercosis, sarcoid, or granulomatous disease.[84]

257. What particular genetic alteration makes malignant gliomas chemoresponsive?

Loss of heterozygosity at 1p and 19p (mainly oligodendrogliomas).[107]

258. What do the terms "communicating" and "noncommunicating" refer to with hydrocephalus?

In communicating hydrocephalus, the ventricular system is in communication with the subarachnoid space of the brain and spinal cord; in the noncommunicating form, there is a block either within the ventricular system (i.e., tumor, blood) or in its outlets to the subarachnoid space, so that the ventricles and subarachnoid space are discontinuous.[123]

259. What are tumor markers and how can they help in diagnosing a brain tumor?

Tumor markers are substances found in the blood, urine, or body tissues that can be elevated in cancer and are identified by immunohistochemical techniques. Identification of certain antigens specific for particular tumors helps in the diagnosis of brain tumors.

- Glial fibrillary acidic protein (GFAP) is a marker for astrocytic tumors.
- S-100 has a distribution similar to that of GFAP, but is more localized in Schwann's cells.
- Cytokeratin is a marker for metastatic carcinoma.
- Synaptophysin is a marker for neuronal tumors.
- HMB45 is a marker for malignant melanoma.
- Ki-67 is a marker of proliferation of various tumors.
- Loss of heterozygosity markers is often important in oligodendrogliomas (1p and 19q).
- AFP and human chorionic gonadotropin are markers for yolk sac tumors and choriocarcinomas, respectively.[94]

260. What tumor marker is useful for differentiating between renal cell carcinoma and hemangioblastoma?

Epithelial membrane antigen is not present in hemangioblastomas, but is present in renal cell carcinoma.[124]

261. What pitfall must be avoided in treating a patient with Parkinson's disease and malignant melanoma?

Levodopa should not be given because dopamine is a precursor of melanin; giving levodopa may stimulate tumor growth.

262. What is gliomatosis cerebri?

Diffusely enlarged cerebral hemisphere filled with tumor. This also refers to diffuse enlargement of the cerebellum or brainstem. There are no focal masses.[125]

263. What is temozolomide?

An oral alkylating agent that penetrates the blood–brain barrier and may be used in patients with recurrent anaplastic astrocytomas and glioblastomas. Temozolomide has a lower toxicity than other chemotherapeutic agents.

264. What is the most common primary brain tumor?

GBM. This is a malignant tumor classified as a grade 4 astrocytoma by the World Health Organization (WHO). Without treatment, patients die within a few months of symptomatic onset.[126]

265. Which factors does the prognosis of gliomas depend on?

1. Age.
2. Karnofsky's score.
3. Degree of neurologic deficit.
4. Histologic findings.
5. Extent of resection.

266. What test can be performed on CSF to diagnose acquired immunodeficiency syndrome (AIDS) lymphoma of the CNS?

An Epstein-Barr test of tumor cells of the CNS will be positive in AIDS lymphoma of the CNS in some cases. PCNSL is also known as high-grade non-Hodgkin B cell lymphoma and is seen in immunocompromised patients. Chemotherapy with methotrexate can improve survival in both AIDS and non-AIDS patients. Radiotherapy is also of some benefit. Because PCNSL appears radiologically similar to toxoplasmosis, a trial of antiprotozoal medications should be done empirically before other more invasive procedures are planned.[127]

267. What is extramedullary hematopoiesis and what are the areas related to the CNS where it may occur?

Extramedullary hematopoiesis is due to chronic stimulation of bone marrow to produce red blood cells. This is seen especially in thalassemia major and other conditions where there is a low hematocrit count. The skull, vertebral bodies, and choroid plexus are sites of extramedullary hematopoiesis. Exuberant tissue that is seen in the spine should be resected in cases of spinal cord compression; radiotherapy is recommended after surgery.[128]

268. What is the most common benign primary intraorbital tumor?

A cavernous hemangioma.

269. In what percentage of cases of hemangioblastoma is polycythemia noted?

Less than 25% of cases. The erythrocytosis is secondary to erythropoietin production by the tumor.

270. What is the goal of surgery for a cerebellar hemangioblastoma?

Complete excision of the mural nodule; the cyst wall need not be removed completely. It is acceptable to cauterize cyst wall that is safe to reach.

271. Patients with what type of tumor of the CNS exhibit polycythemia?

A hemangioblastoma (10%).

272. In patients with von Hippel–Lindau (VHL) syndrome, a CT scan of the abdomen is done to look for what pathology?

Renal cell carcinoma, pancreatic and kidney cysts, pheochromocytoma, and papillary cystadenomas of epididymis and mesosalpinx.

273. Chromosome 22 is associated with which disorders?

Meningiomas, ependymomas, NF2, Ewing's sarcoma, amyotrophic lateral sclerosis, and metachromatic leukodystrophy.

274. Which common pediatric tumor arises from the floor and which one arises from the roof of the fourth ventricle?

- Medulloblastoma: roof of the fourth ventricle (vermis).
- Ependymoma: floor of the fourth ventricle.

275. Name the two most common suprasellar tumors in adults and in children.

- Adults: suprasellar extension of pituitary tumor and meningioma.
- Children: craniopharyngioma and hypothalamic glioma.

276. What percentage of meningiomas are intraventricular?

2%.

277. Which subtype of pituitary tumors is basophilic?

ACTH-secreting adenoma.

278. Describe the main differences between a schwannoma and a neurofibroma.

See **Table 5.1** for details.

279. Which surgical approach is usually appropriate for a pineal region tumor?

Infratentorial supracerebellar.

Table 5.1   Differences between schwannoma and neurofibroma[129]

Schwannoma	Neurofibroma
Eccentric to the nerve	Involves the nerve
Seen in neurofibromatosis 2	Seen in neurofibromatosis 1 (NF1)
Capsulated	No capsule
No mucoid	Mucoid
Biphasic	Monophasic
Malignant change is rare	2% malignant change
Plexiform (unrelated to NF1)	Plexiform (in NF1)
Affects extremities	Affects trunk
Usually solitary	Usually multiple

280. How would you approach an intraventricular tumor located in the lateral ventricle near the foramen of Monro?

- Interhemispheric transcallosal approach if the ventricles are not dilated.
- Endoscopic transventricular approach if there is hydrocephalus.

281. What kind of visual deficit is feared in temporal lobectomy?

Contralateral superior temporal visual field defect.

282. On which chromosome is the VHL gene located?

3p.

283. What are the CNS manifestations of VHL disease?

Hemangioblastomas of the retina, brainstem, cerebellum, spinal cord, and nerve roots; endolymphatic sac tumors.[130]

284. What is the mode of inheritance of VHL?

VHL is autosomal dominant with high penetrance. Almost 100% of the people with the affected gene will develop VHL by age 60.

285. Which skull base tumor ascends into the cranial cavity via perineural spread?

An adenocystic carcinoma.

286. What are the cardinal symptoms of a vestibular schwannoma?

Unilateral hearing loss, tinnitus, vertigo, and unsteadiness.[131]

287. What is the eponym for dysplastic gangliocytoma of the cerebellum?

Lhermitte-Duclos disease.[132]

288. What is the most common genetic mutation associated with astrocytomas?

The P53 gene. This is a tumor suppressor gene on chromosome 17p. Mutations in this gene are seen in one-third of all astrocytomas.[133]

289. The Epstein-Barr virus is associated with which carcinomas?

Burkitt's lymphoma and nasopharyngeal carcinoma.[134]

290. What is the Eaton-Lambert syndrome?

This is a paraneoplastic syndrome in which Ig antibodies to the presynaptic voltage-gated Ca^{2+} are produced. This decreases the number of acetylcholine (ACh) quanta released. It causes proximal limb fatigue. Unlike myasthenia gravis, this syndrome spares ocular muscles. About 60% of cases are associated with pulmonary oat cell (small cell) carcinoma.[135]

291. Where does esthesioneuroblastoma originate from?

The olfactory epithelium. This tumor does not show familial prevalence. It affects all races, occurs in all age groups, and affects males and females equally.[136]

292. What is the most common presenting symptom of esthesioneuroblastoma?

Nasal obstruction, followed by epistaxis.[137]

293. What is the most common cause of death in a patient with low-grade glioma?

Dedifferentiation into a higher-grade glioma.[138]

Endocrine

294. What are symptoms of adrenal insufficiency?

Fatigue, weakness, arthralgia, anorexia, nausea, hypotension, orthostatic dizziness, hypoglycemia, and dyspnea.

295. What does a persistently elevated GH level suggest after transsphenoidal resection for a GH-producing tumor?

Persistent tumor or damage to the pituitary stalk.

296. What suprasellar aneurysm could mimic a pituitary tumor on a CT scan?

A superior hypophyseal artery aneurysm. It arises from the ICA between the origins of the ophthalmic and the PComm arteries and projects medially.

297. What is meant by a prefixed optic chiasm? What is a postfixed optic chiasm?

Because of the normal variation in the length of the optic nerves, the chiasm may lie anterior to the pituitary infundibulum in 10% of cases and posterior to it in a postfixed position in 10% of cases. The optic chiasm is situated immediately above the central portion of the diaphragma sellae and the pituitary gland in most people (80%).[139]

298. If bromocriptine has been used for treating a pituitary tumor and surgical resection still needs to be performed, when is it best to schedule the operation?

During the first 6 months after starting bromocriptine; waiting longer increases the tendency for fibrosis and makes surgery more difficult.[140]

299. Formation of gallstones is an unfortunate complication from what type of treatment for GH tumors?

Octreotide.[140]

300. What parts of the visual fields are affected initially by a suprasellar mass?

Superior temporal quadrants.[140]

301. What is happening when a patient with a known pituitary tumor has a sudden headache, third CN palsy, and a contralateral fourth CN palsy?

Pituitary apoplexy. Expansion of the mass accounts for the CN findings on alternate sides.[140]

302. Which nerve is most commonly involved by a tumor in the cavernous sinus?

The oculomotor nerve (followed by abducens and then trochlear).

303. What is the most common hormone-secreting pituitary tumor?

A prolactinoma.[141]

304. What should be included in a complete endocrine evaluation of a patient with a pituitary tumor?

The following tests are the minimum that should be obtained[142]:

- 24-hour urine free cortisol.
- ACTH.
- Serum cortisol.
- Prolactin.
- Free T4.
- Luteinizing hormone (LH).
- Follicle-stimulating hormone (FSH).
- Gonadotropin-releasing hormone (GnRH).
- Testosterone.
- Insulinlike growth factor (IGF).

305. What are some causes of elevated prolactin besides a pituitary tumor?

Stress, pregnancy, drugs (phenothiazines, estrogens), hypothyroidism, renal disease, hypothalamic lesion (sarcoid, craniopharyngioma), pituitary stalk syndrome (serum prolactin levels rarely exceed 200 mU/L with stalk syndrome), and seizures.[140]

306. What hormone should be drawn to exclude primary hypothyroidism in the setting of a suspected pituitary adenoma?

The thyroid-stimulating hormone (TSH) level should be determined to exclude primary hypothyroidism.[140]

307. What is a combined pituitary stimulation test?

To test the pituitary axis, several tests can be performed simultaneously by injecting insulin, GnRH, and thyrotropin-releasing hormone (TRH). All the anterior pituitary hormones are measured over the next few hours. GH and ACTH are assessed by insulin; FSH and LH are assessed by GnRH; and TSH and prolactin are assessed by TRH.[140]

308. What is an appropriate "stress dose" that should be given to a patient who is taking chronic glucocorticoid therapy?

This can be done with 100 mg IV preoperative and 100 mg IV every 8 hours for the first 24 hours. It avoids the pain from IM shots and a drip, and can later be weaned.[143]

309. What is an easy way to differentiate cerebral salt wasting (CSW) from SIADH?

This can be done by measuring plasma volume and looking for signs and symptoms of dehydration. SIADH patients will have high plasma volumes, increased weight, and high central venous pressure (CVP). CSW patients will have low plasma volumes, decreased weight, and low CVP, and may have orthostatic hypotension. If one cannot determine the cause of hyponatremia, urea (0.5 g per kg IV over 8 hours) may be given as treatment (because it is effective in both SIADH and CSW) until a cause can be determined.[144]

310. What is the most common cause of Cushing's syndrome?

Exogenous administration of glucocorticoids for chronic inflammation.[82]

311. What nerve innervates the diaphragma sellae?

The first division of the trigeminal nerve.

312. What types of lesions can exhibit calcification near the sellar area?

Meningioma, aneurysm, craniopharyngioma, pituitary adenoma, and chondrosarcoma.[84]

313. Describe a pituitary pseudotumor in the setting of thyroid disease.

With chronic primary hypothyroidism, there is secondary hyperplasia of the pituitary, which can mimic a pituitary mass on MRI. Loss of negative feedback from thyroid hormones causes increased TRH release from the hypothalamus producing secondary hyperplasia of thyrotropic cells in the adenohypophysis.[140]

314. What is the most common intrinsic tumor of the hypothalamus?

An astrocytoma.[84]

315. What are the tests that can be used to distinguish between primary Cushing's disease and ectopic ACTH production?

- Measuring serum ACTH.
- High-dose dexamethasone suppression test.
- Overnight 8-mg dexamethasone suppression test.
- Metapyrone test.
- CRH (corticotropin-releasing hormone) stimulation test.
- Inferior petrosal sinus sampling.[82]

316. What is the differential diagnosis for thickening of the pituitary stalk?

Lymphoma, lymphocytic hypophysitis, granulomatous disease, or hypothalamic glioma.

317. What is the "stalk effect"?

Elevation of prolactin due to decreased dopamine from compression on the pituitary stalk from a nonprolactinoma. The prolactin level is usually under 150, whereas in prolactinomas the level is above that.[145]

318. Elevation of prolactin levels can occur through stalk compression and prolactinoma. What stimulation test can be used to differentiate between these two causes of elevated prolactin when the prolactin level is not overwhelmingly high?

A TRH stimulation test can be used, as stalk compression shows a normal prolactin rise with TRH, whereas patients with prolactinomas do not.

319. What is the most common endocrinologic consequence of irradiation for pituitary adenoma?

GH deficiency. Hormonal deficiencies will appear in sequence after radiation treatment: first with GH deficiency, then gonadotropin deficiency, and finally, adrenocorticotropin or thyrotropin deficiency.[140]

320. What percentage of pituitary tumors are biochemically inactive?

About 25%.[140] They are also referred to as nonfunctioning or nonsecretory.

321. What is Nelson's syndrome?

This occurs when there is pituitary enlargement after an adrenalectomy that was performed to treat Cushing's syndrome. Patients usually have hyperpigmentation due to melanin-stimulating hormone that is overproduced along with ACTH.[146]

322. What is the difference between Cushing's syndrome and Cushing's disease?

Cushing's syndrome is a constellation of findings caused by hypercortisolism. The most common cause is exogenous steroid administration. Cushing's disease is endogenous hypercortisolism due to an ACTH-secreting pituitary adenoma.[147,148]

323. What is pituitary apoplexy?

Pituitary apoplexy is acute hemorrhagic necrosis of a pituitary adenoma when it outgrows its blood supply. This can be an emergency as the acute expansion of the tumor that can develop may compress the optic apparatus and may cause blindness. Treatment is with surgery and/or steroids.[149]

324. Which medication is used to temporarily lower cortisol levels?

Ketoconazole. This is an antifungal medication.[150]

325. What serum marker is measured in a GH-secreting pituitary adenoma?

Somatomedin C. It is synthesized in the liver and produces IGF-1.[151]

326. What visual field defect is usually found in suprasellar masses?

Bitemporal hemianopia from compression of the optic chiasm.[152]

Radiation Therapy

327. What is the maximum radiation dose for tumors near the optic nerve?

Less than 8 cGy.[153]

328. What is the usual radiation dose for treatment of trigeminal neuralgia?

80 cGy.

329. Brainstem lesions should receive how much of a radiation dose?

Less than 15 cGy.[153]

330. Lower CNs can tolerate up to how high of a radiation dose?

Less than 25 cGy.[153]

331. Describe the five phases of the cell cycle.

1. G0 phase: resting phase.
2. G1 phase: RNA and protein synthesis.
3. S phase: DNA synthesis.
4. G2 phase: construction of mitotic apparatus.
5. M phase: mitotic phase.

332. Cells are most resistant to radiation therapy in which phase of the cell cycle?

The S phase (DNA synthetic phase). This is thought to be due to the cells' increased ability in this part of the cell cycle to repair the DNA damaged by radiation.[154]

333. At what age is it safe to use brain radiation?

Radiation is avoided in children below 5 years of age.[155]

334. On average, how long after radiation treatment is radiation necrosis seen?

18 months. Radiation necrosis affects mostly the white matter; the neurons are relatively resistant. Treatment is usually with steroids.[156]

335. Besides the risk of radiation necrosis, what is one major drawback to treating AVMs of the brain with stereotactic surgery?

It takes ~2 years for the radiation to obliterate the AVM. During this time, the patient may have an increased risk of hemorrhage[157] (however, this point does remain controversial[158]). Radiation is best reserved for lesions less than 3 cm in size.[159]

Infections

336. What empiric medications should be given to all HIV-positive patients with a CNS mass lesion?

A 2-week trial of toxoplasmosis medications, pyrimethamine, and sulfadiazine.[160]

337. What should be done with a patient if herpes simplex encephalitis is suspected?

Start acyclovir immediately.[161]

338. What is a preferred method to biopsy a hemorrhagic herpes lesion in the temporal lobe?

A subtemporal craniectomy provides a specimen and also mild decompression.

339. How does the administration of acyclovir in the acute phase of herpes infection alter the incidence of postherpetic neuralgia?

The incidence of postherpetic neuralgia is *not* influenced by treatment with acyclovir in the acute phase.[161]

340. What are some organisms involved in shunt infections?

Staphylococcus epidermidis, *Staphylococcus aureus*, streptococci (pyogenes, viridans, pneumoniae), *Propionibacterium acnes*, and rarely gram-negative organisms (associated with higher morbidity and mortality). 90% of possible infections will occur within the first 6 months of shunt insertion.[162] Sterile technique in prepping and draping is important with shunts. Start with clipping hair, then cleaning appropriate fields with alcohol, letting it dry, then applying 10–10 drapes, and finally using two Durapreps or Chloropreps. Sterile towels can then be placed covering the 10–10 drapes. Two gloves should be worn by all in the field. Before irrigating the wounds at the end of the case, hydrogen peroxide can be irrigated first and then saline can rapidly follow.

341. A patient with a ventriculoperitoneal shunt presents with an acute abdomen. Is this a reason to tap the shunt?

Yes. Rarely, patients with shunt infection may present with signs of an acute abdomen. These patients may be treated with catheter externalization and antibiotics. Not performing these maneuvers may expose the patient to an unnecessary abdominal procedure.

342. Why is it prudent from an infectious disease point of view to schedule shunt surgeries early in the day?

The number of airborne microorganisms increases over the course of the day in the operating room. This is the rationale for performing surgery early in the day, as is practiced at some large pediatric centers.[162]

343. When is it appropriate to treat a shunt infection with antibiotics alone?

When the patient is high surgical risk and/or there is a shortage of alternative shunt sites. The standard of care is to remove the shunt, place an external ventricular drain, and start antibiotics once cultures of the CSF are drawn.[162]

344. When can a shunt infection be considered cured?

When three negative cultures are obtained from the external ventricular drain. Once this is observed, the external ventricular drain can be removed and the shunt can be inserted at a different site.[162]

345. What should be at the top of the differential diagnosis in a patient who presents with a suboccipital dimple and an attack of infectious meningitis?

A posterior fossa dermoid cyst with a cutaneous fistula.[163]

346. What type of venous thrombosis may occur with mastoiditis?

Lateral sinus thrombosis may be secondary to mastoiditis due to the proximity of this sinus to the mastoid bone.

347. What is the most frequent neurologic complication of AIDS?

HIV (or AIDS) dementia complex is the most frequent neurologic complication of AIDS. This dementia consists of progressive cognitive decline, motor dysfunction, and behavioral dysfunction. This neurologic disease should be kept separate from the diagnoses of other cerebral infections that may infect patients with AIDS.[161]

348. In what size cerebral abscess is medical therapy not likely to be successful?

Three centimeters is suggested as the cutoff above which surgery for cerebral abscesses should be considered. Smaller lesions may resolve with antibiotics alone. Surgery is indicated for mass effect with neurologic deterioration, and these take precedence over size.

349. What is the proper medical treatment of a Nocardia brain abscess?

Trimethoprim-sulfamethoxazole.[160]

350. What is the most common etiology of subdural empyema?

Frontonasal sinusitis.

351. What are the major clinical signs of sporadic CJD?

Cognitive deficits, myoclonus, pyramidal tract signs, periodic complexes on EEG (bilateral sharp waves 0.5 to 2 per second), cerebellar signs, and extrapyramidal signs.[164]

352. What is the most common cause of hydrocephalus in Latin American countries?

Neurocysticercosis is caused by the larval form of *Taenia solium* and is the most frequent helminthic infection of the CNS.

353. What are the effects of preoperative antibiotics on wound infections and postoperative meningitis?

Preoperative antibiotics decrease wound infections, but have no effect on postoperative meningitis.

Vascular

354. What is the leading cause of death worldwide?

Atherothrombosis, defined as ischemic heart disease and cerebrovascular disease according to the 2001 World Health Organization's Report.[165]

355. What is a stroke?

Stroke is a generic term and does not specifically describe the pathophysiologic process. 85% of strokes are due to infarction; 15% are due to hemorrhage. Stroke can mean an occlusion by thrombus or embolus, rupture of a vessel wall, disease of the vessel wall, or disrupted hemodynamics or blood properties. About one-fourth of ischemic strokes are lacunar (involving small vessels), one-fourth are cardioembolic, one-fourth are cryptogenic, and one-fourth are due to atherothrombotic cerebrovascular disease (such as a diseased carotid artery). About three-fourths of the hemorrhagic strokes are intraparenchymal and one-fourth are SAHs. The peak incidence of hemorrhagic stroke occurs earlier in life than for ischemic stroke.[166]

356. What is the rate of immediate mortality in stroke?

In cerebral hemorrhage, immediate mortality is ~50%; in cerebral infarction, immediate mortality is ~20%.[166]

357. What are the risk factors for stroke?

Risk factors can be described as modifiable and nonmodifiable. Modifiable factors are hypertension, diabetes, cardiac disease, atrial fibrillation, TIA or prior stroke, metabolic syndrome, dyslipidemia, cigarette smoking, alcohol abuse, obesity, physical inactivity, carotid stenosis, and obstructive sleep apnea. Nonmodifiable risk factors are age, gender, race/ethnicity, and heredity.[166]

358. What is the definition of a normal blood pressure?

Equal to or less than 120 mm Hg systolic, and less than 80 mm Hg diastolic. The term prehypertension labels blood pressure just higher than 120/80. It is estimated that ~400,000 strokes can be prevented in the United States each year from better control of hypertension.[167]

359. What are some causes of hemorrhagic stroke?

Hypertension, amyloid vasculopathy, aneurysm, AVM, neoplasm, coagulation disease, anticoagulant therapy, vasculitis, drug abuse, and trauma.[168]

360. What is the meaning of luxury perfusion?

The area adjacent to an ischemic area receives more blood flow than normal due to the vasodilation of the arteriolar bed in response to local lactic acidosis.

361. What is a TIA?

A TIA is caused by inadequate blood supply to the brain resulting in an episodic focal neurologic symptom. Attacks are sudden in onset, resolve within 24 hours or less, and leave no residual deficit. TIAs are important in warning of future cerebral infarction. About 10% of patients who sustain a TIA will suffer from a stroke within 90 days, and ~15% will have a stroke within 1 year. 90% of TIAs involve the anterior circulation, with only ~7% involving the posterior circulation.[169]

362. What is the name given to that area of brain defined as ischemic tissue that is at risk for infarction but is potentially salvageable?

The ischemic penumbra. It is believed that the cerebral blood flow in the penumbra region is ~10 to 20 mL per 100 g per minute. The time for penumbral viability is termed the "therapeutic window," and current therapy is directed toward limiting the damage and salvaging the cells in this border-zone ischemic area within this period. The dense ischemic focus is called the umbra.[169]

363. What is the risk of stroke during the first month after a TIA? What percentage will develop a stroke within 2 years?

5% during the first month. Twenty to 25% are estimated to develop a stroke within 2 years.[169]

364. What is bow hunter's stroke?

Bow hunter's stroke results from vertebrobasilar insufficiency caused by mechanical occlusion or stenosis of the vertebral artery at the C1–C2 level with head rotation.

365. Until proven otherwise, what is a headache in an elderly patient who presents with pain when talking and/or chewing and a high erythrocyte sedimentation rate (ESR)?

Giant cell (temporal) arteritis.[170]

366. Dissecting aneurysms that cause SAH typically arise from which artery?

The vertebral artery.

367. Where is a likely location of a traumatic aneurysm due to previous transsphenoidal surgery?

The anterior aspect of the carotid siphon.[171]

368. What is the name of the test whereby manual compression on the carotid artery is performed with vertebral angiography to assess the size of the PComm artery?

The Allcock test.[172]

369. In what percentage of AVMs are aneurysms also found?

10 to 20%.[173]

370. How often is neither an aneurysm nor an AVM found on an angiogram for SAH?

About 20% of the time. When no lesion is immediately apparent, selective injection of the external carotid arteries may reveal a dural AVM. If neck or back pain or lower extremity neurologic deficit is present, then a search for a spinal AVM, aneurysm, or neoplasm may be indicated.[174]

371. What is a pretruncal nonaneurysmal SAH (also called benign perimesencephalic hemorrhage)?

It is the term given for subarachnoid blood in the prepontine or interpeduncular cisterns from rupture of small perimesencephalic veins and/or capillaries. The blood is inferior to the Liliequist membrane (the membrane that separates the interpeduncular cistern from the chiasmatic cistern). A repeat angiogram may not be needed with this particular type of SAH, and the morbidity and mortality of this type of bleeding is significantly lower than classic SAHs. However, vasospasm or hydrocephalus may still occur.

372. What are the odds of detecting a lesion on a repeat angiogram if the first angiogram was negative?

About 2%.[175]

373. What percentage of patients with aneurysmal SAH have multiple aneurysms confirmed by an angiogram?

About 20 to 30%.[176]

374. What clues can guide the surgeon in determining which aneurysm has bled in a patient with multiple aneurysms?

Looking for the pattern of blood on a CT scan, looking for focal spasm on an angiogram, considering the larger or more irregularly shaped aneurysm, examining the patient for focal neurologic signs, considering repeating the angiogram and looking for changes in size and shape of the aneurysms, and choosing the aneurysm that has the highest chance of rupture (AComm). The most commonly missed aneurysms are also the most common aneurysms (AComm).

375. What size is needed for an aneurysm to be considered a "giant" aneurysm?

2.5 cm and greater.

376. How can one clinically differentiate carotid occlusion from innominate artery occlusion?

The blood pressure in the right arm may be diminished with innominate artery occlusion.

377. If an SAH is suspected, but the CT scan of the brain is normal, what is the next course of action?

Lumbar puncture to determine an SAH. A lumbar puncture has a minimal risk in alert patients with no focal neurologic deficits and no papilledema. A CT scan is important to rule out any cerebral mass lesions before proceeding with a lumbar puncture.

378. What are the odds of rebleeding despite a negative angiogram for SAH?

About 4% over 4 years.[177]

379. What is the cumulative risk of rebleeding in an untreated aneurysm?

20% at 2 weeks and 30% at 1 month after initial rupture.

380. If a CT scan is done for cerebral ischemia, at what time could one expect to see a hyperdense artery sign?

Between 12 and 24 hours.

381. What percentage of patients with an acute MI can be expected to have a cerebrovascular accident (CVA) within 1 to 2 weeks after the MI?

2.5%.[178]

382. What is the rate of stroke per year in the setting of asymptomatic atrial fibrillation without treatment?

4.5%.[179]

383. What is the rate of stroke per year in the setting of symptomatic atrial fibrillation without treatment?

12%.[180]

384. What is the rate of stroke per year in the setting of asymptomatic carotid bruit?

2%.[181,182]

385. What is the rate of stroke per year in the setting of symptomatic carotid stenosis?

13%.[183]

386. What percentage of SAH patients die before reaching the hospital?

10%.[184]

387. Urinary loss of sodium after SAH may mimic SIADH, but what syndrome is it more like in this setting?

CSW.[185]

388. According to the first International Study of Unruptured Intracranial Aneurysms (ISUIA study), what is the quoted annual risk of rupture of an aneurysm less than 10 mm found incidentally on imaging?

The risk is 0.05%. The ISUIA study examined the natural history and the results of treatment of unruptured aneurysms. ISUIA data suggested that the risk of rupture was related to the size of the aneurysm, the site of the aneurysm, and whether there was a previous SAH. For aneurysms greater than 10 mm, the risk is 0.5% annually. If there was a previous SAH, the risk of rupture for an aneurysm less than 10 mm is 0.5% annually, and for an aneurysm greater than 10 mm, the risk is 1% annually. The aneurysms in the posterior circulation have a higher rate of rupture than those in other areas.[186]

389. What does the International Subarachnoid Aneurysm Trial (ISAT) study suggest?

The ISAT study suggested that there was a 7% absolute risk reduction in patients with poor outcome at 2 months and 1 year when coil embolization of aneurysms (23.7% risk) was performed, as opposed to open surgery, which carries greater risk (30.6% risk). There was a greater incidence of rebleeding in the coil group and the coil group required additional treatments four times more frequently than the open surgery group. The ISAT study was almost exclusively restricted to anterior circulation aneurysms (only 2.7% were posterior circulation aneurysms).[187]

390. What is the annual rebleeding rate for SAH from an unknown cause?

0.5%.[177]

391. Following an AComm artery aneurysm clipping from the left side, a patient awakens with hemiparesis and aphasia. What artery was most likely inadvertently coagulated or clipped?

The recurrent artery of Heubner. In the treatment of AComm artery aneurysms, great care must be taken to avoid unnecessary manipulation or occlusion of the Heubner artery. Occlusion may cause hemiparesis with facial and brachial predominance because of compromise of that branch supplying the anterior limb of the internal capsule, and aphasia if the artery is on the dominant side.[188] Johann Otto Leonhard Heubner (1843–1926) was a German pediatrician who first isolated meningococci from CSF in a patient with meningitis. He described the recurrent artery in 1872.

392. During an operation for repair of an MCA aneurysm, temporary clipping is performed, and the anesthesiologist is asked at this time to administer 500 mg of thiopental. What is the purpose of this?

Thiopental is used to reduce cerebral metabolic demand. Temporary clipping is often necessary with complex aneurysms. Intermittent temporary clipping is safer than continuous temporary clipping. Other cerebral protective measures used during aneurysm surgery are the use of isoflurane anesthetic, mannitol, lumbar or ventricular drainage to ensure brain relaxation after the dura is opened, and mild hypothermia.

393. What are some intracranial and extracranial complications of aneurysm rupture?

Intracranial complications include rebleeding, vasospasm (resulting in cerebral ischemia or infarction), hydrocephalus, hematoma formation, and seizures. Extracranial complications include myocardial irritation or infarction, neurogenic pulmonary edema, and gastric ulceration.

394. What area on the circle of Willis is most commonly hypoplastic?

The A1 segment of the anterior cerebral artery.[60]

395. What is the annual stroke rate for patients with a mild neurologic deficit and proven ICA occlusion?

3 to 5%.

396. According to the North American Symptomatic Carotid Endarterectomy Trial (NASCET), carotid endarterectomy (in the setting of greater than 70% stenosis) reduces incidence of stroke and death by what percentages at 18 months?

17% for stroke, 7% reduction in death.[189]

397. According to the Asymptomatic Carotid Atherosclerosis Study (ACAS), carotid endarterectomy is only beneficial when the surgical complication rate is less than what percent?

3%.[190]

398. How is the arterial anatomy defined when the PComm artery is larger than the P1?

Fetal PComm (**Fig. 5.12**).[60]

399. In what percentage of patients are the posterior cerebral arteries supplied on one or both sides by the carotid circulation?

About 20% of patients have a fetal circulation.[60]

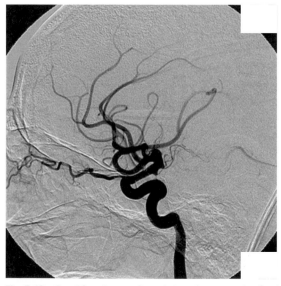

Fig. 5.12 Carotid angiogram, lateral view, demonstrating fetal posterior communicating artery.

400. How can an AComm artery aneurysm result in subarachnoid blood in the third ventricle? What Fisher's grade would this represent?

Rupture through the lamina terminalis, Fisher's grade 4.

401. How can an aneurysm result in fourth ventricular blood?

Rupture of a posterior inferior cerebellar artery aneurysm through the foramen of Luschka.

402. What is the leading cause of death or morbidity after SAH?

Vasospasm is a leading cause of death or morbidity after SAH. If it remains untreated, this may lead to death or permanent disability in ~20% of cases. In addition, reversible clinical deterioration will occur in ~30%. Vasospasm reaches peak severity at about day 7, and in most cases it will resolve by 2 to 3 weeks.[184]

403. What value of MCA velocity in cm per second defines vasospasm?

A value of 120 to 200 cm/s indicates mild vasospasm, and over 200 cm/s indicates severe vasospasm.[191]

404. What is the Lindegaard ratio?

The ratio of velocity of MCA flow to ICA flow, it is used to assess vasospasm. A ratio of greater than 6 indicates severe vasospasm; less than 3 is normal.[191]

405. What is triple-H therapy?

Treatment of vasospasm uses hypervolemia, induced hypertension, and active hemodilution to a hematocrit of ~30%.[191]

406. What is central diabetes insipidus?

Diabetes insipidus is a complication caused by a deficiency of antidiuretic hormone that may occur after an SAH, usually from an aneurysm near the anterior circulation. Polyuria is the most prominent feature; in severe cases, the loss of fluid may exceed 10 L daily. The diagnosis is confirmed by finding high volumes (over 200 mL per hour for over 3 hours) of dilute (specific gravity 1.005 or less) urine of very low osmolality, at the same time as high serum osmolality, with hypernatremia in severe cases. The water deprivation test and aqueous Pitressin (JHP Pharmaceuticals) can help in the diagnosis of equivocal cases.[192]

407. In what neurosurgical situations is diabetes insipidus commonly seen?

Following transsphenoidal surgery, brain death, craniopharyngioma, AComm artery aneurysm, head injury, basal skull fractures, encephalitis, and meningitis.[192]

408. What arteries supply lenticulostriates and thalamoperforators?

Lenticulostriates are from the M1 segment of the MCA; thalamoperforators are from the P1 segment of the PCA.[60]

409. In MCA occlusion in the dominant hemisphere, how can one have hemiplegia without aphasia in one case, and receptive aphasia without hemiplegia in another case?

Occlusion of the superior trunk of the MCA results in a sensory–motor hemiplegia without a receptive aphasia; occlusion of the inferior division results in a receptive aphasia in the absence of hemiplegia.

410. What is the mortality and morbidity from an AVM that hemorrhages?

10% mortality and 30 to 50% morbidity.[193]

411. What are the average annual risk and the lifetime risk of hemorrhage for an unruptured AVM?

The average annual risk of rupture is 2 to 4%. One can use the equation Lifetime Risk $= 1 - (0.97)^{(years\ left\ of\ life)}$ to calculate lifetime risk of AVM rupture. When the AVM ruptures, the risk of rerupture is ~6 to 7% that first year, and then normalizes to 2 to 4% per subsequent year.[193]

412. What are features of AVMs that make for a high operative risk?

A size greater than 3 cm, location in eloquent sites, and drainage to deep veins. Large lesions (greater than 6 cm) have a risk of hyperperfusion syndrome and brain swelling and carry a 40% risk of permanent neurologic deficit (**Fig. 5.13**).[194]

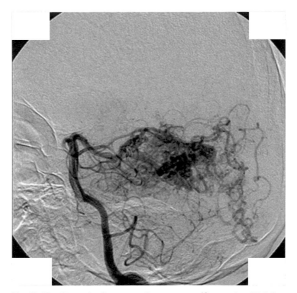

Fig. 5.13 Posterior fossa arteriovenous malformation (AVM) angiogram. The AVM is located in eloquent brain, has deep drainage, and is larger than 3 cm in size.

413. When an AVM is treated by stereotactic radiosurgery, what happens to the annual risk of hemorrhage?

Sometimes, it takes up to 3 years after radiosurgery for the AVM to completely obliterate. During that time, the risk of hemorrhage persists. Some even question whether a partially thrombosed AVM from stereotactic radiosurgery is more likely to bleed because of increased outflow resistance.[195]

414. Is there still a risk of hemorrhage after complete obliteration of the AVM by radiography?

Yes, a *New England Journal of Medicine* article (2005) noted that 6 out of 250 patients bled after a confirmed "cure" of their AVM.[196]

415. What is the annual risk of bleeding with a cavernous malformation (angioma)?

About 0.5 to 1% per year. Those that have not bled in the past have a lower bleeding risk (0.5% per year) than those that have previously bled (5% per year). Brain-stem cavernomas have the highest risk at 6% per year for those that have not bled to up to 34% per year for those that have previously bled in the brainstem. Deep cavernous angiomas are more dangerous than superficial ones. A cavernous malformation (also known as a cavernous angioma) may present with seizures (most common), headaches, or focal neurologic signs. With increasing use of MRI, these angiomas are being diagnosed more frequently in all age groups. Pathologically, cavernous angiomas are composed of sinusoidal vessels that are compact and discrete from the surrounding brain. No intervening brain tissue is present, and hemosiderin-stained parenchyma surrounds the lesion. Almost all cavernous malformations show pathologic evidence of previous hemorrhage.[197]

416. What is the most common vascular malformation found in autopsy specimens?

Venous angiomas. They are frequently diagnosed during evaluation for headaches or unrelated trauma.[197]

417. When is surgery for venous angiomas warranted?

Bleeding or intractable seizures. However, venous angiomas are usually benign and should be managed nonoperatively.[198]

418. How can a vein of Galen aneurysm cause obstructive hydrocephalus?

Compression of the sylvian aqueduct.[199]

419. What types of lesions can cause a pulse-synchronous tinnitus?

Carotid-cavernous fistula, dural AVM, glomus jugulare tumor, and a vascular lesion of the petrous bone/skull base. Pulse-synchronous tinnitus can also be caused by ipsilateral carotid stenosis and idiopathic intracranial hypertension. In 15% of cases, no cause of pulsatile tinnitus can be found.

420. What diagnosis must be excluded when one encounters a red, pulsatile, retrotympanic mass in a patient with conductive hearing loss and pulsatile tinnitus?

Glomus jugulare tumor.

421. What is Vernet's syndrome?

Palsy of CNs IX, X, and XI at one time.[200]

422. Which locations of dural vascular malformations carry a high risk of cerebral hemorrhage?

Dural malformations involving the anterior cranial fossa or the tentorial incisura carry a high risk of cerebral hemorrhage as part of their natural history. In addition, the identification of cortical venous drainage by angiography appears to be predictive of hemorrhage.

423. What percentage of low-flow carotid-cavernous fistulas spontaneously thrombose?

50%; so observe as long as vision is stable and intraocular pressure is not elevated.

424. In carotid endarterectomy, what did the ACAS study show?

The ACAS study showed that in those asymptomatic patients with greater than 60% stenosis, there is a modest benefit to surgery if the complication rate of surgery is less than 3%. The annual risk of stroke is reduced from 0.5 to 0.17%.[190]

425. If one considers absolute risk reduction, what group of patients benefits the most from having a carotid endarterectomy?

Patients with symptomatic carotid stenosis of 70 to 99% realize an absolute risk reduction about eight times greater than the other groups (asymptomatic stenosis of 60–99%, and symptomatic stenosis of 50–59%). Asymptomatic patients, to have a risk reduction, must have an absolute surgical risk of less than 3%.[189,190]

426. What are the major complications from a carotid endarterectomy?

Cerebral infarction, intracerebral hemorrhage, MI, wound hematoma, wound infection, CN injury (vagus, hypoglossal, facial, greater auricular, glossopharyngeal), and recurrent carotid stenosis.[189]

427. What is the most common cause of early and late death after a carotid endarterectomy?

Ischemic heart disease. Thus, preoperative detection and management of coronary artery disease are indispensable to ensure a safe carotid endarterectomy procedure.[189]

428. What are the symptoms of vertebrobasilar insufficiency and what is the risk of a stroke in the first year after a vertebrobasilar TIA?

Drop attack, diplopia, dysarthria, visual defect, and dizziness. The risk of CVA is 22% in the first year after a vertebrobasilar TIA.

429. What is the annual risk of stroke in patients with a known carotid occlusion?

8 to 10%.[166]

430. Until proven otherwise, what is acute retro-orbital pain with a Horner syndrome indicative of?

Carotid artery dissection.

431. According to the ISUIA study, what particular location was most predictive of rupture?

The basilar tip.[186,201]

432. What is the location of the occlusion in a case where TIAs are initiated or aggravated by arm exercise?

The proximal subclavian artery. This results in retrograde flow down the vertebral arteries into the subclavian arteries known as subclavian steal syndrome.

433. What is an EC–IC bypass?

Extracranial–intracranial (EC–IC) bypass aims at enhancing the collateral circulation in patients with carotid or MCA occlusion to lessen the likelihood of further ipsilateral infarction. A randomized multicenter international study demonstrated that EC–IC bypass was no better than conservative treatment.[202]

434. What is Binswanger's encephalopathy?

Subcortical arteriosclerotic encephalopathy, which is a rare disorder in which progressive dementia and pseudobulbar palsy are associated with diffuse hemisphere demyelination. A CT scan shows areas of periventricular low attenuation.

435. What are some atypical dementias that may necessitate a biopsy?

Pick's disease, Binswanger's disease, Niemann-Pick disease, Lewy's body disease.

436. What are some causes of thrombotic occlusion of the cerebral venous system?

Head trauma, infection, dehydration, pregnancy, oral contraceptive pill, coagulation disorders, malignant meningitis, sarcoid, systemic lupus, and Behçet's disease.

437. What are some signs and symptoms of cavernous sinus thrombosis?

Cavernous sinus thrombosis can spread from an infection on the face via draining veins or paranasal sinuses. It is characterized by painful ophthalmoplegia, proptosis, and chemosis with edema of periorbital structures. There may also be facial numbness and fevers.

438. What is the most common tumor of the cavernous sinus?

A meningioma.

439. How does carotid dissection present?

Sudden neck pain, ipsilateral Horner's syndrome, and sometimes lower CN palsies. This should be suspected in patients who have sustained major mechanism trauma, severe stretching, or direct impact on the neck.

440. What are antifibrinolytic agents and how can they help in the setting of an SAH?

The most common antifibrinolytic agents used are tranexamic acid and epsilon-aminocaproic acid. They reduce rebleeding of an aneurysm by delaying clot lysis at the aneurysm fundus, which may be protective. However, they may increase the incidence of cerebral vasospasm and are *not* routinely used.

441. What are common causes of stroke in a young adult?

Trauma, extracranial and intracranial dissections, atherosclerosis, cardiac embolism, fat embolism, patent foramen ovale, vasculopathy, moyamoya disease, lupus, homocystinuria, peripartum, oral contraceptives, venous thrombosis, migraine, and cocaine use. The work-up should include cardiac work-up and routine laboratories including ESR, PT/PTT, venereal disease research laboratory (VDRL) test, lupus anticoagulant, toxicology screen, fasting lipid profile, carotid Doppler, and magnetic resonance angiography (MRA) of the brain.

442. What are the most common causes of PRES (posterior reversible encephalopathy syndrome)?

Hypertensive encephalopathy, immunosuppressive therapy, renal failure, and eclampsia are the most common causes of PRES. Clinically, patients present with seizures and an altered level of consciousness. Radiologically, CT and MRI of the brain show extensive subcortical edema mainly confined to the posterior parietooccipital lobes. PRES affects females more commonly than males. In some cases, hemorrhagic events may occur. Lesions typically disappear in 2 weeks on MRI.

443. What is the incidence of intracerebral aneurysms?

10/100,000 per year.

444. What is the prevalence of intracerebral aneurysms?

About 5%.[203]

445. What is the prevalence of SAH in patients with autosomal dominant polycystic kidney disease (ADPKD) with intracranial aneurysms?

The prevalence of aneurysms in ADPKD is ~15%.[204]

446. Which chromosomes have the ADPKD gene?

- ADPKD has the PKD1 gene and PKD2 gene.
- PKD1 gene is on chromosome 16p (90%).
- PKD2 gene is on chromosome 4q (5–15%).

447. What is the relevance of SAH in patients with ADPKD?

SAH in patients with ADPKD presents about a decade earlier when compared with patients with intracranial aneurysms without ADPKD. Furthermore, there is a relative overrepresentation of MCA aneurysms in patients with ADPKD.[205]

448. What percentage of patients with aneurysms have other family members with aneurysms?

About 7 to 20% of patients with detected aneurysms have other family members with aneurysms, and screening should be considered with two first-degree relatives who have aneurysms.[206]

449. Describe the Borden classification for dural arteriovenous fistulas (AVFs).

- Type I: via meningeal artery → drains anterograde to the venous sinus.
- Type II: via meningeal artery → drains anterograde to venous sinus and sinus drains retrograde to subarachnoid veins.
- Type III: via meningeal artery → drains retrograde to subarachnoid veins.[207]

450. According to the Borden classification, which types of AVFs have a higher chance of bleed?

The fistulas with a retrograde flow into subarachnoid veins have high pressure into veins and carry an increased chance of intracranial bleed and hence require treatment.

451. What is the classification for spinal AVMs?

- Type I: dural AVF (**Fig. 5.14**).
- Type II: intramedullary AVM.
- Type III: juvenile AVM.
- Type IV: perimedullary AVF.
- Type IVa: artery of Adamkiewicz.
- Type IVb: multiple feeders.

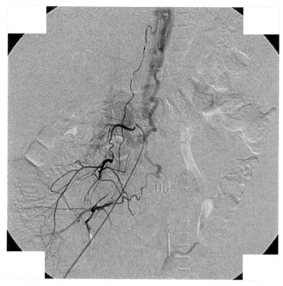

Fig. 5.14 Angiogram demonstrating a type I spinal arteriovenous fistula.

452. Which type of spinal AVM is the most common?

Type I is the most common type of spinal AVM. It is mostly found in males (80–90%) between 40 and 60 years of age and SAH is rare.[208]

453. What is the approximate rate of SAH in patients with intramedullary AVM (type II)?

Both the male:female ratio and the rate of SAH are ~50%.

454. What is the classification for aneurysms associated with AVM?

- Type I: aneurysm is proximally located on an ipsilateral major feeder.
- Type Ia: aneurysm is proximally located on a contralateral major feeder.
- Type II: aneurysm is distally located on a superficial feeder.
- Type III: aneurysm is proximally or distally located on a deep feeder.
- Type IV: aneurysm is on an artery unrelated to the AVM.

455. What percentage of all vascular malformations of brain are cavernous malformations?

About 8 to 16%.

456. What is the usual location of cavernous malformations of brain?

70% are supratentorial and 30% occur in the cerebellum, brainstem, and spinal cord.

457. What percentage of cavernous malformations are radiologically occult?

About 19 to 31% are radiologically occult.[209]

458. What is the usual presentation of cavernous malformations?

- Seizures: 25 to 35%.
- Hemorrhage: 13 to 50%.
- Focal neurologic deficit: 20 to 35%.

459. What is the annual hemorrhage rate of cavernous malformations?

About 1 or 2% per year (rates vary between 0.7 and 6% per year based on a recent meta-analysis).[210]

460. What percentage of cavernous malformations show calcifications?

About 15% of cavernous malformations exhibit calcification, and these exhibit higher epileptogenicity.

461. Describe the genes associated with cavernous malformations.

- CCM1: on chromosome 7q, found in Hispanic Americans.
- CCM2: on chromosome 7p.
- CCM3: on chromosome 3q, found in non-Hispanic Caucasians.[211]

462. What is the sensitivity and specificity of ultrasound in assessing carotid occlusion in neck?

- Sensitivity: 86%.
- Specificity: 87%.

463. What is the restenosis risk after carotid endarterectomy?

- 10% in first year.
- 3% in second year.
- 2% in third year.
- 1% per year thereafter.[212,213]

464. What are some of the causes of carotid dissection?

Chiropractic manipulation, fibromuscular dystrophy, Ehlers-Danlos syndrome, and trauma such as motor vehicle accidents. Chiropractic manipulation of the neck can result in dissection of either carotid or vertebral arteries resulting in death and should be prohibited.

465. What is the mortality associated with carotid dissection?

About 5%.

466. What is the normal cerebral blood flow?

40 to 60 mL/100 g of brain tissue per minute.

467. At what cerebral blood flow do the symptoms start?

- 20 to 30 mL/100 g of brain tissue per minute: neurologic symptoms.
- 16 to 20 mL/100 g of brain tissue per minute: isoelectric EEG and loss of evoked potentials.
- 10 to 12 mL/100 g of brain tissue per minute: Na/K pump failure, cytotoxic edema.
- <10 mL/100 g of brain tissue per minute: infarction.
- 17 to 18 mL/100 g of brain tissue per minute for more than 3 minutes: infarction.

468. All prostaglandins cause vasoconstriction, except?

PGI2.

469. Describe Graeb's classification of intraventricular hemorrhage (IVH).

Maximum score is 12 for two lateral ventricles and the third and fourth ventricles. For lateral ventricles:

1. Trace blood.
2. <50% ventricle filled.

3. >50% ventricle filled.
4. Casting of ventricle.

For third and fourth ventricles:

1. Blood present.
2. Casting of ventricle and expansion.[214]

470. How is mortality associated with IVH?

- Intracerebral hemorrhage with IVH: 32 to 44% mortality.
- All four ventricles IVH: 60 to 90% mortality.
- Primary IVH: 30 to 50% mortality.
- External ventricular drain placement with tissue plasminogen activator: reduced mortality to 30 to 35%.[215,216]

471. How is the neonatal IVH classified?

- Grade I: subependymal hemorrhage.
- Grade II: IVH without dilatation.
- Grade III: IVH with hydrocephalus.
- Grade IV: IVH with intraparenchymal hemorrhage.

472. What is the site of IVH in a premature baby?

The germinal matrix.

473. What is the site of IVH in a full-term newborn baby?

The choroid plexus.

474. What is the risk of progressive hydrocephalus in a premature baby with an IVH?

- Grade I: 0 to 10%.
- Grade II: 15 to 25%.
- Grade III/IV: 65 to 100%.[217,218]

475. What is the mortality associated with a premature baby with an IVH?

- Grade I: 0%.
- Grade II: 5 to 15%.
- Grade III/IV: 50 to 65%.

476. What does "moyamoya" mean in English?

Puff of smoke.

477. What is the effect of the arteriopathy in moyamoya disease?

Progressive occlusion of the terminal ICA as well as the anterior or middle cerebral arteries (ACA or MCA). This occurs while lenticulostriate collateral form (moyamoya vessels) at the base of the brain (**Fig. 5.15**).

478. What are the surgical treatment options of moyamoya disease?

- Direct: EC–IC bypass.
- Indirect: encephalodurosynangiosis, encephalomyosynangiosis, encephalogaleosynangiosis, omental grafts, multiple burr holes.

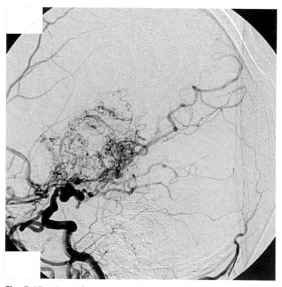

Fig. 5.15 Carotid angiogram demonstrating moyamoya vessels forming as collateral flow, with occlusion of MCA and ACA branches.

Congenital and Pediatric

479. What is the most common type of scalp injury during birth?

Cephalhematoma is the most common type of scalp injury and may occur in 2 to 5% of live births due to shear forces between the pericranium and the skull.

Cephalhematoma is limited by periosteal attachments and does not cross sutures in contradistinction to a subgaleal hematoma. Caput succedaneum is an area of localized scalp edema from compression of the scalp by the cervix.[219,220]

480. What are the common symptoms and signs of a Chiari I malformation?

- Symptoms: headache (sometimes worse with cough), neck pain, weakness, numbness, unsteadiness.[221]
- Signs: hyperactive lower extremity reflexes, downbeat nystagmus, loss of temperature sensation, gait disturbance, hand atrophy, upper extremity weakness.

481. What is often cited as the cutoff below which one may consider tonsillar herniation a Chiari I malformation?

5 mm below the foramen magnum (**Fig. 5.16**).[222] This measurement should be considered in the context of the clinical picture. For example, is the headache daily or once in a while?

482. Chiari II malformation nearly always is associated with what spinal lesion?

Myelomeningocele. All infants with myelomeningocele have magnetic resonance criteria of Chiari II malformation. Hydrocephalus is nearly always present in these patients.[223]

483. What are some common features of Chiari II malformation?

Downward displacement of the medulla, fourth ventricle, and cerebellum into the cervical spinal canal, elongation of the pons and fourth ventricle, dysgenesis of the corpus callosum, and medullary kinking (**Fig. 5.17**).[223]

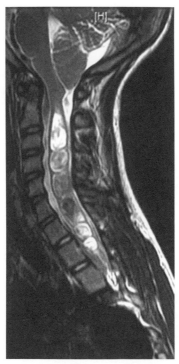

Fig. 5.16 Sagittal T2-weighted magnetic resonance image demonstrating Chiari type I malformation with cervical syrinx.

484. What is the most common type of primary synostosis?

Sagittal synostosis (scaphocephaly). Premature fusion of the sagittal suture accounts for about half of craniosynostosis cases. Most are males. The second most common type is frontal plagiocephaly caused by unilateral coronal suture synostosis.[225,226]

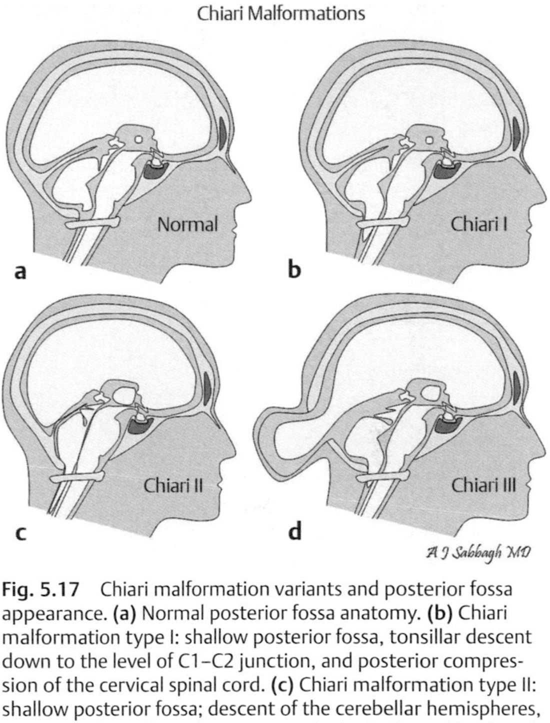

Chiari Malformations

Fig. 5.17 Chiari malformation variants and posterior fossa appearance. **(a)** Normal posterior fossa anatomy. **(b)** Chiari malformation type I: shallow posterior fossa, tonsillar descent down to the level of C1–C2 junction, and posterior compression of the cervical spinal cord. **(c)** Chiari malformation type II: shallow posterior fossa; descent of the cerebellar hemispheres, vermis, and tonsils to the upper cervical spinal canal level; and posterior compression of the brainstem and the cervical spinal cord. **(d)** Chiari malformation type III: shallow posterior fossa, tonsillar herniation, brainstem and cervical spinal cord compression, and associated occipital encephalocele. (Reproduced with permission from Nader and Sabbagh.[224])

485. What is the most common craniofacial deformity?

Crouzon's syndrome (autosomal dominant). It is characterized by calvarial deformity, facial deformity, and exophthalmos. The calvarial deformities always involve more than one suture. Hydrocephalus is more common in Crouzon's syndrome than in simple craniosynostosis. The second most common craniofacial deformity is Apert's syndrome, which is characterized by turricephaly, mental retardation, maxillary hypoplasia, orbital hypertelorism, syndactyly, and vertebral and skeletal abnormalities.[227]

486. How does one make the diagnosis of "shaken baby syndrome"?

The parents or caregivers typically give no history or an inappropriate history for the degree of trauma observed. A CT scan of the head shows interhemispheric or tentorial subdural blood. Physical examination reveals retinal hemorrhages, which is evidence of acceleration–deceleration injury.[228]

487. What is the most common suprasellar tumor in children?

A craniopharyngioma.[229]

488. What hereditary conditions are associated with cerebral aneurysms?

Marfan's syndrome, Ehlers-Danlos syndrome, pseudoxanthoma elasticum, polycystic kidney disease, tuberous sclerosis, hereditary hemorrhagic telangiectasia, Anderson-Fabry disease, neurofibromatosis.[230]

489. What are the inheritance and clinical manifestation of NF1?

The gene on chromosome 17 is transmitted in an autosomal dominant fashion; however, it has a very high spontaneous mutation rate. About 50% of people with NF1 do not have a family history of the disorder. NF1 is characterized by 100% penetrance; all patients with this genetic defect have at least some manifestation of the disorder. Skin lesions are the most common manifestations: café au lait spots, cutaneous neurofibromas, intertriginous freckling, Lisch's nodules (which are very sensitive for NF1), optic gliomas, and osseous abnormalities. Patients with six café au lait spots larger than 15 mm fulfill the criteria for NF1. Plexiform neurofibromas in NF1 patients have about a 5 to 10% rate of malignant transformation and should be suspected in a patient with rapid growth of a subcutaneous lesion.[231]

490. What are the features of NF1?

A good mnemonic is POOR CLAN: plexiform neurofibroma, osseous lesions, optic nerve gliomas, relative with the disease, café au lait spots, Lisch's nodule, axillary freckling, neurofibromas.[231]

491. Before operating on a cranial neurofibroma, what imaging study is necessary before positioning?

An MRI of the cervical spine is imperative as it may disclose intraspinal tumors that can cause cord injury.

492. What disease should be considered in a child who presents with a schwannoma or meningioma?

NF2.[231]

493. What is the most common presenting symptom of ataxia telangiectasia?

Cerebellar ataxia, often noted within the first 2 years of life.[232]

494. What genetic disorder is associated with an imperfection of the vessel wall and increased incidence of cerebral AVMs?

Rendu-Osler-Weber disease (also known as hereditary hemorrhagic telangiectasia).[233,234]

495. What disease should be considered in a child with multiple cerebral AVMs, recurrent epistaxis, and/or cerebral abscesses?

Hereditary hemorrhagic telangiectasia. Pulmonary fistulas also occur in this disorder and render the patient susceptible to cerebral abscesses.[235]

496. What congenital diseases may present with seizures?

Tuberous sclerosis and Sturge-Weber syndrome.[236]

497. What are the manifestations of Sturge-Weber syndrome?

Unilateral port-wine stain in the ophthalmic division of the trigeminal nerve (look for upper eyelid involvement), seizures, contralateral hemisensory and motor deficit, and cortical tramline calcification on CT scan. Hemispherectomy on appropriately selected patients has been shown to decrease or alleviate seizures and possibly improve intellectual capacity.[237]

498. What is the most common cancer in children?

Leukemia. Brain malignancies are the second most common, and ~70% of those are infratentorial. This is in contrast to adults where 70% of primary brain tumors are supratentorial.[238,239]

499. Where is the most common location of germ cell tumors in the CNS?

The pineal region. These are most common in children and adolescents, with a peak incidence around 12 years.[240]

500. What is the most common presenting symptom in patients with choroid plexus papillomas?

Headache from increased ICP. These tumors produce communicating hydrocephalus by overproducing CSF. Other symptoms of increased ICP may be present, such as nausea/vomiting and craniomegaly.[241]

501. What classic radiographic signs are seen in a CT scan of a patient with Sturge-Weber disease?

Tram-track cortical calcifications and ipsilateral calvarial thickening.[129]

502. What is the mode of inheritance of Sturge-Weber syndrome?

Sporadic.

503. What is the most common brain tumor that arises from patients with tuberous sclerosis?

Giant cell astrocytoma. It occurs in ~10% of patients.[114]

504. What is the classic triad seen in patients with tuberous sclerosis?

Mental retardation, seizures, and adenoma sebaceum. This triad is seen in less than 50% of patients.[39] Adenoma sebaceum appears as red papules on the face sometimes confused with acne.

505. What is the most common cutaneous manifestation of tuberous sclerosis?

Ash-leaf hypopigmented macules. By 12 years of age, 90% of the patients develop skin lesions.[242]

506. What is the most common childhood orbital lesion?

Retinoblastoma. 90% of these lesions are diagnosed before the age of 5. These tumors arise from photoreceptor precursors.[243]

507. How can the maternal AFP test be normal in a woman carrying a child with a large encephalocele?

The AFP test can be normal if the encephalocele is fully epithelialized; it is necessary for the lesion to be leaking tissue fluid and CSF to produce an abnormal level of AFP.[244]

508. What is the diagnosis (until proven otherwise) of a nasal polypoid mass in a newborn?

Encephalocele.[245]

509. How can one differentiate a nasal polyp from a sincipital encephalocele?

An encephalocele pulsates, presents medially from the nasal septum, and widens the nasal bridge; a polyp does not pulsate, is located laterally, emanates from the turbinates, and does not widen the nasion.[245]

510. A child with Dandy-Walker syndrome undergoes ventriculoperitoneal shunt placement. While inserting the shunt via a posterior occipital burr hole, the surgeon encounters brisk venous bleeding. What may be happening in this scenario?

The transverse sinus has been penetrated. In cases of posterior fossa malformations (such as Dandy-Walker and posterior fossa arachnoid cysts), the transverse sinus may reside at a higher level than usual. It is necessary to get a preoperative MRI-MRV (magnetic resonance venography) to prevent this complication.[246]

511. How can one differentiate a Dandy-Walker cyst from a posterior fossa arachnoid cyst?

Asymmetry of cystic formation and visualization of the cerebellar vermis on the midsagittal slice of an MRI point toward an arachnoid cyst. Dandy-Walker malformation and Dandy-Walker variant are both characterized by partial agenesis of the cerebellar vermis.[246]

512. What is the most common primary CNS tumor to exhibit extraneural spread?

Medulloblastoma (cerebellar primitive neuroectodermal tumor).[247] Much more common is intraneural spread; imaging of the whole neuraxis is recommended to identify drop metastases and leptomeningeal spread.

513. What is a malignant tumor of childhood arising from the cerebellar vermis?

A medulloblastoma. In 30% of cases, spread occurs through the CSF to the spinal area or lateral ventricles. Destruction of the cerebellar vermis results in truncal and gait ataxia. The 5-year survival rate ranges from 50 to 85% depending on the extent of tumor removal, dissemination, and age. Radiotherapy is the most effective postoperative treatment with radiation of the entire neuraxis in patients greater than 3 years of age. During the operation, care must be taken to ensure that the vital structures at the floor of the fourth ventricle are preserved. Medulloblastomas account for ~25% of all childhood intracranial malignancies.[247]

514. What is the difference in the location of a medulloblastoma in an adolescent (or adult) from that of a very young child?

Medulloblastomas may be present in the cerebellar hemisphere more often in adolescents and adults; they are more often found in the midline in children.[247]

515. What are the most common location and presentation for supratentorial arachnoid cysts?

The sylvian fissure is the most common location for supratentorial arachnoid cysts. Headache is the most common presenting symptom; however, seizures and symptoms of increased ICP may be present. Males are affected more commonly than females, and the left hemisphere is more commonly affected than the right. Treatment of sylvian fissure arachnoid cysts involves excision of the cyst membranes and/or placement of a cystoperitoneal shunt.[248,249]

516. What is a "harlequin" orbit?

It is the shape seen on radiography of the orbit from a fused coronal suture found in a unilateral coronal synostosis. The elevation of the greater and lesser wings of the sphenoid ipsilateral to the fused suture gives the eye this unusual shape.[250]

517. What are the four normal embryologic arterial connections in the cerebral vascular system that may persist after birth?

Four normal embryologic arterial connections may persist after birth in some individuals. These arteries are the *trigeminal artery*, which connects the intracavernous portion of the carotid artery to the basilar artery; the *otic artery*, which joins the intrapetrous carotid artery to the midportion of the basilar artery; the *hypoglossal artery*, which connects the extracranial ICA to the intracranial vertebral artery; and the *proatlantal artery*, which links the extracranial ICA to the extracranial vertebral artery at the C2 level. The trigeminal artery is purely subarachnoid and is easy to identify intracranially. The otic artery is partly intrapetrous, coursing through the vidian canal to become subarachnoid and join the midportion of the basilar artery. The hypoglossal artery is initially extracranial in origin and gains access to the intracranial cavity through the hypoglossal canal. The proatlantal artery is entirely extracranial.[251]

518. What is the name of the persistent frontal suture that is continuous with the sagittal suture?

The metopic suture.[252]

519. How does one perform a subdural tap in an infant?

Prep with alcohol and let it dry, then use betadine or Duraprep over the intended field. A 20-gauge spinal needle is introduced at a right angle to the scalp's surface and at least 2 cm lateral to the midline within the coronal suture. The needle is advanced until free flow of fluid is obtained. Forceful aspiration is to be avoided.[253]

520. What type of arachnoid cyst may present with "bobble-head doll syndrome"?

Suprasellar arachnoid cysts may present with hydrocephalus, endocrine problems, head bobbing, and vision problems.[254]

521. What is the accepted lower limit of weight for placement of a ventriculoperitoneal shunt in an infant?

2,500 g.[255]

522. What is a Pott puffy tumor?

A Pott puffy tumor is a subperiosteal abscess of the frontal bone that appears as a localized swelling of the overlying region of the forehead associated with frontal osteomyelitis. This condition is associated with a high risk of meningitis, intracranial abscess, and venous sinus thrombosis; aggressive medical and surgical treatment is essential for a good outcome.[256]

523. What is the most common cause of a Pott puffy tumor?

Frontal sinusitis.[256]

524. What is positional posterior plagiocephaly?

An oblique skull shape with unilateral flattening of the occiput with frontal bossing due to persistent head positioning to one side, in the absence of lambdoid synostosis.[257]

525. What is the treatment of positional posterior plagiocephaly?

Most cases are treated with conservative positional maneuvers, with helmet therapy reserved for severe or nonrefractory cases.[257]

526. What is a frequently encountered muscular deformity in patients with positional plagiocephaly?

Congenital torticollis.[258]

527. What is a common systemic dysfunction in newborns with a vein of Galen malformation at the time of presentation?

Congestive heart failure.[259]

528. What is a growing skull fracture?

Also known as posttraumatic leptomeningeal cyst, it is a rare entity almost exclusively seen before 3 years of age that consists of a fracture line that widens over time and has an underlying dural tear.[260]

529. What are the common findings in McCune-Albright syndrome?

- Endocrine abnormalities.
- Unilateral café au lait spots with jagged edges.
- Fibrous dysplasia.
- Precocious puberty (in females).[261]

530. What is the success rate of endoscopic third ventriculostomy in children less than 2 years of age?

50%.[262]

531. What is the rate of tumor recurrence in children with cerebellar pilocytic astrocytomas after radiologically confirmed complete tumor resection?

Less than 10%.[263]

532. Which location of benign childhood pilocytic astrocytoma has the highest incidence of leptomeningeal spread?

The optic-hypothalamic pathway.[264]

533. How does a cerebellar pilocytic astrocytoma appear on a nonenhanced CT scan?

It appears as a hypodense mass lesion in almost three-fourths of the cases and is isodense to the white matter in the rest. This is a helpful differentiating feature from medulloblastomas that are hyperdense on a nonenhanced CT scan.[265]

534. What is the survival rate of children with diffuse brainstem gliomas?

The median survival rate of children with diffuse brainstem gliomas is between 11 and 12 months.[266]

535. What are the classic triad on neurologic examination at presentation in children with brainstem gliomas?[266]

- Ataxia.
- Long tract signs.
- CN palsies.

536. What are the features of Aicardi syndrome?[267]

- Agenesis of corpus callosum.
- Infantile spasms.
- Mental retardation.
- Chorioretinopathy.

537. What is the incidence of hydrocephalus in patients with myelomeningocele?

Up to 85% of patients with myelomeningocele develop hydrocephalus.[268]

538. What is the incidence of calcification in pediatric craniopharyngiomas on a CT scan?

90%.[269]

539. Which pediatric brain tumor typically exhibits high serum and CSF levels of placental alkaline phosphatase?

Germinoma.[270]

540. What is the Mt. Fuji sign?

A characteristic finding of two frontal poles surrounded by air on a CT scan indicative of pneumocephalus.[271]

541. Describe some features of Apert's syndrome.

- Autosomal dominant.
- Involvement of coronal suture.
- Syndactyly.
- Cleft palate.
- Associated gastrointestinal, cardiovascular, and genitourinary abnormalities.
- Frontal encephalocele.

Pain and Functional

542. What are the technique and location for an occipital nerve block?

Greater occipital nerve block is both diagnostic and therapeutic. A 23-gauge needle is inserted 3.5 cm inferolaterally to the occipital protuberance, and the nerve is infiltrated with a local anesthetic agent (1–2% lidocaine hydrochloride) or, occasionally, with a corticosteroid (e.g., triamcinolone acetonide).[272] If an occipital nerve block does not relieve the pain, the differential diagnosis should be expanded to cervicogenic headache.

543. What are the typical causes of occipital neuralgia?

Occipital neuralgia attacks are similar to trigeminal and glossopharyngeal neuralgias, except the pain of occipital neuralgia involves the occipital and periauricular areas. Similar to other neuropathic pain syndromes, occipital neuralgia can be provoked by palpating a trigger point. Trauma of the C2 root during exercise or through injury with or without arthritic changes to the atlantoaxial joint is the main cause of occipital neuralgia. Chiari malformation, cervical cord tumors, ligamentous hypertrophy, and neck spasms may also be involved.[273]

544. What disorders may present with occult occipital neuralgia where the second or third cervical dorsal roots are tethered or stretched?

Chiari malformation, cerebellar tumor, spinal tumor, arachnoiditis, bony abnormalities in the atlantoaxial region, vertebral artery ectasia.[273]

545. What diagnosis must be kept in mind when a young woman presents with bilateral trigeminal neuralgia?

MS.[274]

546. What is the procedure of choice for deafferentation pain from nerve root avulsion?

Dorsal root entry zone lesioning.[275]

547. What is meant by the term allodynia?

Pain caused by normally nonnoxious stimuli.

548. What percentage of MS patients have trigeminal neuralgia?

About 2%.[274]

549. What is most often the offending vessel in trigeminal neuralgia?

The superior cerebellar artery. Other nonvascular causes are a posterior fossa tumor and an MS plaque.[274]

550. What are the appropriate landmarks for proper positioning of an electrode at the foramen ovale?

Under methohexital anesthesia, insert the electrode needle 3 cm lateral to the orbital commissure. Using a gloved finger inside the mouth to palpate the buccal mucosa, aim toward a plane intersecting a point 3 cm anterior to the external acoustic meatus and the medial aspect of the pupil.[276]

551. What is the most common neurologic complication seen with electrode implantation in the periaqueductal-periventricular gray region?

Diplopia.

552. What areas are targeted in DBS to help with essential tremor and parkinsonian tremor?

DBS of the VIM thalamic nucleus (Hassler's classification) helps to improve essential tremor. DBS of the subthalamic nucleus helps with parkinsonian tremor.[277]

553. What are the clinical coordinates most frequently used to locate the VIM?

In relation to the AC–PC (anterior commissure–posterior commissure) line: (1) 3 to 7 mm anterior to the PC, (2) 11 to 12 mm lateral to the wall of the third ventricle, and (3) at the level of the intercommissural plane.[277]

554. What is considered the best target for dystonia?

Globus pallidus internus.[278]

555. What are some uses for Botox (BTX-A) in neurosurgery?

Hemifacial spasm, strabismus, blepharospasm, hyperhidrosis, and occipital neuralgia. Spasticity is treated also (off-label).

556. What is the most reliable electrodiagnostic measurement to quantitate spasticity?

The H-reflex.

557. What are the only involuntary movement disorders that persist during sleep?

Hemifacial spasm and palatal myoclonus.[279]

558. What is the main difference between facial myokymia and hemifacial spasm?

Facial myokymia is a continuous facial spasm and may be a manifestation of an intrinsic brainstem glioma or MS. Hemifacial spasm is intermittent and unilateral, and starts in the orbicularis oculi and slowly progresses down the entire side of the face.[280]

559. How can a posterior fossa AVF result in hemifacial spasm?

Compression of the facial nerve occurs through arterialized leptomeningeal veins. Microsurgical obliteration by ligation of the draining vein at the site of the fistula can cure the hemifacial spasm in most cases.[280]

Cases

■ Case 1

A 5-year-old boy presents with the tumor shown in **Fig. 5.18**. What is the most likely diagnosis? What radiologic factors can potentially determine the behavior of such a tumor?

■ Case 1 Answer

The most likely diagnosis is pilocytic astrocytoma. Favorable factors suggestive of a lower-grade tumor include the cervicomedullary location and the nondiffuse well-circumscribed cystic appearance with a mural nodule. Most of these tumors bulge into the fourth ventricle and some may have a dorsal exophytic component.[281]

■ Case 2

A 28-year-old pregnant woman is referred to you at 25 weeks of gestation due to an abnormal finding in the antenatal ultrasound (**Fig. 5.19**). Describe the MRI finding. What are important features to be examined on fetal imaging in a case of fetal hydrocephalus and how do they impact prognosis? What is the perspective classification of congenital hydrocephalus?

■ Case 2 Answer

The in utero fetal sagittal MRI shows ventricular dilatation with vermian agenesis. Important features to examine on imaging include the cortical mantle thickness (at the coronal suture). There is a reported worse prognosis if it measures less than 10 mm. In addition, the lateral ventricle atrial width, if greater than or equal to 15 mm, is suggestive of hydrocephalus. Neonatal uncomplicated hydrocephalus with a frontal mantle of less than 2 cm typically results in severe developmental delay. Posthemorrhagic hydrocephalus has a worse prognosis than congenital hydrocephalus.

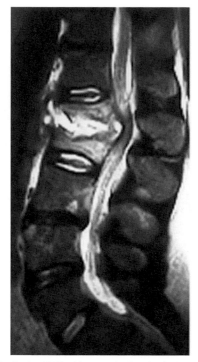

Fig. 5.18 Sagittal MRI with contrast showing lesion in the brainstem of a 5-year-old boy with a brain tumor.

The perspective classification of congenital hydrocephalus classifies hydrocephalus in three clinicopathologic types:

- Primary (31%): communicating hydrocephalus, aqueductal atresia, foramen atresia.
- Dysgenetic (56%): hydrocephalus with spina bifida, bifid cranium, Dandy-Walker cyst, holoprosencephaly.
- Secondary (13%): due to brain tumor, hemorrhage, infection, or trauma.[282,283]

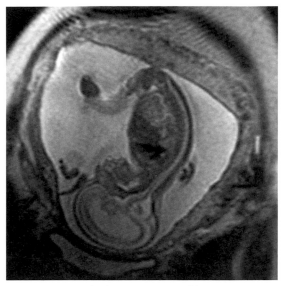

Fig. 5.19 In utero fetal MRI in a 28-year-old pregnant woman.

■ Case 3

A 50-year-old woman presents with the worse headache of her life. She is currently lethargic and difficult to arouse and has blurred vision. A CT scan and angiogram are obtained and shown in **Figs. 5.20** and **5.21**. What are the Hunt-Hess and Fisher grades? She undergoes surgical repair and develops severe vasospasm postoperatively. What are some common options to treat this condition in the postoperative setting?

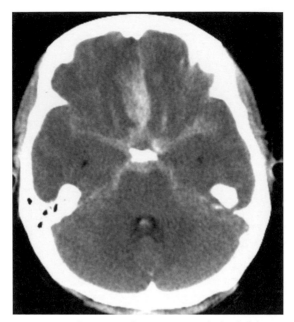

Fig. 5.20 Axial CT scan without contrast at the level of the basal cisterns in a 50-year-old woman with subarachnoid hemorrhage.

■ Case 3 Answer

Hunt-Hess grade 3 and Fisher grade 4. Treatment of vasospasm includes the "triple-H" therapy, which comprises hypervolemia, hypertension, and hemodilution.[284] Alternatively, normovolemia can be used, as hypervolemia can increase the risk of cardiorespiratory complications (CVP is kept around 6 mm Hg). Pressors such as norepinephrine bitartrate can be used to maintain elevated blood pressure and/or to induce hypertension. Angioplasty[285] and/or injection of intra-arterial papaverine or verapamil may be performed in refractory cases. Other medications used intra-arterially include nicardipine.

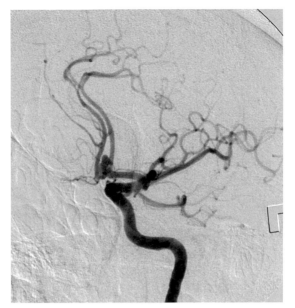

Fig. 5.21 Cerebral angiogram showing anterior communicating artery aneurysm in 50-year-old woman with subarachnoid hemorrhage.

■ **Case 4**

A 41-year-old man presents with retinal hemangioma, pheochromocytoma, renal cell carcinoma, and multiple lesions as seen in **Fig. 5.22**. What is the diagnosis?

■ **Case 4 Answer**

This appears to be VHL syndrome with CNS hemangioblastomas, retinal hemangiomas, renal cell carcinoma, pheochromocytoma, and liver pancreas and liver cysts. These lesions tend to be on the surface of the spinal cord or in a posterior fossa near the sigmoid transverse junction. A complete resection is usually achievable.

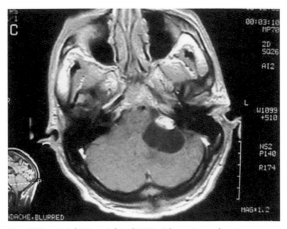

Fig. 5.22 Axial T1-weighted MRI with contrast showing posterior fossa mass in patient with von Hippel–Lindau syndrome.

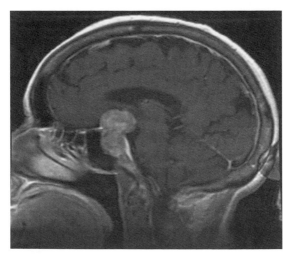

Fig. 5.23 Sagittal MRI showing pituitary mass in patient with elevated prolactin.

■ Case 5

A 30-year-old woman has the tumor noticed in **Fig. 5.23**. The prolactin level is elevated at 100. What is the likely diagnosis?

■ Case 5 Answer

Prolactinomas usually cause prolactin levels over 150. Mildly elevated prolactin is due to stalk effect from compression on the pituitary stalk causing decreased dopamine input that normally inhibits prolactin secretion. Prolactinomas can usually be treated with medications such as cabergoline or bromocriptine that act as a dopamine agonist and decrease tumor size by as much as 75% over 8 weeks. This could be nonsecreting macroadenoma since prolactin level is not markedly elevated.

■ Case 6

A 14-year-old girl presents with these lesions bilaterally (**Fig. 5.24**). What is the diagnosis?

■ Case 6 Answer

These are bilateral vestibular schwannomas. Bilateral lesions are most often seen with an NF2. Other lesions associated with NF2 include meningiomas, astrocytomas, hamartomas, spinal ependymomas (spinal astrocytomas are more common in NF1), and nerve root schwannomas.

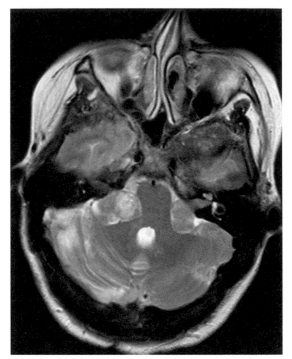

Fig. 5.24 Axial T2-weighted MRI showing posterior fossa lesions in patient with bilateral vestibular schwannomas.

■ Case 7

What is the lesion seen in **Fig. 5.25**?

■ Case 7 Answer

This is a colloid cyst. It frequently will cause headaches and possibly hydrocephalus. Management is typically via an open transcallosal resection or endoscopic removal (other options include shunt placement or stereotactic aspiration). The key in surgery is to avoid damaging the internal cerebral veins or fornix, which can cause memory problems.

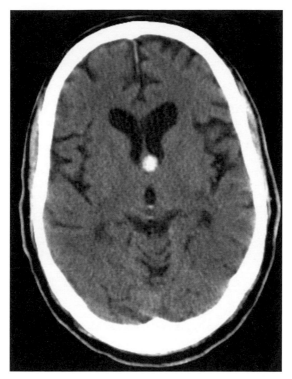

Fig. 5.25 CT scan at the level of the foramen of Monro in patient with colloid cyst.

■ References

1. Jacobson DM, Warner JJ, Choucair AK, Ptacek LJ. Trochlear nerve palsy following minor head trauma. A sign of structural disorder. J Clin Neuroophthalmol 1988;8(4):263–268
2. Jacobs L, Kaba S, Pullicino P. The lesion causing continuous facial myokymia in multiple sclerosis. Arch Neurol 1994;51(11):1115–1119
3. Papapetropoulos S, Gallo BV, Guevara A, et al. Objective tremor registration during DBS surgery for essential tremor. Clin Neurol Neurosurg 2009;111(4):376–379

4. Pahwa R, Lyons KE, Wilkinson SB, et al. Long-term evaluation of deep brain stimulation of the thalamus. J Neurosurg 2006;104(4):506–512

5. Spertell RB, Ransom BR. Dysarthria—clumsy hand syndrome produced by capsular infarct. Ann Neurol 1979;6(3):263–265

6. Leavitt JA, Wayman LL, Hodge DO, Brubaker RF. Pupillary response to four concentrations of pilocarpine in normal subjects: application to testing for Adie tonic pupil. Am J Ophthalmol 2002;133(3):333–336

7. Tsementzis SA. Differential Diagnosis in Neurology and Neurosurgery. Stuttgart: Georg Thieme Verlag; 2000

8. Bartalena L, Tanda ML. Clinical practice. Graves' ophthalmopathy. N Engl J Med 2009;360(10):994–1001

9. Wall M, Wray SH. The one-and-a-half syndrome—a unilateral disorder of the pontine tegmentum: a study of 20 cases and review of the literature. Neurology 1983;33(8):971–980

10. Ropper AH, Brown RH. Disorders of ocular movement and pupillary function. In: Adams and Victor's Principles of Neurology. 8th ed. New York, NY: McGraw-Hill; 2005:234–235

11. Cook M. Differential diagnosis of epilepsy. In: Perucca E, Fish D, Dodson E, Shorvon S, eds. The Treatment of Epilepsy. Oxford: Blackwell Science; 2004:64–73

12. Rohkamm R. Epilepsy: seizure types. In: Color Atlas of Neurology. Stuttgart: Georg Thieme Verlag; 2004:192–196

13. Liu WW, Chen A. Diagnosing myasthenia gravis with an ice pack. N Engl J Med 2016;375(19):e39

14. Recker D, Amann J, Lang GK. Ocular motility and strabismus. In: Lang GK, ed. Ophthalmology: A Short Textbook. Stuttgart: Georg Thieme Verlag; 2000:459–496

15. Fauci AS, Braunwald E, Kasper DL, et al. Hypertension. In: Harrison's Manual of Medicine. 17th ed. New York, NY: McGraw-Hill; 2009:693–698

16. Rohkamm R. Disturbances of memory. In: Color Atlas of Neurology. Stuttgart: Georg Thieme Verlag; 2004:134–135

17. Hellige JB. Hemispheric asymmetry. Annu Rev Psychol 1990;41:55–80

18. Ropper AH, Brown RH. Disturbances of cerebrospinal fluid and its circulation. In: Adams and Victor's Principles of Neurology. 8th ed. New York, NY: McGraw-Hill; 2005:529–545

19. Parent A. Carpenter's Human Neuroanatomy. 9th ed. Baltimore, MD: Williams & Wilkins; 1996

20. Haines DE. Synopsis of functional components, tracts, pathways, and systems: pupillary pathways. In: Neuroanatomy—Atlas of Structures, Sections, Systems. 6th ed. Philadelphia, PA: Lippincott Williams & Wilkins; 2003:220–225

21. Ropper AH, Brown RH. Adams and Victor's Principles of Neurology. 8th ed. New York, NY: McGraw-Hill; 2005:973, 1033, 1084

22. Sajjadi H, Paparella MM. Meniere's disease. Lancet 2008;372(9636):406–414

23. Ropper AH, Brown RH. Myasthenia gravis and related disorders of the neuromuscular junction. In: Adams and Victor's Principles of Neurology. 8th ed. New York, NY: McGraw-Hill; 2005:1250–1264

24. Rohkamm R. Vertigo. In: Color Atlas of Neurology. Stuttgart: Georg Thieme Verlag; 2004:58

25. Ropper AH, Brown RH. Cerebrovascular diseases. Lateral medullary syndrome. In: Adams and Victor's Principles of Neurology. 8th ed. New York, NY: McGraw-Hill; 2005:678–670

26. Gareis O, Lang GK. Pupil. In: Lang GK, ed. Ophthalmology: A Short Textbook. Stuttgart: Georg Thieme Verlag; 2000:219–232

27. Wagner P, Lang GK. The eyelids. In: Lang GK, ed. Ophthalmology: A Short Textbook. Stuttgart: Georg Thieme Verlag; 2000:17–48

28. Ropper AH, Brown RH. Cerebrovascular diseases. Familial subcortical infarction. In: Adams and Victor's Principles of Neurology. 8th ed. New York, NY: McGraw-Hill; 2005:707–708

29. Rohkamm R. Stroke: ischemia. In: Color Atlas of Neurology. Stuttgart: Georg Thieme Verlag; 2004:166–181

30. Feneis H, Dauber W. Sense organs: retinal blood vessels. In: Pocket Atlas of Human Anatomy. 4th ed. Stuttgart: Georg Thieme Verlag; 2000:360

31. Ropper AH, Brown RH. Multiple sclerosis and allied demyelinative diseases. In: Adams and Victor's Principles of Neurology. 8th ed. New York, NY: McGraw-Hill; 2005:771–796

32. Ropper AH, Brown RH. Neurovascular syndromes. The carotid artery. In: Adams and Victor's Principles of Neurology. 8th ed. New York, NY: McGraw-Hill; 2005:667–671

33. Murie JA, Sheldon CD, Quin RO. Carotid artery bruit: association with internal carotid stenosis and intraluminal turbulence. Br J Surg 1984;71(1):50–52

34. Brunton L, Blumenthal D, Buxton I, Parker K. Pharmacotherapy of the epilepsies. In: The Goodman & Gilman Manual of Pharmacology and Therapeutics. New York, NY: McGraw-Hill; 2008:319–336

35. Alvestad S, Lydersen S, Brodtkorb E. Rash from antiepileptic drugs: influence by gender, age, and learning disability. Epilepsia 2007;48(7):1360–1365

36. Ropper AH, Brown RH. Deafness, dizziness, and disorders of equilibrium. In: Adams and Victor's Principles of Neurology. 8th ed. New York, NY: McGraw-Hill; 2005:261–262

37. Tsementzis SA. Diplopia. In: Differential Diagnosis in Neurology and Neurosurgery. Stuttgart: Georg Thieme Verlag; 2000:91–94

38. Brackmann DE. Excision of acoustic neuromas by the middle fossa approach. In: Rengachary S, Wilkins R, eds. Neurosurgical

268 Neurosurgery Rounds ▬▬▬▬▬▬▬▬▬▬▬▬

Operative Atlas. Vol 1. Chicago, IL: American Association of Neurological Surgeons; 1991:240–248

39. Greenberg MS, ed. Handbook of Neurosurgery. 6th ed. New York, NY: Thieme Medical Publishers; 2006

40. Alp H, Yavuz H, Alp E. Melkersson-Rosenthal syndrome: a case report on a child [in Turkish]. Kulak Burun Bogaz Ihtis Derg 2009;19(2):99–102

41. Tamme T, Leibur E, Kulla A. Sarcoidosis (Heerfordt syndrome): a case report. Stomatologija 2007;9(2):61–64

42. Patten JP. Neurological Differential Diagnosis. 2nd ed. New York, NY: Springer-Verlag; 1996

43. Panayiotopoulos CP, Michael M, Sanders S, Valeta T, Koutroumanidis M. Benign childhood focal epilepsies: assessment of established and newly recognized syndromes. Brain 2008;131(pt 9):2264–2286

44. De Monte F, Anand VK, Al-Mefty O. Surgery for tumors affecting the cavernous sinus. In: Rengachary SS, Wilkins, RH, eds. Neurosurgical Operative Atlas. Vol 4. Chicago, IL: American Association of Neurological Surgeons; 1991:199–207

45. Badie B. Neuro-oncology. New York, NY: Thieme Medical Publishers; 2007

46. Rhoton AL Jr. The lateral and third ventricles. Neurosurgery 2002;51(4, suppl):S207–S271

47. Sekhar L, Fessler R. Atlas of Neurosurgical Techniques: Brain. New York, NY: Thieme Medical Publishers; 2006

48. Tatter SB, Wilson CB. Harsh GRIV Neuroepithelial tumors of the adult brain. In: Youmans JR, ed. Neurological Surgery. 4th ed. Philadelphia, PA: WB Saunders; 1996:2612–2684

49. Mesiwala AH, Newell DW, Britz GW. Surgical management of moyamoya disease in adults. In: Schmidek HH, Roberts DW, eds. Schmidek & Sweet Operative Neurosurgical Techniques. Indications, Methods and Results. Vol 1. 5th ed. Philadelphia, PA: Saunders Elsevier; 2006:1075–1083

50. Rhoton AL Jr. Anatomy and surgical approaches of the temporal bone and adjacent areas. Neurosurgery 2007;61 (4, suppl):1–250

51. Hendelman WJ. Basal ganglia. In: Functional Neuroanatomy. 2nd ed. Boca Raton, FL: Taylor & Francis Group; 2006:76–77

52. Awasthi D, Kruse JJ. Excision of colloid cyst via the transcallosal approach. In: Rengachary S, Wilkins R, eds. Neurosurgical Operative Atlas. Chicago, IL: American Association of Neurological Surgeons; 1991:227–233

53. Krisht AF, Kadri PA. Surgical clipping of complex basilar apex aneurysms: a strategy for successful outcome using the pretemporal transzygomatic transcavernous approach. Neurosurgery 2005;56(2, suppl):261–273, discussion 261–273

54. Kawase T, Toya S, Shiobara R, Mine T. Transpetrosal approach for aneurysms of the lower basilar artery. J Neurosurg 1985;63(6):857–861

55. Ryken TC, Loftus CM. Surgical management of anterior communicating artery aneurysm. In: Rengachary S, Wilkins R, eds. Neurosurgical Operative Atlas. Vol 2. Chicago, IL: American Association of Neurological Surgeons; 1991:273–281

56. Camarata PJ, Haines SJ. Ventriculoatrial shunting. In: Rengachary S, Wilkins R, eds. Neurosurgical Operative Atlas. Vol 1. Chicago, IL: American Association of Neurological Surgeons; 1991:247–255

57. Piatt JH, Burchiel KJ. Technique of ventriculostomy. In: Rengachary S, Wilkins R, eds. Neurosurgical Operative Atlas. Vol 1. Chicago, IL: American Association of Neurological Surgeons; 1991:171–175

58. Rhoton AL Jr. The sellar region. Neurosurgery 2002;51(4, suppl):S335–S374

59. Greenberg MS. Handbook of Neurosurgery. 6th ed. New York, NY: Thieme Medical Publishers; 2006:171–179

60. Rhoton AL Jr. The supratentorial arteries. Neurosurgery 2002;51(4, suppl):S53–S120

61. Yasuda A, Campero A, Martins C, Rhoton AL Jr, de Oliveira E, Ribas GC. Microsurgical anatomy and approaches to the cavernous sinus. Neurosurgery 2008;62(6, suppl 3):1240–1263

62. Brunton L, Blumenthal D, Buxton I. Goodman and Gilman's Manual of Pharmacology and Therapeutics. New York, NY: McGraw-Hill Professional; 2007

63. Hopf NJ, Grunert P, Fries G, Resch KD, Perneczky A. Endoscopic third ventriculostomy: outcome analysis of 100 consecutive procedures. Neurosurgery 1999;44(4):795–804, discussion 804–806

64. Gruen P. Management of head injury. In: Demetriades D, Asensio JA, eds. Trauma Management. Austin, TX: Landes Biosciences; 2000:84–93

65. Wise SK, Schlosser RJ. Evaluation of spontaneous nasal cerebrospinal fluid leaks. Curr Opin Otolaryngol Head Neck Surg 2007;15(1):28–34

66. Smith DH, Meaney DF, Shull WH. Diffuse axonal injury in head trauma. J Head Trauma Rehabil 2003;18(4):307–316

67. Yamashita DR, Urata MM. Maxillofacial trauma. In: Demetriades D, Asensio JA, eds. Trauma Management. Austin, TX: Landes Biosciences; 2000:94–113

68. Pauwels LW, Akesson EJ, Stewart PA, Spacey SD. Cranial Nerves in Health and Disease. 2nd ed. Ontario: BC Decker Inc; 2002

69. Pak J, Pedley TA. Status epilepticus. In: Loftus CM, ed. Neurosurgical Emergencies. Vol I. Chicago, IL: American Association of Neurological Surgeons; 1994:217–222

70. Juul N, Morris GF, Marshall SB, Marshall LF; Executive Committee of the International Selfotel Trial. Intracranial hypertension and cerebral perfusion pressure: influence on neurological deterioration and outcome in severe head injury. J Neurosurg 2000;92(1):1–6

71. Greenberg M. Intracranial pressure. In: Handbook of Neurosurgery. 6th ed. Stuttgart: Georg Thieme Verlag; 2006:647–663

72. Quality Standards Subcommittee of the American Academy of Neurology. Practice parameters for determining brain death in adults (summary statement). Neurology 1995;45(5):1012–1014

73. Infection in Neurosurgery Working Party of the British Society for Antimicrobial Chemotherapy. Antimicrobial prophylaxis in neurosurgery and after head injury. Lancet 1994;344(8936):1547–1551

74. Greenberg M. Head trauma. In: Handbook of Neurosurgery. 6th ed. New York, NY: Thieme Medical Publishers; 2006:632–697

75. Ebisu T, Naruse S, Horikawa Y, Tanaka C, Higuchi T. Nonacute subdural hematoma: fundamental interpretation of MR images based on biochemical and in vitro MR analysis. Radiology 1989;171(2):449–453

76. Schutzman SA, Barnes PD, Mantello M, Scott RM. Epidural hematomas in children. Ann Emerg Med 1993;22(3):535–541

77. Stallmeyer MJ, Morales RE, Flanders AE. Imaging of traumatic neurovascular injury. Radiol Clin North Am 2006;44(1):13–39, vii

78. Mendelow AD, Teasdale G, Jennett B, Bryden J, Hessett C, Murray G. Risks of intracranial haematoma in head injured adults. Br Med J (Clin Res Ed) 1983;287(6400):1173–1176

79. Greenberg M. Myxedema coma. In: Handbook of Neurosurgery. 6th ed. Stuttgart: Georg Thieme Verlag; 2006:454–455

80. Sawin PD. Spontaneous subarachnoid hemorrhage in pregnancy and the puerperium. In: Loftus CM, ed. Neurosurgical Aspects of Pregnancy. Chicago, IL: American Association of Neurological Surgeons; 1996:85–100

81. Greenberg M. Addisonian crisis. In: Handbook of Neurosurgery. 6th ed. Stuttgart: Georg Thieme Verlag; 2006:11

82. Kaye AH. Craniopharyngioma. In: Essential Neurosurgery. Malden, MA: Blackwell Publishing; 2005:210–212

83. Greenberg M. Cushing's disease. In: Handbook of Neurosurgery. 6th ed. Stuttgart: Georg Thieme Verlag; 2006:441–442

84. Osborn AG, Salzman KL, Barkovich AJ. Neoplasms and tumorlike lesions. In: Diagnostic Imaging: Brain. Salt Lake City, UT: Amirsys; 2004

85. Nakamura Y, Becker LE, Marks A. S-100 protein in tumors of cartilage and bone. An immunohistochemical study. Cancer 1983;52(10):1820–1824

86. Almefty K, Pravdenkova S, Colli BO, Al-Mefty O, Gokden M. Chordoma and chondrosarcoma: similar, but quite different, skull base tumors. Cancer 2007;110(11):2457–2467

87. Slotman BJ, Mauer ME, Bottomley A, et al. Prophylactic cranial irradiation in extensive disease small-cell lung cancer: short-term health-related quality of life and patient reported symptoms: results of an international Phase III randomized controlled trial by the EORTC Radiation Oncology and Lung Cancer Groups. J Clin Oncol 2009;27(1):78–84

88. Greenlee JD, Teo C, Ghahreman A, Kwok B. Purely endoscopic resection of colloid cysts. Neurosurgery 2008;62(3, suppl 1): 51–55, discussion 55–56

89. Alnaghmoosh N, Alkhani A. Colloid cysts in children, a clinical and radiological study. Childs Nerv Syst 2006;22(5):514–516

90. Bouguila J, Yacoub K, Bouguila H, Neji NB, Sahtout S, Besbes G. Intraorbital cavernous hemangioma [in French]. Rev Stomatol Chir Maxillofac 2008;109(5):312–315

91. Chang KC, Chang Y, Jones D, Su IJ. Aberrant expression of cyclin A correlates with morphogenesis of Reed-Sternberg cells in Hodgkin lymphoma. Am J Clin Pathol 2009;132(1):50–59

92. Haberland C. Common neurohistologic stains. In: Clinical Neuropathology: Text and Color Atlas. New York, NY: Demos Medical Publishing; 2007:2–7

93. Greenberg M. Magnetic resonance spectroscopy. In: Greenberg M, ed. Handbook of Neurosurgery. 6th ed. New York, NY: Thieme Medical Publishers; 2006:137–138

94. Haberland C. Major tumor-related immunohistologic stains. In: Clinical Neuropathology: Text and Color Atlas. New York, NY: Demos Medical Publishing; 2007:214–216

95. Jabbour SK, Zhang Z, Arnold D, Wharam MD. Risk of second tumor in intracranial germinoma patients treated with radiation therapy: the Johns Hopkins experience. J Neurooncol 2009;91(2):227–232

96. Osborn A, Blaser S, Salzman K, et al. Primary CNS lymphoma. In: Diagnostic Imaging: Brain. Salt Lake City, UT: Amirsys; 2004:124–126

97. Cairncross JG, Ueki K, Zlatescu MC, et al. Specific genetic predictors of chemotherapeutic response and survival in patients with anaplastic oligodendrogliomas. J Natl Cancer Inst 1998;90(19):1473–1479

98. Antunes JL. Management of tumors of the anterior third and lateral ventricles. In: Sindou M, ed. Practical Handbook of Neurosurgery from Leading Neurosurgeons. New York, NY: Springer; 2009:256–270

99. Gudinaviciene I, Pranys D, Juozaityte E. Impact of morphology and biology on the prognosis of patients with gliomas. Medicina (Kaunas) 2004;40(2):112–120

100. Greenberg M. Pilocytic astrocytomas. In: Handbook of Neurosurgery. 6th ed. Stuttgart: Georg Thieme Verlag; 2006:417–422

101. Sutherland GR, Sima AAF. Incidence and clinicopathological features of meningioma. In: Schmidek HH, ed. Meningiomas and Their Surgical Management. Philadelphia, PA: WB Saunders; 1991:10–21

102. Chason JL. Origin and classification of meningiomas. In: Schmidek HH, ed. Meningiomas and Their Surgical Management. Philadelphia, PA: WB Saunders; 1991:3–9

103. Scott EW, Rhoton AL Jr. Foramen magnum meningiomas. In: Al-Mefty O, ed. Meningiomas. New York, NY: Raven Press; 1991:543–568

104. Chaparro MJ, Young RF, Smith M, Shen V, Choi BH. Multiple spinal meningiomas: a case of 47 distinct lesions in the absence of neurofibromatosis or identified chromosomal abnormality. Neurosurgery 1993;32(2):298–301, discussion 301–302

105. Al-Mefty O, ed. Meningiomas. New York, NY: Raven Press; 1991

106. Acebes X, Arruga J, Acebes JJ, Majos C, Muñoz S, Valero IA. Intracranial meningiomatosis causing Foster Kennedy syndrome by unilateral optic nerve compression and blockage of the superior sagittal sinus. J Neuroophthalmol 2009;29(2):140–142

107. Marsh H. Low grade gliomas in adults. In: Moore AJ, Newell DW, eds. Neurosurgery: Principles and Practice. New York, NY: Springer-Verlag; 2005:155–166

108. Leeman SA. From sound to silence: a case study of neurofibromatosis type II. Am J Electroneurodiagn Technol 2005;45(3):186–191

109. Greenberg M. Neurosarcoidosis. In: Handbook of Neurosurgery. 6th ed. Stuttgart: Georg Thieme Verlag; 2006:56–57

110. Greenberg M. Osteoma. In: Handbook of Neurosurgery. 6th ed. Stuttgart: Georg Thieme Verlag; 2006:481

111. Wu R, López-Correa C, Rutkowski JL, Baumbach LL, Glover TW, Legius E. Germline mutations in NF1 patients with malignancies. Genes Chromosomes Cancer 1999;26(4):376–380

112. Alwan S, Tredwell SJ, Friedman JM. Is osseous dysplasia a primary feature of neurofibromatosis 1 (NF1)? Clin Genet 2005;67(5):378–390

113. Hoang-Xuan K, Merel P, Vega F, et al. Analysis of the NF2 tumor-suppressor gene and of chromosome 22 deletions in gliomas. Int J Cancer 1995;60(4):478–481

114. Ellison D, Love S, Chimell L, Harding B, Lowe JS, Vinters HV. Neuropathology—A Reference Text to CNS Pathology. St. Louis, MO: Mosby; 2004

115. Doorenbosch X, Santoreneos S, Molloy CJ, David DJ, Anderson PJ. Modified transoral approach for resection of skull

base chordomas in children. Childs Nerv Syst 2009;25(11): 1481–1483

116. Bruneau M, Polivka M, Cornelius JF, George B. Progression of an osteoid osteoma to an osteoblastoma. Case report. J Neurosurg Spine 2005;3(3):238–241

117. Raizer JJ, Hwu WJ, Panageas KS, et al. Brain and leptomeningeal metastases from cutaneous melanoma: survival outcomes based on clinical features. Neuro Oncol 2008;10(2):199–207

118. Waldau B, McLendon RE, Fuchs HE, George TM, Grant GA. Few isolated neurons in hypothalamic hamartomas may cause gelastic seizures. Pediatr Neurosurg 2009;45(3):225–229

119. Greenberg M. Glomus jugulare. In: Greenberg M, ed. Handbook of Neurosurgery. 6th ed. Stuttgart: Georg Thieme Verlag; 2006:468–470

120. Bratt GW, Bess FH, Miller GW, Glasscock ME III. Glomus tumor of the middle ear: origin, symptomatology, and treatment. J Speech Hear Disord 1979;44(1):121–134

121. Ravon R, Pelissou I, Bessede JP, Lasjaunias P, Moreau JJ, Sauvage JP. Excision of a glomus jugulare tumor after embolization [in French]. Neurochirurgie 1983;29(6):429–433

122. Coles MC. Glomus jugulare tumor presentation and management: a case study. J Neurosci Nurs 2004;36(4):221–223, 235

123. Chazal J. Management of hydrocephalus in childhood. In: Sindou M, ed. Practical Handbook of Neurosurgery from Leading Neurosurgeons. New York, NY: Springer-Verlag/Wien; 2009:525–540

124. Haberland C. Capillary hemangioblastomas. In: Clinical Neuropathology: Text and Color Atlas. New York, NY: Demos Medical Publishing; 2007:244–245

125. Kaloshi G, Guillevin R, Martin-Duverneuil N, et al. Gray matter involvement predicts chemosensitivity and prognosis in gliomatosis cerebri. Neurology 2009;73(6):445–449

126. Adamson C, Kanu OO, Mehta AI, et al. Glioblastoma multiforme: a review of where we have been and where we are going. Expert Opin Investig Drugs 2009;18(8):1061–1083

127. Greenberg M. CNS lymphoma. In: Handbook of Neurosurgery. 6th ed. Stuttgart: Georg Thieme Verlag; 2006:461–464

128. Greenberg M. Extramedullary hematopoiesis. In: Handbook of Neurosurgery. 6th ed. Stuttgart: Georg Thieme Verlag; 2006:27

129. Osborn AG. Diagnostic Neuroradiology. St. Louis, MO: Mosby; 1994:465

130. Matsukawa Y, Hattori R, Komatsu T, Yoshino Y, Ono Y, Gotoh M. Two cases of bilateral renal cell carcinoma in patients with Von Hipple-Lindau disease [in Japanese]. Hinyokika Kiyo 2007;53(1):61–65

131. Haapaniemi J, Laurikainen E, Johansson R, Miettinen S, Varpula M. Cochleovestibular symptoms related to the site of vestibular schwannoma. Acta Otolaryngol Suppl 2000;543:14–16

132. Prestor B. Dysplastic gangliocytoma of the cerebellum (Lhermitte-Duclos disease). J Clin Neurosci 2006;13(8):877–881

133. Kleihues P, Cavanee WK. Pathology and Genetics of Tumors of the Nervous System. Lyon: World Health Organization; 2000

134. Levine PH. Immunologic markers for Epstein-Barr virus in the control of nasopharyngeal carcinoma and Burkitt lymphoma. Cancer Detect Prev Suppl 1987;1:217–223

135. Sandyk R. The Eaton-Lambert syndrome. S Afr Med J 1983;63(9):323–325

136. Tseng J, Michel MA, Loehrl TA. Peripheral cysts: a distinguishing feature of esthesioneuroblastoma with intracranial extension. Ear Nose Throat J 2009;88(6):E14

137. Bragg TM, Scianna J, Kassam A, et al. Clinicopathological review: esthesioneuroblastoma. Neurosurgery 2009;64(4):764–770, discussion 770

138. Unal E, Koksal Y, Cimen O, Paksoy Y, Tavli L. Malignant glioblastomatous transformation of a low-grade glioma in a child. Childs Nerv Syst 2008;24(12):1385–1389

139. Renn WH, Rhoton AL Jr. Microsurgical anatomy of the sellar region. J Neurosurg 1975;43(3):288–298

140. Nemergut EC, Dumont AS, Barry UT, Laws ER. Perioperative management of patients undergoing transsphenoidal pituitary surgery. Anesth Analg 2005;101(4):1170–1181

141. Kars M, Roelfsema F, Romijn JA, Pereira AM. Malignant prolactinoma: case report and review of the literature. Eur J Endocrinol 2006;155(4):523–534

142. Simard MF. Pituitary tumor endocrinopathies and their endocrine evaluation. Neurosurg Clin N Am 2003;14(1):41–54

143. Greenberg M. Steroids. In: Handbook of Neurosurgery. 6th ed. Stuttgart: Georg Thieme Verlag; 2006:7–12

144. Greenberg M. Electrolyte abnormalities. In: Handbook of Neurosurgery. 6th ed. Stuttgart: Georg Thieme Verlag; 2006:13–25

145. Skinner DC. Rethinking the stalk effect: a new hypothesis explaining suprasellar tumor-induced hyperprolactinemia. Med Hypotheses 2009;72(3):309–310

146. Munir A, Newell-Price J. Nelson's syndrome. Arq Bras Endocrinol Metabol 2007;51(8):1392–1396

147. Gatta B, Chabre O, Cortet C, et al. Reevaluation of the combined dexamethasone suppression-corticotropin-releasing hormone test for differentiation of mild Cushing's disease from pseudo-Cushing's syndrome. J Clin Endocrinol Metab 2007;92(11):4290–4293

148. Greenberg MS, ed. Handbook of Neurosurgery. 6th ed. Stuttgart: Georg Thieme Verlag; 2006

149. Murad-Kejbou S, Eggenberger E. Pituitary apoplexy: evaluation, management, and prognosis. Curr Opin Ophthalmol 2009;20(6):456–461

150. Dash RJ, Khandekar S, Lata V, Bhansali A. Circulating cortisol & related steroids following ketoconazole challenge in Cushing's disease. Indian J Med Res 1990;92:167–168

151. Furlanetto RW, Underwood LE, Van Wyk JJ, D'Ercole AJ. Estimation of somatomedin-C levels in normals and patients with pituitary disease by radioimmunoassay. J Clin Invest 1977;60(3):648–657

152. Overly C. Bitemporal hemianopia arising from a suprasellar craniopharyngioma. Optometry 2009;80(11):621–629

153. Flickinger JC, Kondziolka D, Niranjan A, Lunsford LD. Dose selection in stereotactic radiosurgery. Prog Neurol Surg 2007;20:28–42

154. Wilson GD. Radiation and the cell cycle, revisited. Cancer Metastasis Rev 2004;23(3–4):209–225

155. Radcliffe J, Bunin GR, Sutton LN, Goldwein JW, Phillips PC. Cognitive deficits in long-term survivors of childhood medulloblastoma and other noncortical tumors: age-dependent effects of whole brain radiation. Int J Dev Neurosci 1994;12(4):327–334

156. Alexiou GA, Tsiouris S, Kyritsis AP, Voulgaris S, Argyropoulou MI, Fotopoulos AD. Glioma recurrence versus radiation necrosis: accuracy of current imaging modalities. J Neurooncol 2009;95(1):1–11

157. Wedderburn CJ, van Beijnum J, Bhattacharya JJ, et al; SIVMS Collaborators. Outcome after interventional or conservative management of unruptured brain arteriovenous malformations: a prospective, population-based cohort study. Lancet Neurol 2008;7(3):223–230

158. Laakso A, Dashti R, Seppänen J, et al. Long-term excess mortality in 623 patients with brain arteriovenous malformations. Neurosurgery 2008;63(2):244–253, discussion 253–255

159. Dion JE, Mathis JM. Cranial arteriovenous malformations. The role of embolization and stereotactic surgery. Neurosurg Clin N Am 1994;5(3):459–474

160. Ropper AH, Brown RH. Protozoal diseases. In: Adams and Victor's Principles of Neurology. 8th ed. New York, NY: McGraw-Hill; 2005:623–624

161. Ropper AH, Brown RH. Viral infections of the nervous system. In: Adams and Victor's Principles of Neurology. 8th ed. New York, NY: McGraw-Hill; 2005:631–660

162. Choux M, Genitori L, Lang D, Lena G. Shunt implantation: reducing the incidence of shunt infection. J Neurosurg 1992;77(6):875–880

163. Doczi TP. Epidermoid and dermoid cysts. In: Sindou M, ed. Practical Handbook of Neurosurgery from Leading Neurosurgeons. New York, NY: Springer-Verlag/Wien; 2009:301–318

164. Ropper AH, Brown RH. Creutzfeldt-Jacob disease. In: Adams and Victor's Principles of Neurology. 8th ed. New York, NY: McGraw Hill; 2006:653–656

165. Expert Panel on Detection, Evaluation, and Treatment of High Blood Cholesterol in Adults. Executive Summary of the Third Report of the National Cholesterol Education Program (NCEP) Expert Panel on Detection, Evaluation, and Treatment of High Blood Cholesterol in Adults (Adult Treatment Panel III). JAMA 2001;285(19):2486–2497

166. Feigin VL, Lawes CM, Bennett DA, Anderson CS. Stroke epidemiology: a review of population-based studies of incidence, prevalence, and case-fatality in the late 20th century. Lancet Neurol 2003;2(1):43–53

167. Zanchetti A, Grassi G, Mancia G. When should antihypertensive drug treatment be initiated and to what levels should systolic blood pressure be lowered? A critical reappraisal. J Hypertens 2009;27(5):923–934

168. Anderson CS. Medical management of acute intracerebral hemorrhage. Curr Opin Crit Care 2009;15(2):93–98

169. Easton JD, Saver JL, Albers GW, et al. American Heart Association; American Stroke Association Stroke Council; Council on Cardiovascular Surgery and Anesthesia; Council on Cardiovascular Radiology and Intervention; Council on Cardiovascular Nursing; Interdisciplinary Council on Peripheral Vascular Disease. Definition and evaluation of transient ischemic attack: a scientific statement for healthcare professionals from the American Heart Association/American Stroke Association Stroke Council; Council on Cardiovascular Surgery and Anesthesia; Council on Cardiovascular Radiology and Intervention; Council on Cardiovascular Nursing; and the Interdisciplinary Council on Peripheral Vascular Disease. The American Academy of Neurology affirms the value of this statement as an educational tool for neurologists. Stroke 2009;40(6):2276–2293

170. Ropper AH, Brown RH. Mechanisms of cranial pain. In: Adams and Victor's Principles of Neurology. 8th ed. New York, NY: McGraw-Hill; 2005:145–147

171. Ciceri EF, Regna-Gladin C, Erbetta A, et al. Iatrogenic intracranial pseudoaneurysms: neuroradiological and therapeutical considerations, including endovascular options. Neurol Sci 2006;27(5):317–322

172. Pelz DM, Viñuela F, Fox AJ, Drake CG. Vertebrobasilar occlusion therapy of giant aneurysms. Significance of angiographic morphology of the posterior communicating arteries. J Neurosurg 1984;60(3):560–565

173. Kim EJ, Halim AX, Dowd CF, et al. The relationship of coexisting extranidal aneurysms to intracranial hemorrhage in patients harboring brain arteriovenous malformations. Neurosurgery 2004;54(6):1349–1357, discussion 1357–1358

174. Fassett DR, Rammos SK, Patel P, Parikh H, Couldwell WT. Intracranial subarachnoid hemorrhage resulting from cervical spine dural arteriovenous fistulas: literature review and case presentation. Neurosurg Focus 2009;26(1):E4

175. Topcuoglu MA, Ogilvy CS, Carter BS, Buonanno FS, Koroshetz WJ, Singhal AB. Subarachnoid hemorrhage without evident cause on initial angiography studies: diagnostic yield of subsequent angiography and other neuroimaging tests. J Neurosurg 2003;98(6):1235–1240

176. Ostergaard JR, Høg E. Incidence of multiple intracranial aneurysms. Influence of arterial hypertension and gender. J Neurosurg 1985;63(1):49–55

177. Berdoz D, Uske A, de Tribolet N. Subarachnoid haemorrhage of unknown cause: clinical, neuroradiological and evolutive aspects. J Clin Neurosci 1998;5(3):274–282

178. Behar S, Tanne D, Abinader E, et al; SPRINT Study Group. Cerebrovascular accident complicating acute myocardial infarction: incidence, clinical significance and short- and long-term mortality rates. Am J Med 1991;91(1):45–50

179. Kannel WB, Wolf PA, Benjamin EJ, Levy D. Prevalence, incidence, prognosis, and predisposing conditions for atrial fibrillation: population-based estimates. Am J Cardiol 1998;82(8A):2N–9N

180. Finsterer J, Stöllberger C. Strategies for primary and secondary stroke prevention in atrial fibrillation. Neth J Med 2008;66(8):327–333

181. Gutierrez IZ, Barone DL, Makula PA, Currier C. The risk of perioperative stroke in patients with asymptomatic carotid bruits undergoing peripheral vascular surgery. Am Surg 1987;53(9):487–489

182. Gutierrez IZ, Makula PA, Gage AA. The asymptomatic carotid bruit. Am Surg 1985;51(7):388–391

183. Rothwell PM, Howard SC, Spence JD; Carotid Endarterectomy Trialists' Collaboration. Relationship between blood pressure and stroke risk in patients with symptomatic carotid occlusive disease. Stroke 2003;34(11):2583–2590

184. van Gijn J, Rinkel GJE. Subarachnoid haemorrhage: diagnosis, causes and management. Brain 2001;124(pt 2):249–278

185. Greenberg MS. Hyponatremia following SAH. In: Handbook of Neurosurgery. 6th ed. Stuttgart: Georg Thieme Verlag; 2006:788–789

186. International Study of Unruptured Intracranial Aneurysms Investigators. Unruptured intracranial aneurysms—risk of rupture and risks of surgical intervention. N Engl J Med 1999;340(9):744

187. Molyneux AJ, Kerr RS, Yu LM, et al; International Subarachnoid Aneurysm Trial (ISAT) Collaborative Group. International

Subarachnoid Aneurysm Trial (ISAT) of neurosurgical clipping versus endovascular coiling in 2143 patients with ruptured intracranial aneurysms: a randomised comparison of effects on survival, dependency, seizures, rebleeding, subgroups, and aneurysm occlusion. Lancet 2005;366(9488):809–817

188. Rhoton AL Jr. Aneurysms. Neurosurgery 2002;51(4, suppl): S121–S158

189. Clinical alert: benefit of carotid endarterectomy for patients with high-grade stenosis of the internal carotid artery. National Institute of Neurological Disorders and Stroke Stroke and Trauma Division. North American Symptomatic Carotid Endarterectomy Trial (NASCET) investigators. Stroke 1991;22(6):816–817

190. Endarterectomy for asymptomatic carotid artery stenosis. Executive Committee for the Asymptomatic Carotid Atherosclerosis Study. JAMA 1995;273(18):1421–1428

191. Greenberg MS. Vasospasm. In: Handbook of Neurosurgery. 6th ed. Stuttgart: Georg Thieme Verlag; 2006:791–799

192. Loh JA, Verbalis JG. Disorders of water and salt metabolism associated with pituitary disease. Endocrinol Metab Clin North Am 2008;37(1):213–234, x

193. Morgan MK, Rochford AM, Tsahtsarlis A, Little N, Faulder KC. Surgical risks associated with the management of grade I and II brain arteriovenous malformations. Neurosurgery 2007;61(1, suppl):417–422, discussion 422–424

194. Hashimoto N, Nozaki K, Takagi Y, Kikuta K, Mikuni N. Surgery of cerebral arteriovenous malformations. Neurosurgery 2007;61(1, suppl):375–387, discussion 387–389

195. Veznedaroglu E, Andrews DW, Benitez RP, et al. Fractionated stereotactic radiotherapy for the treatment of large arteriovenous malformations with or without previous partial embolization. Neurosurgery 2008;62(suppl 2):763–775

196. Maruyama K, Kawahara N, Shin M, et al. The risk of hemorrhage after radiosurgery for cerebral arteriovenous malformations. N Engl J Med 2005;352(2):146–153

197. Al-Shahi Salman R, Berg MJ, Morrison L, Awad IA; Angioma Alliance Scientific Advisory Board. Hemorrhage from cavernous malformations of the brain: definition and reporting standards. Stroke 2008;39(12):3222–3230

198. Rammos SK, Maina R, Lanzino G. Developmental venous anomalies: current concepts and implications for management. Neurosurgery 2009;65(1):20–29, discussion 29–30

199. Jones BV, Ball WS, Tomsick TA, Millard J, Crone KR. Vein of Galen aneurysmal malformation: diagnosis and treatment of 13 children with extended clinical follow-up. AJNR Am J Neuroradiol 2002;23(10):1717–1724

200. Ropper AH, Brown RH. The main clinical syndromes caused by tumors at the base of the skull. In: Adams and Victor's Principles of Neurology. 8th ed. New York, NY: McGraw Hill; 2005:581–582

201. Wiebers DO, Whisnant JP, Huston J III, et al; International Study of Unruptured Intracranial Aneurysms Investigators. Unruptured intracranial aneurysms: natural history, clinical outcome, and risks of surgical and endovascular treatment. Lancet 2003;362(9378):103–110

202. EC/IC Bypass Study group. The International Cooperative Study of Extracranial/Intracranial Arterial Anastomosis (EC/IC Bypass Study): methodology and entry characteristics. The EC/IC Bypass Study group. Stroke 1985;16(3):397–406

203. Rinkel GJ, Djibuti M, Algra A, van Gijn J. Prevalence and risk of rupture of intracranial aneurysms: a systematic review. Stroke 1998;29(1):251–256

204. Hughes RL, Chapman A, Rubinstein D, Stears J, Johnson A, Gabow P. Recurrent intracranial aneurysms (ICA) in autosomal dominant polycystic kidney disease (ADPKD). Stroke 1996;27:178

205. Belz MM, Fick-Brosnahan GM, Hughes RL, et al. Recurrence of intracranial aneurysms in autosomal-dominant polycystic kidney disease. Kidney Int 2003;63(5):1824–1830

206. Ronkainen A, Hernesniemi J, Puranen M, et al. Familial intracranial aneurysms. Lancet 1997;349(9049):380–384

207. Borden JA, Wu JK, Shucart WA. A proposed classification for spinal and cranial dural arteriovenous fistulous malformations and implications for treatment. J Neurosurg 1995;82(2):166–179

208. Klopper HB, Surdell DL, Thorell WE. Type I spinal dural arteriovenous fistulas: historical review and illustrative case. Neurosurg Focus 2009;26(1):E3

209. Dillon WP. Cryptic vascular malformations: controversies in terminology, diagnosis, pathophysiology, and treatment. AJNR Am J Neuroradiol 1997;18(10):1839–1846

210. Washington CW, McCoy KE, Zipfel GJ. Update on the natural history of cavernous malformations and factors predicting aggressive clinical presentation. Neurosurg Focus 2010;29(3):E7

211. Stahl S, Gaetzner S, Voss K, et al. Novel CCM1, CCM2, and CCM3 mutations in patients with cerebral cavernous malformations: in-frame deletion in CCM2 prevents formation of a CCM1/CCM2/CCM3 protein complex. Hum Mutat 2008;29(5):709–717

212. AbuRahma AF, Hopkins ES, Robinson PA, Deel JT, Agarwal S. Prospective randomized trial of carotid endarterectomy with polytetrafluoroethylene versus collagen-impregnated dacron (Hemashield) patching: late follow-up. Ann Surg 2003;237(6):885–892, discussion 892–893

213. AbuRahma AF, Hannay RS. A study of 510 carotid endarterectomies and a review of the recent carotid endarterectomy trials. W V Med J 2001;97(4):197–200

214. Graeb DA, Robertson WD, Lapointe JS, Nugent RA, Harrison PB. Computed tomographic diagnosis of intraventricular hemorrhage. Etiology and prognosis. Radiology 1982;143(1):91–96

215. Andrews CO, Engelhard HH. Fibrinolytic therapy in intraventricular hemorrhage. Ann Pharmacother 2001;35(11):1435–1448

216. Engelhard HH, Andrews CO, Slavin KV, Charbel FT. Current management of intraventricular hemorrhage. Surg Neurol 2003;60(1):15–21, discussion 21–22

217. Kazan S, Güra A, Uçar T, Korkmaz E, Ongun H, Akyuz M. Hydrocephalus after intraventricular hemorrhage in preterm and low-birth weight infants: analysis of associated risk factors for ventriculoperitoneal shunting. Surg Neurol 2005;64 (suppl 2):S77–S81, discussion S81

218. Ment LR, Duncan CC, Scott DT, Ehrenkranz RA. Posthemorrhagic hydrocephalus. Low incidence in very low birth weight neonates with intraventricular hemorrhage. J Neurosurg 1984;60(2):343–347

219. Doumouchtsis SK, Arulkumaran S. Head injuries after instrumental vaginal deliveries. Curr Opin Obstet Gynecol 2006;18(2):129–134

220. Hughes CA, Harley EH, Milmoe G, Bala R, Martorella A. Birth trauma in the head and neck. Arch Otolaryngol Head Neck Surg 1999;125(2):193–199

221. Steinbok P. Clinical features of Chiari I malformations. Childs Nerv Syst 2004;20(5):329–331

222. Caldarelli M, Di Rocco C. Diagnosis of Chiari I malformation and related syringomyelia: radiological and neurophysiological studies. Childs Nerv Syst 2004;20(5):332–335

223. Stevenson KL. Chiari type II malformation: past, present, and future. Neurosurg Focus 2004;16(2):E5

224. Nader R, Sabbagh AJ. Neurosurgery Case Review: Questions and Answers. New York, NY: Thieme Medical Publishers; 2010

225. Slater BJ, Lenton KA, Kwan MD, Gupta DM, Wan DC, Longaker MT. Cranial sutures: a brief review. Plast Reconstr Surg 2008;121(4):170e–178e

226. Blaser SI. Abnormal skull shape. Pediatr Radiol 2008; 38(suppl 3):S488–S496

227. Section of Pediatric Neurosurgery of the American Association of Neurological Surgeons. Pediatric neurosurgery. In: Surgery of the Developing Nervous System. 2nd ed. Philadelphia, PA: WB Saunders; 1989:120–141

228. Gerber P, Coffman K. Nonaccidental head trauma in infants. Childs Nerv Syst 2007;23(5):499–507

229. Al-Mefty O, Hassounah M, Weaver P, Sakati N, Jinkins JR, Fox JL. Microsurgery for giant craniopharyngiomas in children. Neurosurgery 1985;17(4):585–595

230. Schievink WI. Genetics and aneurysm formation. Neurosurg Clin N Am 1998;9(3):485–495

231. Boyd KP, Korf BR, Theos A. Neurofibromatosis type 1. J Am Acad Dermatol 2009;61(1):1–14, quiz 15–16

232. Boder E, Sedgwick RP. Ataxia-telangiectasia. (Clinical and immunological aspects). Psychiatr Neurol Med Psychol Beih 1970;13–14:8–16

233. Juares AJ, Dell'Aringa AR, Nardi JC, Kobari K, Gradim Moron Rodrigues VL, Perches Filho RM. Rendu-Osler-Weber syndrome: case report and literature review. Rev Bras Otorrinolaringol (Engl Ed) 2008;74(3):452–457

234. Begbie ME, Wallace GM, Shovlin CL. Hereditary haemorrhagic telangiectasia (Osler-Weber-Rendu syndrome): a view from the 21st century. Postgrad Med J 2003;79(927):18–24

235. Bergler W, Götte K. Hereditary hemorrhagic telangiectasias: a challenge for the clinician. Eur Arch Otorhinolaryngol 1999;256(1):10–15

236. Obeid M, Wyllie E, Rahi AC, Mikati MA. Approach to pediatric epilepsy surgery: state of the art, Part II: Approach to specific epilepsy syndromes and etiologies. Eur J Paediatr Neurol 2009;13(2):115–127

237. Di Rocco C, Tamburrini G. Sturge-Weber syndrome. Childs Nerv Syst 2006;22(8):909–921

238. Dearlove JV, Fisher PG, Buffler PA. Family history of cancer among children with brain tumors: a critical review. J Pediatr Hematol Oncol 2008;30(1):8–14

239. Rendón-Macías ME, Mejía-Aranguré JM, Juárez-Ocaña S, Fajardo-Gutiérrez A. Epidemiology of cancer in children under one year of age in Mexico City. Eur J Cancer Prev 2005;14(2):85–89

240. Diez B, Balmaceda C, Matsutani M, Weiner HL. Germ cell tumors of the CNS in children: recent advances in therapy. Childs Nerv Syst 1999;15(10):578–585

241. Sharma R, Rout D, Gupta AK, Radhakrishnan VV. Choroid plexus papillomas. Br J Neurosurg 1994;8(2):169–177

242. Umeoka S, Koyama T, Miki Y, Akai M, Tsutsui K, Togashi K. Pictorial review of tuberous sclerosis in various organs. Radiographics 2008;28(7):e32

243. Ellsworth RM. Orbital retinoblastoma. Trans Am Ophthalmol Soc 1974;72:79–88

244. Nørgaard-Pedersen B, Bagger P, Bang J, et al. Maternal-serum-alphafetoprotein screening for fetal malformations in 28 062 pregnancies. A four-year experience from a low-risk area. Acta Obstet Gynecol Scand 1985;64(6):511–514

245. Boseley ME, Tami TA. Endoscopic management of anterior skull base encephaloceles. Ann Otol Rhinol Laryngol 2004;113(1):30–33

246. Nelson MD Jr, Maher K, Gilles FH. A different approach to cysts of the posterior fossa. Pediatr Radiol 2004;34(9):720–732

247. Zakhary R, Keles GE, Aldape K, Berger MS. Medulloblastoma and primitive neuroectodermal tumors. In: Laws ER, Kaye AH, eds.

Brain Tumors—An Encyclopedic Approach. 2nd ed. Edinburgh: Churchill Livingstone; 2001:605–615

248. Sommer IE, Smit LM. Congenital supratentorial arachnoidal and giant cysts in children: a clinical study with arguments for a conservative approach. Childs Nerv Syst 1997;13(1):8–12

249. Rengachary SS, Watanabe I. Ultrastructure and pathogenesis of intracranial arachnoid cysts. J Neuropathol Exp Neurol 1981;40(1):61–83

250. Selber JC, Brooks C, Kurichi JE, Temmen T, Sonnad SS, Whitaker LA. Long-term results following fronto-orbital reconstruction in nonsyndromic unicoronal synostosis. Plast Reconstr Surg 2008;121(5):251e–260e

251. ten Donkelaar JT, van der Vliet T. Overview of the development of the human brain and spinal cord. In: Lammens M, Hori A, ten Donkelaar HJ, eds. Clinical Neuroembryology: Development and Developmental Disorders of the Human Central Nervous System. Berlin: Springer-Verlag; 2006:31–37

252. Gallucci M, Capoccia S, Catalucci A. Radiographic Atlas of Skull and Brain Anatomy. Berlin: Springer-Verlag; 2007:2–23

253. Yamini B, Gupta N. Bedside procedures. In: Gupta N, Frim DM, eds. Pediatric Neurosurgery. Georgetown, TX: Landes Bioscience; 2006:241–242

254. Fioravanti A, Godano U, Consales A, Mascari C, Calbucci F. Bobble-head doll syndrome due to a suprasellar arachnoid cyst: endoscopic treatment in two cases. Childs Nerv Syst 2004;20(10):770–773

255. Jamjoom AB, Khalaf NF, Mohammed AA, et al. Factors affecting the outcome of foetal hydrocephaly. Acta Neurochir (Wien) 1998;140(11):1121–1125

256. Kombogiorgas D, Solanki GA. The Pott puffy tumor revisited: neurosurgical implications of this unforgotten entity. Case report and review of the literature. J Neurosurg 2006;105 (2, suppl):143–149

257. Vernet O, de Ribaupierre S, Cavin B, Rilliet B. Treatment of posterior positional plagiocephaly [in French]. Arch Pediatr 2008;15(12):1829–1833

258. Rekate HL. Occipital plagiocephaly: a critical review of the literature. J Neurosurg 1998;89(1):24–30

259. McElhinney DB, Halbach VV, Silverman NH, Dowd CF, Hanley FL. Congenital cardiac anomalies with vein of Galen malformations in infants. Arch Dis Child 1998;78(6):548–551

260. Lende RA, Erickson TC. Growing skull fractures of childhood. J Neurosurg 1961;18:479–489

261. Mauras N, Blizzard RM. The McCune-Albright syndrome. Acta Endocrinol Suppl (Copenh) 1986;279:207–217

262. Buxton N, Macarthur D, Mallucci C, Punt J, Vloeberghs M. Neuroendoscopic third ventriculostomy in patients less than 1 year old. Pediatr Neurosurg 1998;29(2):73–76

263. Due-Tønnessen BJ, Helseth E, Scheie D, Skullerud K, Aamodt G, Lundar T. Long-term outcome after resection of benign cerebellar astrocytomas in children and young adults (0-19 years): report of 110 consecutive cases. Pediatr Neurosurg 2002;37(2):71–80

264. Mamelak AN, Prados MD, Obana WG, Cogen PH, Edwards MS. Treatment options and prognosis for multicentric juvenile pilocytic astrocytoma. J Neurosurg 1994;81(1):24–30

265. Fernandez C, Figarella-Branger D, Girard N, et al. Pilocytic astrocytomas in children: prognostic factors—a retrospective study of 80 cases. Neurosurgery 2003;53(3):544–553, discussion 554–555

266. Farmer JP, Montes JL, Freeman CR, Meagher-Villemure K, Bond MC, O'Gorman AM. Brainstem gliomas. A 10-year institutional review. Pediatr Neurosurg 2001;34(4):206–214

267. Renier W, Gabreëls F, Mol L, Korten J. Agenesis of the corpus callosum, chorioretinopathy and infantile spasms (Aicardi syndrome). Psychiatr Neurol Neurochir 1973;76(1):39–45

268. Stein SC, Schut L. Hydrocephalus in myelomeningocele. Childs Brain 1979;5(4):413–419

269. Samii M, Bini W. Surgical treatment of craniopharyngiomas. Zentralbl Neurochir 1991;52(1):17–23

270. Shinoda J, Yamada H, Sakai N, Ando T, Hirata T, Miwa Y. Placental alkaline phosphatase as a tumor marker for primary intracranial germinoma. J Neurosurg 1988;68(5):710–720

271. Ishiwata Y, Fujitsu K, Sekino T, et al. Subdural tension pneumocephalus following surgery for chronic subdural hematoma. J Neurosurg 1988;68(1):58–61

272. Gauthier-Lafaye P, Muller A. Regional anesthesia of head and neck. In: Anesthesie loco-regionale et traitment de la douleur. 3rd ed. Paris: Masson; 1996:115–120

273. Cohen DB, Oh MY, Whiting DM. Occipital neuralgia. In: Lozano AM, Gildenberg PL, Tasker RR, eds. Textbook of Stereotactic and Functional Neurosurgery. Berlin: Springer-Verlag; 2009:2507–2516

274. Hurt RW. The pathophysiology of trigeminal neuralgia. In: Lozano AM, Gildenberg PL, Tasker RR, eds. Textbook of Stereotactic and Functional Neurosurgery. Berlin: Springer-Verlag; 2009:2359–2420

275. Cosman ER Sr, Cosman ER Jr. Radiofrequency lesions. In: Lozano AM, Gildenberg PL, Tasker RR, eds. Textbook of Stereotactic and Functional Neurosurgery. Berlin: Springer-Verlag; 2009: 1359–1370

276. Taub E. Radiofrequency rhizotomy for trigeminal neuralgia. In: Lozano AM, Gildenberg PL, Tasker RR, eds. Textbook of Stereotactic and Functional Neurosurgery. Berlin: Springer-Verlag; 2009:2421–2428

277. Lee JYK, Kondziolka D. Thalamic deep brain stimulation for management of essential tremor. J Neurosurg 2005;103(3): 400–403

278. Vayssiere N, Hemm S, Cif L, et al. Comparison of atlas- and magnetic resonance imaging-based stereotactic targeting of the globus pallidus internus in the performance of deep brain stimulation for treatment of dystonia. J Neurosurg 2002;96(4):673–679

279. Kumagami H. Neruopathological findings of hemifacial spasm and trigeminal neuralgia. Arch Otolaryngol 1974;99(3):160–164

280. Han IB, Chang JH, Chang JW, Huh R, Chung SS. Unusual causes and presentations of hemifacial spasm. Neurosurgery 2009;65(1):130–137, discussion 137

281. Fisher PG, Breiter SN, Carson BS, et al. A clinicopathologic reappraisal of brain stem tumor classification. Identification of pilocystic astrocytoma and fibrillary astrocytoma as distinct entities. Cancer 2000;89(7):1569–1576

282. Oi S. Diagnosis, outcome, and management of fetal abnormalities: fetal hydrocephalus. Childs Nerv Syst 2003;19(7–8):508–516

283. Cochrane DD, Myles ST, Nimrod C, Still DK, Sugarman RG, Wittmann BK. Intrauterine hydrocephalus and ventriculomegaly: associated anomalies and fetal outcome. Can J Neurol Sci 1985;12(1):51–59

284. Origitano TC, Wascher TM, Reichman OH, Anderson DE. Sustained increased cerebral blood flow with prophylactic hypertensive hypervolemic hemodilution ("triple-H" therapy) after subarachnoid hemorrhage. Neurosurgery 1990;27(5):729–739, discussion 739–740

285. Higashida RT, Halbach VV, Cahan LD, et al. Transluminal angioplasty for treatment of intracranial arterial vasospasm. J Neurosurg 1989;71(5, pt 1):648–653

6 Spine

Spinal Anatomy and Surgical Technique

1. What percentage of people will experience low back pain at some point in their lives?

80%.[1]

2. What is the definition of acute low back pain?

Pain of 6 weeks' or less duration.[2]

3. What are some of the nonsurgical treatments for spinal stenosis?

- Nonsteroidal anti-inflammatory drugs (NSAIDs), such as aspirin, naproxen,[2,3] ibuprofen, and indomethacin, to reduce inflammation and relieve pain.
- Analgesics, such as acetaminophen, to relieve pain.
- Corticosteroid injections into the outermost of the membranes covering the spinal cord and nerve roots to reduce inflammation and treat acute pain that radiates to the hips or down a leg.
- Anesthetic injections, known as nerve blocks, near the affected nerve to temporarily relieve pain.
- Restricted activity (varies depending on extent of nerve involvement).
- Prescribed exercises and/or physical therapy to maintain motion of the spine, strengthen abdominal and back muscles, and build endurance, all of which help stabilize the spine. Some patients may be encouraged to try slowly progressive aerobic activity such as swimming or using exercise bicycles.
- A lumbar brace or corset to provide some support and help the patient regain mobility. This approach is sometimes used for patients with weak abdominal muscles or older patients with degeneration at several levels of the spine.
- Spinal manipulative therapies such as traction.[4]

4. Define radiculopathy.

Irritation of the lower motor neuron due to a mechanical or chemical insult to the nerve root in a single spinal level. It can result in burning pain and numbness accompanied by weakness and loss of reflex in the corresponding nerve's motor and sensory distribution.

5. What is the name given for compression when more than one nerve root is affected?

Polyradiculopathy.

6. What is the Lasègue sign?

The straight leg raise (SLR) test. This test is done during the physical examination and is positive when pain is elicited on lifting the leg passively off the table by the examiner.[5]

7. In the cervical spine, which nerve root will be affected in case of a disk herniation?

The lower nerve root will be affected. For example, if there is a disk herniation at C4–C5, then the C5 nerve root will be affected.

8. What is a Spurling test?

In cases of radiculopathy, cervical extension with axial compression and rotation of the head to the pathology side decreases the size of the neural foramen and compresses the exiting nerve root resulting in increased pain or symptoms along the arm. A Spurling test is positive if the maneuver results in arm symptoms along the specific nerve distribution.[6]

9. What is cervical myelopathy?

It is caused by chronic pressure on the cervical spinal cord mostly due to a degenerative process. Myelopathy presents with the lower motor neuron signs in the upper extremity, such as loss of manual dexterity and muscular atrophy, especially in the intrinsics. It can be accompanied by upper motor neuron signs in the lower and upper extremities such as hyperreflexia and spasticity. Neck pain and stiffness along with shuffling or waddling gait might also be present. Other physical signs may include clonus greater than three to four beats and positive Hoffman's or Babinski's signs.[7]

10. What are the red flag symptoms in spinal evaluation?

Red flags indicate that further evaluation is needed and there might be a serious underlying pathology. The red flags include fever, pain in recumbent position, unexplained weight loss, bowel or bladder dysfunction, trauma, history of cancer, saddle anesthesia, osteoporosis, age > 50 years, failure to respond to standard treatment, and drug abuse.[8]

11. What is a Schober test?

It measures the movement of the lumbar spine eliminating the hip flexion: 10 cm proximal and 5 cm distal to the line between the posterior superior iliac spines in the midline are marked. The distance between these points in flexion should be at least 5 cm more than in extension.[9]

12. What is the appropriate test to perform in a malnourished patient with symmetric paresthesias in the feet and hands and poor proprioception on physical examination?

Vitamin B_{12} level to rule out subacute combined degeneration.[10]

13. The L4 reflex is elicited by which joint?

The knee.

14. The Achilles reflex and sensation on the sole of the foot is supplied by which nerve root?

S1.

15. In lateral recess stenosis, is an SLR test positive or negative?

Negative, usually.

16. Can a positive SLR test exclude the diagnosis of Guillain-Barré syndrome (GBS)?

No. The SLR test is often positive in GBS. Typically, a patient presents with back pain, radiculopathic symptoms, and a positive SLR test. A history of a viral antecedent event, peak of symptoms at 4 weeks, ascending paralysis, areflexia, autonomic dysfunction, and high cerebrospinal fluid (CSF) protein help to make the diagnosis of GBS.[11]

17. What is a Patrick test used for in the examination of the lower extremities?

A test for arthritis of the hip. The thigh and knee of the supine patient are flexed and the external malleolus of the ankle is placed over the patella of the opposite leg. The test is positive if depression of the knee produces pain. It is also called the FABER test for **f**lexion, **ab**duction, and **e**xternal **r**otation.

18. What nerve roots are tensed by an SLR maneuver?

L5 and S1.

19. What types of nerves are contained in the dorsal ramus of the nerve root?

The dorsal ramus contains nerves that serve the dorsal portions of the trunk carrying visceral motor, somatic motor, and sensory information to and from the skin and muscles of the back.[12]

20. What type of nerve is located in the ventral ramus of the nerve root?

The ventral ramus contains nerves that serve the remaining ventral parts of the trunk and the upper and lower limbs carrying visceral motor, somatic motor, and sensory information to and from the ventrolateral body surface, structures in the body wall, and the limbs.[12]

21. How is the pain from lateral recess stenosis and herniated lumbar disk affected by sitting?

Lateral recess stenosis pain is relieved by sitting, whereas herniated lumbar disk pain is exacerbated by sitting.

22. Why does a C5 radiculopathy follow anterior or posterior decompression in a minority of cases even if the case was done without obvious complication?

A C5 radiculopathy (deltoid weakness) may be related to traction on the nerve root from posterior migration of the cord after decompression because the C5 nerve has the shortest length from the foramen to muscle ending.

23. What urinary metabolite is elevated in Paget's disease?

Hydroxyproline. The majority of pagetic lesions are symptomatic with lesions detected on radiographs for unrelated issues. The most common complaint in patients is back pain. Pagetic vascular steal is the compromise of vascular supply to the nerves of the spinal cord due to reactive vasodilatation of nearby vessels.[13]

24. Which spinal tract is most responsible for lower limb subconscious proprioception from muscles, joints, and skin?

The spinocerebellar pathways.

25. What is the significance of the intercristal line on anteroposterior (AP) and lateral X-rays?

It usually confirms the location of L5 and often the L4–L5 disk level.

26. What conditions may have Lhermitte's phenomenon as part of the patient's history?

Multiple sclerosis, cervical myelopathy, and subacute combined degeneration.[14]

27. What type of nystagmus is present in compressive lesions of the craniocervical border?

Downbeat nystagmus.

28. What type of traumatic spinal lesion results in a cap-elike sensory deficit?

A central cord lesion damages the second sensory neuron crossing to join the lateral spinothalamic tract in the anterior commissure. Pain and temperature sensations are impaired bilaterally. Because sacral fibers are located most peripherally in the lateral spinothalamic tract, there is sometimes sacral sparing with central cord lesions. As the lesion expands, anterior horn cells may become involved and weakness may result.[15]

29. How can it be possible for a C5–C6 disk to cause C7 symptoms?

This may be attributable to a prefixed brachial plexus in which normal levels of innervation are aberrant by one level. Normally, a C5–C6 disk herniation results in C6 nerve root compression and/or symptoms.

30. How can one differentiate mechanical back pain from ankylosing spondylitis–related back pain?

Rest usually relieves mechanical back pain; however, mild activity relieves the pain of ankylosing spondylitis. Patients with ankylosing spondylitis are frequently young men with the HLA-B27 genetic marker; they also have morning stiffness (sometimes nocturnal pain) and sacroiliitis.[16]

31. Why are disk herniations usually posterolateral?

The presence of thicker posterior longitudinal ligament in the center prevents the disk from herniating directly posteriorly (**Fig. 6.1**).

32. What makes up the anulus fibrosus?

Layers of fibrocartilage.

33. What is the most common extra-articular manifestation of ankylosing spondylitis?

Acute anterior uveitis.[16]

34. What are the types of spondylolisthesis?

Congenital, isthmic, degenerative, traumatic, pathologic, and iatrogenic/postsurgical.[17]

35. Which type of spondylolisthesis is thought to result from a stress fracture of the pars interarticularis?

Isthmic spondylolisthesis.[18]

36. What are the main causes of thoracic myelopathy from degenerative disease?

Herniated disks, ossification of the posterior longitudinal ligament, ossification of the ligamentum flavum, and posterior bone spurs.[19]

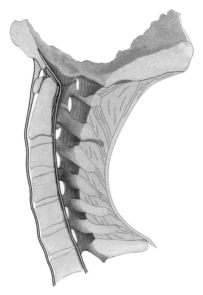

Fig. 6.1   A diagram showing the posterior and anterior longitudinal ligaments. These ligaments are strongest in the midline.

37. What are some musculoskeletal conditions that can mimic lumbar spine problems?

Osteoarthritis of the hip joint can mimic anterior thigh pain due to L2–L3–L4 radiculopathies. This can be distinguished by a hip range of motion examination especially with internal rotation as well as by a Stinchfield test. Vascular insufficiency of the lower limb can cause claudication similar to spinal stenosis. This can be diagnosed by a peripheral vascular examination and differentiating the exacerbating and ameliorating factors between vascular and neurogenic claudication. Piriformis syndrome and inflammatory sacroiliitis can mimic S1 radiculopathy with buttocks pain and radicular pain in the S1 distribution.

38. How long must elective surgery wait for a patient who has been taking clopidogrel?

At least 7 days.

39. What is the laboratory test needed to test coagulation for a patient taking clopidogrel?

Bleeding time. Remember that prothrombin time/partial thromboplastin time/international normalized ratio (PT/PTT/INR) are normal in a patient taking clopidogrel; therefore, a bleeding time is necessary.

40. What is the cervical level of the inferior edge of mandible, the hyoid bone, thyroid cartilage, and cricoid ring?

Inferior edge of mandible: C2; hyoid bone: C3; thyroid cartilage: C4–C5; and cricoid ring: C6.

41. Which is the largest and strongest cervical vertebra?

C2.

42. Which vertebra has no body?

C1.

43. Which vertebra is considered the cervicothoracic inflection point (the point where cervical lordosis becomes thoracic kyphosis)?

T3.

44. What is the best way to verify (using anatomical landmarks) the T7 area when the patient is positioned prone on the operating table?

Drawing a line from one scapular tip to another best approximates the T7 lamina when radiographs cannot be used due to patient size or poor X-ray quality.[20]

45. What is the normal range of motion in the cervical spine?

- Flexion: 45 degrees.
- Extension: 55 degrees.
- Lateral bending: 40 degrees.
- Rotation to each side: 70 degrees.

46. Describe the sensory (s) and motor (m) distribution and reflex (r) of the cervical nerve roots.

- C5 = s: lateral arm; m: deltoid; r: none.
- C6 = s: lateral forearm; m: wrist extension, biceps; r: brachioradialis.
- C7 = s: middle finger; m: triceps, wrist flex, finger extension; r: triceps.
- C8 = s: small finger; m: finger flexors; r: none.
- T1 = s: medial arm; m: interossei; r: none.

47. Which nerves arise from the lateral cord?

The lateral pectoral nerve to the pectoralis major muscle, the musculocutaneous nerve that innervates the biceps muscle, brachialis, and coracobrachialis, and partly the median nerve.

48. Which nerves arise from the posterior cord?

The upper subscapular nerve (C7 and C8) to the subscapularis muscle, the lower subscapular nerve (C5 and C6) to the teres major muscle and subscapularis muscle, the thoracodorsal nerve (C6, C7, and C8) to the latissimus dorsi muscle, the axillary nerve (sensation to the shoulder and motor to the deltoid muscle and teres minor), and the radial nerve (the triceps brachii muscle, the brachioradialis muscle or musculus brachioradialis, the extensor muscles of the fingers and wrist).

49. What is the general motor and sensory distribution of each lumbar nerve?

- L1: sensation of the anterior thigh and innervation of the psoas muscle.
- L2: sensation of the anterior thigh and groin and innervation of the quadriceps muscle.
- L3: sensation of the anterior and lateral thigh and innervation of the quadriceps muscle.
- L4: sensation of the medial leg and foot and innervation of the tibialis anterior muscle.
- L5: sensation of the lateral leg and dorsal foot and innervation of the extensor hallucis longus muscle.
- S1: sensation of the lateral and plantar foot and innervation of the gastrocnemius and peronealis muscles.

50. During a thoracolumbar spine procedure, dissection of the psoas muscle should take into account which nerve on the anterior surface of the muscle?

The genitofemoral nerve.

51. Where and how does a disk herniation cause radiculopathy?

The exiting nerve root courses beneath the pedicle of the corresponding cephalad vertebra and above the caudad intervertebral disk. The traversing nerve root courses medial to the pedicle of the cephalad vertebra over the intervertebral disk and then below the pedicle of the caudad vertebra. Thus, a posterolateral disk herniation will compress the traversing nerve root of the motion segment, whereas a lateral herniation will compress the exiting nerve root. Large central disk herniation can affect a single or multiple caudal nerve roots and is a common cause of cauda equina syndrome. A central disk bulge can be asymptomatic and is different than a central disk herniation. For example, a posterolateral L4–L5 disk herniation affects the L5 root and a lateral L4–L5 disk herniation affects the L4 root (**Fig. 6.2**).

52. What is a superficial abdominal reflex?

It is performed by stroking each of the four quadrants of the abdomen, and the normal response is the movement of the umbilicus toward the stroked segment. It is an upper motor neuron reflex, and asymmetry suggests intraspinal (upper motor neuron) pathology. It should be evaluated with thoracic magnetic resonance imaging (MRI).[21]

53. What anatomical landmarks are used to verify the location of a lumbar pedicle?

The crest of the transverse process is a good approximation of the center of the lumbar pedicle. Using a Leksell rongeur over this area will expose some cancellous bone that will confirm the center of the pedicle. After a laminectomy is done, feeling the pedicle from inside the canal with a Penfield #3 dissector will confirm the location of the pedicle. When a wide laminectomy is done, seeing the course of the nerve root is reassuring when placing the pedicle screw.

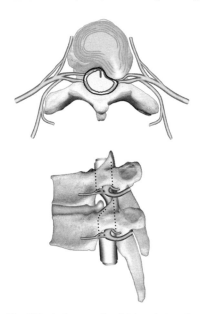

Fig. 6.2 A diagram of a disk herniation. For example, an L4–L5 disk usually compresses the L5 nerve root.

54. What ligaments serve as the ventral extent of safe dissection to avoid injury to the spinal nerve root during exposure and decortication of the transverse processes?

The intertransverse ligaments.

55. What is the first vertebra that can safely accommodate a pedicle screw?

C7; there is usually no vertebral artery in the transverse foramen at this level, which often permits safe placement of a pedicle screw (**Fig. 6.3**).

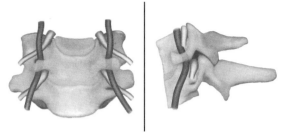

Fig. 6.3 A diagram showing the entrance of the vertebral artery in the foramen transversarium.

56. How can the correct placement of a pedicle screw be determined?

- By making sure that the screw is aimed medially.
- By confirming placement with an X-ray (AP and lateral) before the screw is placed. Many spine device companies have a tool shaped like a gearshift to perform the initial localization.
- By using neuronavigation while the screw is being placed and its tract determined.
- By feeling with a ball probe that bone is present in all areas surrounding the initial pilot hole.
- By using neurophysiologic monitoring to test the pedicle screw once placed. The stimulation threshold should be greater than 8 mA.[22,23]

57. The sympathetic plexus lies slightly ventral to what joint?

The costovertebral joint.

58. Sympathetic outflow arises from what nucleus of the cord? At what spinal cord levels?

Sympathetic outflow arises from the intermediolateral nucleus of the spinal cord from T1 to L2.

59. Where is the best place near the nerve root to expose an intervertebral herniated disk?

The shoulder of the nerve root is the best place to expose and remove the disk. An extruded disk may sometimes be found in the axilla of the nerve root.

60. What are the general clinical indications for surgery in the lumbar spine?[24]

- Emergent: cauda equina syndrome, progressive motor deficit(s).
- Elective: incapacitating leg pain in the distribution of a specific nerve root.
- Nerve root tension signs with or without neurologic signs.
- Failure to respond to conservative treatment for 4 to 8 weeks.

61. What are the general clinical indications for surgery in the cervical spine?[24]

- Significant radicular pain or radiculopathy (persistent or recurrent) refractory to conservative treatments.
- Progressive neurologic deficit(s).
- Progressive or profound myelopathy.

62. When is surgical intervention needed for spinal infection?[25]

- Open biopsy to obtain tissue when closed biopsy has failed.
- Failure of medical management with persistent pain and increased erythrocyte sedimentation rate and/or C-reactive protein.
- Drainage of abscess.
- Decompression of spinal cord or nerve root with neurologic deficit(s).
- Correction of progressive or unacceptable spine deformity or instability.

63. What are the surgical indications for primary spine tumor?[26]

- Open biopsy for diagnosis.
- Failure of chemotherapy or radiation.
- Decompression of spinal cord or nerve roots with neurologic deficit(s).
- Tumors resistant to medical treatment.
- Correction of progressive or unacceptable spine deformity or instability.

64. What are the surgical indications for metastatic spine tumor?[26]

- Open biopsy for diagnosis.
- Failure of chemotherapy or radiation.
- Tumors resistant to medical treatment.
- Correction of progressive or unacceptable spine deformity or instability.
- Decompression of spinal cord or nerve roots with neurologic deficit(s).
- Intractable pain or neurologic deficit(s) during radiation therapy despite steroids.

65. What are the general indications for surgery for adult spine scoliosis?

Progressive deformity, intractable pain, cardiopulmonary symptoms, neurologic dysfunction, and cosmesis.[27]

66. When is revision surgery indicated?

The pathology should be correctable and the symptoms should be explained by this pathology. There is usually some correlation between the imaging findings and patient's symptoms.

Surgery is recommended in the following situations: recurrent or persistent disk herniation or spinal stenosis, postlaminectomy instability, lumbar disk space infection following lumbar diskectomy, symptomatic lumbar pseudoarthrosis, and flatback syndrome.

67. What areas of bone does a C1–C2 transarticular screw pass through if properly placed?

The inferior C2 facet (3 mm from the medial edge), the C2 pars interarticularis, and the C1 lateral mass. In 30% of patients, the position of the vertebral artery will preclude this type of surgery.

68. What are the landmarks for a C1–C2 puncture?

1 cm caudal and 1 cm posterior to the tip of the mastoid (aiming for the posterior third of the bony spinal canal under fluoroscopy).

69. What is another name for the dorsal ramus of the C1 nerve root?

The suboccipital nerve.

70. Successful odontoid screw placement requires preservation of which ligament?

The transverse ligament.[28]

71. In an anterior cervical diskectomy, what structures must be verified and retracted?

- The platysma is the first muscle incised to gain access to the structures in the anterior neck area.
- The carotid artery should be palpated and the pulse appreciated. The carotid artery should be carefully displaced laterally.
- The esophagus needs to be identified and carefully placed medially. The esophagus can be confirmed by having anesthesia move the nasogastric tube if one is available.
- The anterior spine can be exposed with blunt dissection and the first disk space encountered should be radiographed.

72. In which groove is the recurrent laryngeal nerve located?

The tracheoesophageal groove.[29]

73. On what side of the neck does the recurrent laryngeal nerve have a more variable course?

The recurrent laryngeal nerve has a more variable course on the right side of the neck and theoretically has an increased risk of injury on the right side.

74. What is the upper limit of traction that should be used in cervical spine injuries?

Ten pounds per level is the upper limit.

75. What are some possible complications that can happen from an anterior cervical diskectomy and fusion (ACDF)?

The most common complications are the development of isolated postoperative dysphagia, postoperative hematoma (sometimes requiring surgical intervention), symptomatic recurrent laryngeal nerve palsy, dural penetration, esophageal perforation, worsening of preexisting myelopathy, Horner's syndrome, instrumentation failure/back-out, and superficial wound infection.[30,31]

76. How can a patient develop Horner's syndrome after a routine ACDF?

Disruption of the sympathetic plexus due to dissection too far lateral on the longus colli muscles—best to dissect laterally within 1 cm of the medial edge of the muscle.[32] Limiting use of Bovie cautery (setting < 20) is also important to avoid nerve damage.

77. In an occipitocervical fusion, where is a safe area to drill a hole and place a screw in the occiput?

Halfway between the foramen magnum and the transverse sinus, and ~3 cm off the midline.

78. What are some drugs that inhibit bony fusion?

Steroids, NSAIDs, immunosuppressive drugs, and nicotine. It is important that a patient stop or decrease smoking before and after undergoing a spinal fusion.

79. What postoperative devices and maneuvers can increase the chances of a quality fusion?

- Use of a bone stimulator in the postoperative period.
- Use of bracing intermittently (using a brace constantly will promote muscle atrophy).
- Cessation of smoking.
- Maintaining a proper diet with adequate protein intake.
- Maintaining proper glucose control in diabetic patients.

80. Because a laminectomy cannot access the spaces lateral and anterior in the thoracic spine, what other options does the surgeon have for thoracic stenosis, tumor, or disk herniation?

Transthoracic, transpedicular, and costotransversectomy are potential approaches in the thoracic spine. Unlike the lumbar spine, the thoracic neural elements should not be manipulated or retracted, as severe neurologic injury can result.[33]

81. What does "ligamentotaxis" refer to in the setting of spinal stabilization?

Using posterior instrumentation to distract burst fractures to indirectly decompress the spinal canal. Intact ligaments can reimpact the bone fragments into the vertebral body following distraction.[34]

82. What do SSEPs, TcMEPs, and pedicle screw stimulation measure?

The SSEP (somatosensory evoked potential) gives direct feedback on the integrity of the posterior columns by stimulating the posterior tibial nerve at the ankle and recording the responses from the popliteal fossa, cervical spine, and somatosensory cortex. In general, manipulations of the spinal cord and ischemic events will usually affect dorsal column function; thus, SSEPs correlate well with overall spinal cord function, but they do not indicate changes in motor pathways. The TcMEPs (transcranial motor evoked potentials) are determined by stimulating the scalp over the motor cortex; this gives direct feedback on the integrity of the corticospinal tracts of the spinal cord. Pedicle screw stimulation evaluates the integrity of the pedicle. Because bone is an insulator, an intact pedicle requires a threshold of 8 mA to activate the nerve. Anything less than this means that there is a possibility of a pedicle breach.[35]

83. What spinous process of the cervical spine is the lowest bifid spine?

Usually C6.

84. What is the average distance between the transverse foramina containing the vertebral arteries?

Three centimeters. Thus, it is imperative during an anterior diskectomy to ensure that one is aware of where midline is at all times. Complications of anterior cervical diskectomy of operating too lateral result in vertebral artery injury; likewise, operating too far laterally on the longus colli muscles can result in injury to the cervical sympathetic chain resulting in Horner's syndrome.[36]

85. Unilateral ligation of the vertebral artery usually has what consequences?

None. Unilateral ligation of the vertebral artery (if absolutely necessary) is usually well tolerated.

86. Where are the proper entry point and trajectory for lateral mass screws?

The entry point for lateral mass screws is 1 mm medial to the exact center of the lateral mass. The appropriate trajectory for lateral mass screws is 10 to 30 degrees in the cephalad direction (use the spinous process as a guide) and 10 to 30 degrees lateral, which facilitates the avoidance of the anterior neurovascular structures. There are different techniques and trajectories. It is recommended to study the preoperative films and determine the best trajectory for each patient. This is best done with an axial computed tomography (CT) scan.

87. What is BMP?

Bone morphogenetic protein (BMP) is a bone growth factor with osteoinductive properties to help promote bone formation. Target cells for BMP are primarily undifferentiated mesenchymal stem cells. Recombinant BMP2 is currently the only FDA-approved BMP product for spinal fusion.[37]

88. What is the definition of pseudoarthrosis?

Pseudoarthrosis is the persistence of a motion segment resulting from the incomplete development of a rigid osseous construct after attempted bony fusion.[38]

89. When is an intertransverse (Jane) procedure utilized?

A Jane intertransverse procedure through a Wiltse intermuscular approach is used to resect far lateral disk herniations. It involves removal of the most superolateral aspect of the facet joint while carefully preserving the pars interarticularis. A far lateral disk herniation often results in compression of the more cephalad (or exiting) nerve root rather than the traversing nerve root as in a posterolateral disk herniation.[39,40]

90. How is a far lateral disk herniation identified and where is the most common location?

A far lateral disk herniation is located lateral to a line drawn between two adjacent pedicles. The most common level is L4–L5. Due to its location, the far lateral disk can compress the ganglion as well as the exiting and the traversing nerve root. The terrible pain that patients experience is from this ganglionic irritation.[39,40]

91. Where is the best place to insert an intrathecal baclofen pump?

The tip of the catheter is placed at the level corresponding with the therapeutic indication: T10–T12 for spastic diplegia, C5–T2 for spastic tetraplegia, and C1–C4 for generalized secondary dystonia.[41]

92. Compare the fusion potential in anterior and posterior spinal fusions.

Because 80% of the body's weight passes through the anterior spinal column, whereas only 20% passes through the posterior column, the bone graft placed in the anterior column is subject to compression, which promotes fusion. Additionally, the wide bony surface area and high vascularity of the vertebral end plates promote anterior interbody fusion. The bone graft placed in the posterior column is subject to tensile forces; therefore, fusion is more dependent on biologic factors such as osteogenic cells and the quality of the soft tissue bed into which the graft is inserted posteriorly.

93. What types of bone graft are recommended for posterior spinal fusion?

Autologous, cancellous iliac crest bone graft is considered the gold standard in posterior spinal fusion. Although allograft alone does not achieve a high fusion rate in adults, it is used frequently in pediatric patients with good success for scoliosis fusion. If enough autogenous graft is not available, then autograft extenders such as β-tricalcium phosphate, allograft, and biologics such as BMP and demineralized bone matrix can be used with good success if a meticulous decortication and a bone grafting technique are employed.[37]

94. What is the difference between nonstructural and structural bone grafts?

Nonstructural bone grafts typically consist of particulate corticocancellous bone that can be used to promote arthrodesis between adjacent vertebral bodies, but the graft itself does not provide any stability to the anterior column. Structural grafts such as a femoral allograft ring with cortical bone provide mechanical support anteriorly during the process of fusion through the disk space.[42]

95. How do you diagnose a pseudoarthrosis?

Localized pain over the fusion site after 6 to 12 months post-operatively should prompt imaging studies such as flexion and extension radiographs, technetium bone scan, or CT scan (the gold standard for imaging). Pseudoarthrosis is suggested by radiographic findings such as progressive spinal deformity, displacement in flexion and extension, broken screws, screws with halo effect, and discontinuity in the fusion mass. Surgical exploration of the fusion bed is the most accurate method to determine if a pseudoarthrosis is present.[38]

96. What is the difference between a laminotomy, a laminectomy, and a laminoplasty?

A posterior approach is utilized for all three procedures with the surgical goal to decompress the neural elements. A laminotomy is usually unilateral, and partial removal of the lamina or facet joint to decompress the ipsilateral nerve root or dural sac is performed. In a laminectomy, the spinous process and the entire lamina are removed. In a laminoplasty, the area for the neural elements is widened through the lamina but without removal of the posterior spinal elements.

97. When is the posterior surgical approach employed for cervical decompression?

If three or more levels require surgical decompression, a posterior surgical approach is frequently recommended. To perform a posterior laminectomy or laminoplasty for decompression, a neutral to lordotic sagittal alignment of the cervical spine should be present, which permits dorsal migration of spinal cord away from the anterior pathology. Multilevel posterior laminectomy for decompression is often combined with instrumented fusion to avoid postlaminectomy kyphosis. A cervical laminoplasty can provide central decompression without fusion with the caveat that the patient does not have significant preoperative neck pain because postoperative neck pain can occur. A unilateral cervical keyhole laminoforaminotomy is utilized to decompress for unilateral arm pain caused by a soft posterolateral disk herniation or foraminal stenosis from facet hypertrophy.[43]

98. When is an anterior surgical approach indicated for decompression of the cervical spine?

In patients with cervical spinal stenosis who have three or fewer involved levels. In this approach—regardless of the lordotic, neutral, or kyphotic sagittal plane alignment—the decompression can be successful. If neural compression is localized to the level of disk space, multilateral diskectomy and interbody fusion might be used. When cord compression extends beyond the disk level or when a significant kyphotic deformity is present, an anterior corpectomy and a strut graft are performed.[43]

99. When should anterior and posterior approaches be combined in the cervical spine?

In multilevel conditions, such as cervical stenosis, which requires three or more levels of anterior surgical approach decompression; two or more levels of corpectomies when associated with kyphotic deformity; and in rigid posttraumatic or postlaminectomy kyphosis (**Fig. 6.4**).[44]

100. What nerve root injury is the most common after cervical laminectomy or laminoplasty?

C5 nerve root. Dysfunction may appear immediately following surgery, but can appear in a delayed fashion several days after the surgery. It is believed that because the C5 nerve has a short length, tension is produced as the spine is decompressed in this area. This tension deprives the nerve of oxygen and nutrients and may be a cause of the dysfunction.[45]

101. Should a laminectomy be performed for the treatment of a thoracic disk herniation?

In the thoracic spine, a midline laminectomy and midline approaches should be avoided because they are associated with a high rate of complications such as paraplegia. This approach provides poor access to the central lateral aspect of this space; due to the risk of paraplegia, retraction of the spinal cord is not advised.

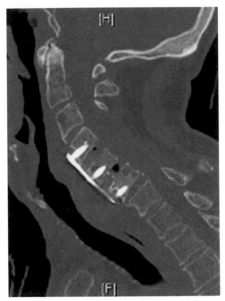

Fig. 6.4 An example of postlaminectomy kyphosis. This patient eventually needed posterior fixation via lateral mass screws.

102. What are the indications for performing a corpectomy in the thoracic or lumbar spine?

Burst fractures with retropulsed bone causing anterior cord compression, tumor extending from the posterior part of the vertebral body into the spinal canal, osteomyelitis, and in cases of collapsed vertebral body with retropulsed material in the canal. It is also indicated for drainage of a vertebral abscess.

103. What are some intraoperative maneuvers that can decrease the postoperative pain of a lumbar laminectomy?

- Injecting bupivacaine in the paraspinal musculature at the end of the procedure.
- Placing an epidural pain catheter.
- Minimizing the muscle dissection during exposure.
- Releasing the retractors periodically to prevent venous congestion and skin necrosis.

104. What are the proper ways to deal with an inadvertent dural breach?

1. Place a cottonoid on the dural breach and remove some CSF to allow the nerves to descend in the thecal sac.
2. Under magnified vision, place a 4–0 suture starting at the beginning of the breach and continue to the end. This can be done in a running or interrupted fashion depending on the nature of the tear. A patch of muscle may be used to augment the closure. If no dural edges are available, then using a dural substitute is an option. More bone may have to be removed to expose the edges of the dural breach and facilitate its primary closure.
3. Ask the anesthetist to perform a Valsalva maneuver to verify the quality of the sutured area.
4. Use a fibrin sealant over the sutured area. Apply the sealant in layers alternating with surgical patches rather than placing the entire amount at one time.
5. During closure of the incision, perform a watertight closure of the fascial layer and a thorough closure of the skin edges using a 2–0 or 3–0 nylon suture (running or interrupted). If a JP drain is necessary, it is best to place this under the fascia.
6. Place the patient on at least 3 days of antibiotics and remove the drains promptly. Drains are best placed suprafacial.

105. If a wound continues to leak CSF even though all the above maneuvers were employed at surgery, what is the accepted next step?

Insertion of a lumbar drain at a site away from the incision can help the wound to seal by creating a path of least resistance. Ten to 15 mL per hour can be drained for up to 5 days. At that time, the drain can be clamped for 12 to 24 hours and discontinued thereafter. If this drainage maneuver fails, it is prudent to reexplore and close the leak.

106. When is accepted antibiotic usage preoperatively, intraoperatively, and postoperatively?

- Preoperative: 30 minutes before skin incision.
- Intraoperatively: every 6 hours of operating time antibiotics should be repeated.
- Postoperatively: three to six doses of antibiotics (24–48 hours) or antibiotics for as long as a drain is in place.

107. What are the main ligaments in the subaxial cervical spine and what is their primary role?

- Anterior longitudinal ligament: reinforces anterior aspect of the disks, limits extension.
- Posterior longitudinal ligament: reinforces posterior aspect of the disks, limits flexion.
- Ligamentum nuchae or supraspinous ligament: thicker in the thoracic/lumbar regions, limits flexion.
- Interspinous/intertransverse ligaments: limit flexion and rotation/limits lateral flexion.
- Ligamentum flavum: attaches lamina of one vertebra to another, reinforces articular facets, limits flexion and rotation.

108. How many intervertebral disks are there and what percentage of height of the spine do they account for?

There are 23 intervertebral disks, which are interposed between the vertebral bodies. The most rostral is the C2–C3 disk and the most distal is the L5–S1 disk. They account for one-third to one-fifth of the height of the vertebral column.

109. Describe the different types of sacroiliac ligaments and their course.

The short sacroiliac ligaments: these are composed of horizontal fibers extending from the sacrum to the posterior part of the iliac bone.

The long sacroiliac ligaments: these are composed of fibers extending vertically from the sacrum to the posterior superior iliac spine.

110. What is the lumbosacral ligament?

The lumbosacral ligament is a thick, fibrous band that extends from the anterior inferior aspect of the transverse process of L5 and attaches to the lateral surface of the sacrum.[46]

111. What is the iliolumbar ligament?

The iliolumbar ligament is a thick, fibrous band that extends from the transverse processes of L4 and L5 to the iliac crest.

112. Describe the main ligaments essential for stability that are in relation to the odontoid process.

- Apical ligament: it extends from the tip of the dens up to the anterior margin of the foramen magnum.
- Alar ligament: it extends from the back of the dens and courses to the occipital condyles.
- Cruciate ligament (vertical part): extends from the back of the dens to the anterior margin of the foramen magnum.
- Tectorial membrane: this is an extension of the posterior longitudinal ligament (up to the posterior aspect of the clivus).

113. Describe the most common complications of bone graft harvesting from the iliac crest and ways in which to avoid them.

Common complications of iliac crest bone graft harvesting include pain (in up to 29% of patients), hematoma or seroma formation, lateral femoral cutaneous nerve syndrome, infection, and gluteal lurch gait due to excessive stripping of gluteus medius muscle (posterior approach).[47]

Avoidance of some of these complications includes maneuvers such as performing the opening incision for an anterior harvest at least 3 cm behind the anterior superior iliac spine before exposing bone, achieving good hemostasis or leaving a drain behind should there be persistent sanguineous ooze (e.g., JP drain), utilizing preoperative antibiotics, and avoiding excessive muscle dissection.

114. List all the nerves that may be damaged during an anterior approach to the cervical spine.

- Recurrent laryngeal nerve (more common with right-sided approaches).
- Vagus nerve.
- Superior laryngeal nerve.
- Sympathetic chain.
- Stellate ganglion.
- C5 nerve root.
- Phrenic nerve.
- Ansa cervicalis.
- Hypoglossal nerve.
- Mental branch of mandibular nerve.

115. What is the sagittal vertical axis?

The sagittal vertical axis is a measurement obtained by the following method: a vertical plumb line is drawn from the center of the C7 vertebral body on a lateral X-ray of the thoracolumbar spine and measurements are taken from the posterosuperior corner of the S1 end plate. The plumb line is normally within 5 cm of the posterosuperior corner of the S1 end plate. If it deviates from that position, then the patient is in sagittal imbalance. This is believed to be a key element in assessing patients with kyphoscoliosis as it relates to their outcome and clinical status.[48]

116. List complications associated with scoliosis surgery.[49]

- Dural tear.
- Wound infections.
- Pulmonary insufficiency.
- Renal complications.
- Neurologic deficits.
- Gastrointestinal problems.
- Cardiac issues.
- Pseudarthrosis.
- Proximal junctional kyphosis.
- Proximal junctional failure.
- Distal junctional kyphosis.
- Death.

Trauma

117. What are the most common areas of the spine that are injured?

The most common levels of injury are the middle and lower cervical areas, which are the most mobile and flexible regions of the spine. The second most common level is the thoracolumbar junction.[50,51]

118. In the cervical spine, what vertebral level is most frequently fractured or dislocated?

The C2 is the level most frequently injured due to trauma in young people, and there are increasing numbers of odontoid fractures in the elderly. The most common C2 fracture is the type II odontoid fracture (**Figs. 6.5** and **6.6**). C2 (bilateral) fractures at the pedicles or pars interarticularis are called hangman fractures and are classified on the degree of angulation. Axis fractures are seen with C1 fractures in combination, and a careful search for an associated C1 fracture is mandatory with an axis fracture. Most C2 nondisplaced fractures can be managed nonoperatively.[50,51]

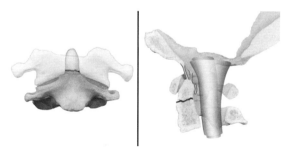

Fig. 6.5 An artist's rendition of a type II odontoid fracture showing the ligamentous attachments to the dens.

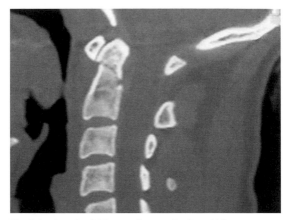

Fig. 6.6 A sagittal CT scan of a type II odontoid fracture treated with a collar.

119. What percentage of spinal column injuries involve multiple noncontinuous levels?

Approximately 20%. Therefore, survey of the entire spine is necessary in the trauma patient.[52,53]

120. When there is a C1 fracture, what are the chances of having an associated C2 fracture?

This occurs 41% of the time.[52,53]

121. Has there ever been a case of an occult cervical spine injury in an alert, asymptomatic, sober patient, with a non-tender neck to palpation, and with full range of motion?

Not to our knowledge. A collar would not be mandatory in these cases, but could be used for the patient's comfort.

122. What is the accepted and safest way to provide spinal immobilization at the scene of an accident?

A rigid cervical collar with supportive blocks on a rigid backboard with straps provides safe and effective spinal immobilization for transport.[54]

123. What type of injury is most likely in a patient with known spinal stenosis who sustained a hyperextension injury and presents with marked upper extremity weakness?

Central cord syndrome. This is a classic presentation. Often, prevertebral soft tissue swelling may be the only radiologic sign in central cord syndrome. During hyperextension, the ligamentum flavum bulges forward in the canal causing spinal cord injury.

124. What are the types of odontoid fractures and what are the treatments?

Type I fractures involve the tip of the dens; type II are through the base of the dens; type III are through the body of C2. Treatment is controversial and external immobilization may be used for most cases of type III fractures and nondisplaced type II fractures. Indications for surgery are in patients older than 7 years, displacement of greater than 6 mm, instability while in a halo vest, or nonunion especially if accompanied by myelopathy. Surgical fusion may at times be necessary in type I fractures, but this is rare.[55,56]

125. What percentage of odontoid type III fractures will eventually need surgery?

Ten percent. Odontoid type III fractures (those extending through the vertebral body or C2) are usually best treated in an external orthosis (cervical collar or halo).[57]

126. What is the critical distance of dens displacement above which open reduction and internal fixation should be considered?

Six millimeters. If the dens is displaced 6 mm or more, internal fixation is recommended because of the high rate of nonunion associated with widely displaced type II fractures. If the dens is displaced less than 6 mm, a halo brace is adequate.

127. What is the critical displacement distance in a hangman fracture where conservative therapy usually fails?

4 mm.

128. MRI should be taken to assess the competence of which ligament in atlantoaxial dislocation?

The transverse ligament.

129. What particular sequence of MRI is good to visualize disruption of the transverse ligament?

Gradient-echo sequences and contrast images assess soft tissue pathology and the integrity of the ligaments of the C1–C2 complex.

130. What sensations are lost and retained in syringomyelia?

Pain and temperature sensations are lost; light touch, vibration, and position sensibilities are retained. This is termed a "dissociated sensory loss."[58]

131. What condition constitutes the triad of cephalgia, hyperhidrosis, and cutaneous vasodilation, and at what level of the spinal cord is the injury?

Autonomic hyperreflexia occurs with a spinal cord lesion above T6.[59]

132. What disease should be considered in a spinal cord injury patient with new neurologic defects or changes in previously stable voiding patterns?

Syringomyelia; in children, consider tethered cord.

133. What are the types of hangman fractures and what is the best treatment?[60,61]

A hangman fracture is a bilateral fracture through the pars interarticularis of the pedicle of C2. Categorization of hangman fractures is based on the Effendi classification:

- Type I fractures have 3 mm or less of subluxation of C2 on C3.
- Type II fractures have increased subluxation ($\geq$ 4 mm) with angulation over 11 degrees.
- Type III fractures have disrupted facet capsules and possibly locked C2/C3 facets (if locked facets are present, do not place the patient in traction).

Type I fractures are treated best with external orthosis. Type II fractures may be reduced with gentle cervical traction and placed in a halo vest. Type III fractures may need open reduction and internal fixation. Other reasons to perform surgery are traumatic disk at C2–C3, failure to heal with external orthosis, and movement on flexion-extension film taken several weeks after injury. Motion can be preserved by performing an anterior diskectomy and fusion of C2–C3.

134. What are the most important structures in maintaining atlantooccipital stability?

The tectorial membrane and the alar ligaments (**Fig. 6.7**).

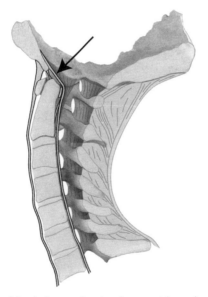

Fig. 6.7 A diagram showing the tectorial membrane merging into the posterior longitudinal ligament.

135. How can Collet-Sicard syndrome occur from trauma?

Lower cranial nerve (CN) injury (CNs IX–XII) from an occipital condyle fracture, infection, carotid artery dissection, gunshot wound, and possibly neoplasia. Collet-Sicard syndrome is a collective term for involvement of CNs IX, X, XI, and XII producing paralysis of the vocal cords, palate, trapezius muscle, and sternocleidomastoid muscle and secondary loss of the sense of taste in the back of the tongue and anesthesia of the larynx, pharynx, and soft palate.[62,63,64]

136. How can one tell if a locked facet is unilateral or bilateral from a lateral cervical spine film?

With a bilateral locked facet, there is a greater translation of one vertebral body on the other and the same degree of obliquity of the facets above and below the level of the lesion. With a unilateral locked facet, there is less subluxation and there is rotation across the injured level (as evidenced by changes in the obliquity of the facets above and below the injury) (**Fig. 6.8**).

137. On plain films, subluxation of less than 50% of the width of the vertebral body is usually indicative of what cervical traumatic pathology?

Unilateral locked facets.[65]

138. On plain films, subluxation of greater than 50% of the width of the vertebral body is usually indicative of what cervical traumatic pathology?

Bilateral locked facets.

139. What is the Powers ratio and what is it used for?

The ratio of the distance between the basion and the posterior arch of the atlas to the distance from the posterior margin of the foramen magnum to the anterior arch of the atlas. The Powers ratio is used in a diagnosis of occipitocervical dislocation. Atlantooccipital dislocation is suggested by a ratio greater than 1.0.[66]

140. Many months after an accident, the appearance of upper extremity symptoms in a paraplegic patient should raise suspicion of what?

Posttraumatic syringomyelia.[67]

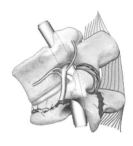

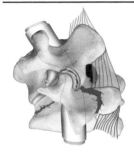

Fig. 6.8   A case of bilateral locked facets.

141. What is a central cord syndrome?

It is seen in a hyperextension injury in the elderly and in cases with preexisting spinal stenosis. The upper extremity is weaker than the lower extremity. Both sensory and motor functions are affected bilaterally. Signs of hyperreflexia are present in the lower extremity. For a partial injury, the prognosis is good; however, the recovery in the hands will be poor. Decompression is indicated in general early in the course of this condition.[68]

142. What is the most common type of incomplete spinal cord injury?

Central cord syndrome.

143. What does one clinically find in Brown-Séquard syndrome?

Ipsilateral loss of dorsal column functions (proprioception, touch, and vibration) and motor function, and contralateral loss of pain and temperature. There are lower motor neuron signs ipsilaterally at the level of the lesion and upper motor neuron signs ipsilaterally below the level of the lesion. This syndrome is usually the result of a penetrating spinal cord injury, resulting in hemisection of the cord. Prognosis is good with some ambulatory capacity. Common causes are stab wounds and tumors.[69]

144. What is an anterior cord syndrome and how does it occur?

Anterior cord syndrome is the second most common cervical syndrome (central cord syndrome is the most common). The syndrome results from a flexion or axial loading mechanism, or both, and is often associated with a vertebral fracture, dislocation, and/or disk herniation. It is due to ischemia of the anterior two-thirds of the spinal cord because of retropulsed vertebral fracture or compression of the anterior spinal artery. Findings include motor and sensory loss (including pain and temperature) below the injury level, and preservation of proprioception, touch, and vibration sensations.[70]

145. What is posterior cord syndrome?

It involves injury to the posterior columns of the spinal cord resulting in loss of vibration, proprioception, and touch sensations (deep pressure), along with a foot-slapping gait. Common causes are posterior spinal artery occlusion and syphilis.[70]

146. Where do conus medullaris and cauda equina syndromes occur?

Patients with conus medullaris syndrome usually have injuries from T11 to L1 where the spinal cord is usually terminating into the cauda equina. Therefore, cauda equina syndrome is seen in injuries from L1 down through the sacral levels that centrally involve the canal and compress or compromise the nerve roots of the cauda equina.[71]

147. What are the main clinical differences between conus medullaris and cauda equina syndrome?

Conus medullaris syndrome involves a symmetric motor deficit and preserved knee reflex; cauda equina patients have asymmetric motor and sensory loss with decreased knee reflex. Pain is prominent in cauda equina syndrome and rare in conus medullaris syndrome. Both conditions have a flaccid bladder with overflow incontinence.[71]

148. What condition carries a worse prognosis, conus medullaris or cauda equina syndrome?

Conus medullaris syndrome.

149. What are the most common contributors to secondary injury in spinal cord trauma?

Untreated hypotension, hypoxia, and patient mishandling with regard to spinal instability and immobilization.

150. What are some associated conditions seen with acute transverse myelitis?

Trauma, systemic lupus erythematosus, Sjögren's syndrome, herpes zoster, cytomegalovirus, and schistosomiasis.[72,73]

151. What is the most common cranial neuropathy seen with atlantooccipital dislocation?

Seventh cranial nerve neuropathy, probably due to concomitant head injury.

152. What type of diagnostic evaluation is important in evaluating atlantoaxial rotatory subluxation?

"Three-position" CT scans of the cervical spine: one in the presenting position, one in the anatomical zero position, and one in the extreme corrected position. These patients have a painful neck that is laterally flexed and the chin is rotated to the contralateral side; this is called the "cock robin deformity."[74]

153. What is the most common type of injury to the thoracic spine?

Wedge compression fracture. Only 10% of thoracic vertebral body injuries are associated with a concurrent spinal cord injury. The thoracic spinal cord is very susceptible to trauma and has the poorest prognosis for functional recovery of any of the spinal regions. What differentiates a wedge compression fracture from a burst fracture is disruption of the middle column in the latter (the anterior column is fractured in both) (**Fig. 6.9**).

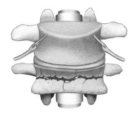

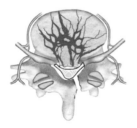

Fig. 6.9 A diagram of a wedge compression fracture with moderate retropulsion into the thoracic spinal cord.

154. Increased interpediculate distance indicates failure of which column?

The middle column. Recall that the middle column is the posterior half of the disk and vertebral body and the posterior longitudinal ligament.

155. Due to the normal kyphosis of the thoracic spine, an axial compression load is converted into what type of injury to the vertebral body?

An axial compression load to the spinal column is converted into an anterior flexion load to the individual vertebral body. Note that the thoracic levels T1 to T10 are behind the spine's center of gravity.

156. What is SCIWORA?

SCIWORA is an acronym for spinal cord injury without radiographic abnormality. This is typically a finding in patients 1.5 to 16 years of age. It is attributed to the increased elasticity of the spinal ligaments in the young population. MRI may show increased signal within the spinal cord on T2 sequences.[75]

157. What are the most common instances where a neck fracture is treated with a halo?

An unstable Jefferson fracture, type II and III odontoid fracture, an unstable hangman fracture (**Figs. 6.10** and **6.11**).

158. What have cadaveric studies shown regarding ligamentous instability?

Horizontal subluxation of greater than 3.5 mm of one vertebra on another or angulation of 11 degrees of one vertebral body relative to the next one indicates ligamentous instability.

159. Where is the axis of spinal loading in a Chance fracture?

The axis of spinal loading in a Chance fracture is anterior to the spine. Chance fractures are seen with high-speed motor vehicle accidents where the lower half of the torso is relatively fixed (as with a seatbelt). There is a predominant force of flexion with an element of shear injury to the vertebra.[76]

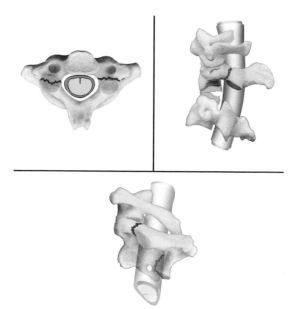

Fig. 6.10 A diagram of a Jefferson fracture.

160. Why do children under 8 years of age have a higher incidence of injuries at the craniovertebral border and more ligamentous injuries than older children?

Children younger than 8 years have a high fulcrum of neck motion and trauma to the spine will result in a greater proportion of ligamentous injuries and craniovertebral injuries than in older children.

161. What should be considered in a patient who presents less than 48 hours after intrathecal treatment with methotrexate with paraplegia, leg pain, sensory level, and bladder dysfunction?

Transverse myelitis from a rare idiosyncratic reaction to the intrathecal methotrexate. Also, consider a traumatic spinal subdural hematoma from the procedure.[77]

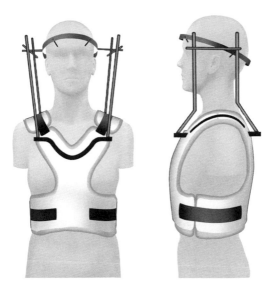

Fig. 6.11 Proper application and alignment of a halo vest device used for high cervical fractures.

162. A patient who is 2 hours postoperative from a routine lumbar laminectomy develops perineal numbness, extraordinary pain, and weakness in multiple muscle groups. Until proven otherwise, what is happening to this patient?

A spinal epidural hematoma.

163. What is the significance of the NASCIS trial?

The National Acute Spinal Cord Injury Studies (NASCIS) published in the 1990s demonstrated significant benefit in administering high doses of methylprednisolone early after spinal cord injury. The dose is 30 mg/kg IV (intravenous) over 15 minutes, a 45-minute pause, and then 5.4 mg/kg/h via continuous IV infusion over the next 23 hours. Sometimes the infusion can run 47 hours after the bolus if the therapy was started from 3 to 8 hours after injury.[78] The relative benefits of steroids following blunt spinal cord trauma have since been disproven with several more recent studies. Currently it is no longer considered a standard.

164. What is the emergent treatment of spinal cord compression from a tumor?

When the diagnosis is made, dexamethasone should be given immediately and a decompression should be considered if indicated.

165. What are the recent recommendations regarding the use of methylprednisolone in acute spinal cord injury (SCI)?

There is level 1a evidence (including four randomized control trials) that methylprednisolone is not effective in promoting neurologic recovery in acute SCI patients. There is also similar evidence that its use is associated with the development of medical complications in acute SCI.[79,80,81]

166. What is the emergent treatment of hypercalcemia from bone metastases?

Initial treatment involves hydration to improve urinary calcium output. Isotonic sodium chloride solution is used, because increasing sodium excretion increases calcium excretion as well. Addition of a loop diuretic inhibits tubular reabsorption of calcium, with furosemide having been used up to every 2 hours. Attention should be paid to other electrolytes (i.e., magnesium and potassium) during saline diuresis. These treatments work within hours and can lower serum calcium levels by 1 to 3 mg/dL within a day. Bisphosphonates (such as etidronate, pamidronate, alendronate, tiludronate, and risedronate) serve to block bone resorption over the next 24 to 48 hours by absorbance into the hydroxyapatite and by shortening the life span of osteoclasts.

167. What is autonomic hyperreflexia?

Exaggerated autonomic response to normally innocuous stimuli occurring in patients with spinal cord lesions above the T6 level (above the origin of the splanchnic outflow). Stimuli for autonomic hyperreflexia are bladder distension, colorectal stimulation (from fecal impaction), skin infections, and deep venous thromboses (DVTs). The classic triad is seen in 85% of cases and includes headache, hyperhidrosis, and cutaneous vasodilation. Treatment involves resolution of the offending stimulus, aggressive control of blood pressure, and anxiolytics to relieve muscle spasms and relax the bladder in some cases.[59]

168. Why is sacral sparing important in the setting of spinal cord injury?

It signifies that there is a partial, rather than complete, injury of the spinal cord with potential for some neurologic recovery. On exam, there is some sensation preserved in the perineal region. In the spinal cord, the caudad sensory and motor fibers are located more peripherally. Spinal cord contusion and ischemia usually damage the central tracts of the cord more so than the peripheral tracts.

169. What is spinal shock?

It occurs after acute spinal trauma when all the reflex activities of the spinal cord are depressed below the injured level, and it usually presents for 24 to 48 hours after the injury. Return of the reflexes below the injury level signifies the end of spinal shock. A physical examination cannot reliably distinguish an incomplete injury from a complete one until spinal shock has ended.[82]

170. The return of which reflex usually indicates the end of the spinal shock?

Bulbocavernous: contraction of the anal sphincter after digital pressure on the penis or clitoris or pulling on the Foley catheter.[82]

171. What is the American Spinal Injury Association (ASIA) scale for assessment of motor strength?[83,84,85,86,87]

- 0: no contraction or movement.
- 1: minimal movement.
- 2: Active movement, but not against gravity.
- 3: active movement against gravity.
- 4: active movement against partial resistance.
- 5: active movement against full resistance.

172. What is the Frankel classification of a spinal cord injury?

No function (A), sensory only (B), some sensory and motor preservation (C), useful motor function (D), and normal (E).[88]

173. What is nociceptive pain?

Nociceptive pain is pain that occurs when nociceptors are stimulated. The pain is typically well localized and constant, and it often has an aching or throbbing quality. A structural disorder, such as foraminal stenosis and disk herniation, typically stimulates the nerve endings.

174. What is neuropathic pain?

It is due to nerve damage or injury. The nerve is a source of pain itself although it is not stimulated. Pain increases with little stimulation. Examples are arachnoiditis and battered root.[89,90]

175. What drugs are best for nociceptive pain?

- Mild to moderate pain: NSAIDs and weak opioids.
- Moderate to severe pain: strong opioids.

176. What are the best medications for neuropathic pain?

Tricyclic antidepressants (TCAs), anticonvulsants, and cannabidiol (CBD).[89,90]

177. Which medications are best for chronic pain?

TCAs, anticonvulsants, opioids, and CBD.

178. Do opioids cause organ toxicity?

They might cause respiratory depression in patients with pulmonary disease and sleep apnea, but they are not organ toxic.[91]

179. For which spine problems can opioids be used?

They should not be used for nonspecific spine pain. They might be used if there is a well-defined stimulus that cannot be treated definitively, conservative treatment failure, and absence of significant psychologic illness or history of addiction or drug abuse. The drugs should not be refilled by phone.

180. What are the side effects of TCAs?

Daytime sedation, dry mouth, urinary retention, constipation, weight gain, blurry vision, and orthostatic hypotension. Selective serotonin reuptake inhibitors (SSRIs) might cause sexual dysfunction and irritability.

181. What is the role of muscle relaxants in chronic low back pain (LBP)?

They have a limited role. If there is an acute LBP in the setting of a chronic LBP, they can be used. However, they can be sedating or cause dependence; there is little evidence supporting that they can relax tight muscles.[92]

182. What is the role of sedative-hypnotics in chronic LBP?

In occasional sleep disturbance due to flares of chronic LBP they can be used (zolpidem). For chronic sleep problems of chronic LBP, trazodone or TCAs can be used.[92]

183. Which muscle relaxant is helpful for short-term use?

Cyclobenzaprine is similar to amitriptyline and is useful for sleep disturbance. Baclofen is effective for painful muscle spasm and acts centrally. Orphenadrine, methocarbamol, and tizanidine are also useful. Diazepam is too sedating and lorazepam is effective occasionally for spasm.[92]

184. Is there any role for antihistamines in spine pain?

They can be used for nausea, vomiting, and itching of opioids. They should not be used for sedation because there are better medications available.

185. What is meant by the term "reducible" when describing a fracture?

The term "reducible" refers to the ability to achieve normal osseous alignment and relieve compression on neural structures. Ligamentous reducible pathology such as inflammatory states or recent trauma must be given a trial of immobilization.[93]

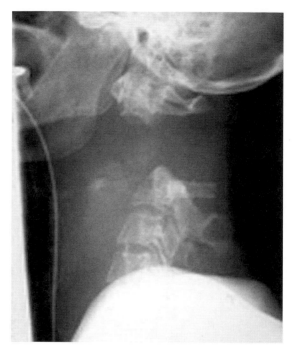

Fig. 6.12 An extreme case of atlantoaxial dislocation in a 14-year-old boy involved in an all-terrain vehicle accident.

186. In what traumatic condition is a cervical collar and/ or traction contraindicated and can actually precipitate additional neurologic injury?

Occipitoatlantal dislocation is usually caused by high-velocity accidents and a cervical collar should not be used because it reproduces the distractive mechanism of the injury. Likewise, cervical traction is contraindicated. Atlantoaxial dislocation is a condition that can be worsened with traction (**Figs. 6.12** and **6.13**).[94,95]

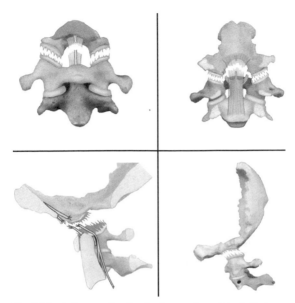

Fig. 6.13 A diagram showing the ligaments and facets that need to be disrupted in order for this type of dislocation to occur.

187. What is the purpose of awake fiberoptic intubation in a patient with cervical spine injury?

The awake fiberoptic intubation is to confirm that no new neurologic deficits have been incurred during the intubation process.

188. What are some other pharmacologic agents that show promising results in the treatment of acute SCI?

There is level 1b evidence that erythropoietin is effective and thyrotropin-releasing hormone may be effective in promoting neurologic recovery in acute SCI individuals.

There is level 2 evidence that a moderate dose (10 µg/kg/d) of granulocyte colony-stimulating factor (G-CSF) and riluzole may be effective in promoting motor and sensory recovery in acute SCI individuals.[96–101]

189. What are the main indications for thoracic or lumbar X-rays in a trauma patient?

A trauma patient should undergo thoracic or lumbar X-rays if they were thrown from a vehicle, fell from a height greater than 6 feet to the ground, complain of back pain, are unconscious or are unable to reliably describe their back pain, have altered mental status preventing the completion of an adequate examination, have an unknown mechanism of injury, or have other injuries that cast suspicion of a potential spine injury. Note that a CT scan through the area of bony abnormality or level of neurologic deficit should follow the completion of these X-rays.

190. What are the main indications for a spine MRI in a trauma patient?[102]

An MRI should be obtained on a trauma patient in the presence of the following conditions:

- Incomplete SCI with normal alignment seen on X-rays.
- Neurologic deterioration after closed reduction of a fracture.
- Neurologic deficit(s) not explained by radiographic findings, such as when the fracture level is different from the level of deficit, when no bony injury can be identified on X-rays or CT scan, or when there is a possible arterial dissection.
- Indications for nonemergent MRI include:
  - Inconclusive cervical spine radiography.
  - Significant midline paraspinal tenderness and inability to have flexion-extension X-rays.
  - Obtunded or comatose patients.

191. What are the main purpose of and requirement criteria for flexion and extension cervical spine X-rays in a trauma patient?

The main purpose of flexion and extension cervical spine X-rays is to disclose occult ligamentous instability. In cases of limited flexion due to paraspinal muscle spasm, a rigid collar should be prescribed and worn at all times. If the pain persists 2 to 3 weeks after the injury, the flexion-extension films should be repeated.

The required criteria for flexion and extension cervical spine X-rays include the presence of a cooperative patient free of mental impairment; there should be no subluxation greater than 3.5 mm at any level on cervical spine X-rays; and the patient should also be neurologically intact. Please note that this modality is no longer recommended in obtunded patients.[103]

192. What are some of the secondary injury mechanisms that may be involved in SCI patients?

Systemic shock caused by profound hypotension and bradycardia (often lasting for days) following cord injury can lead to compromise of an already damaged cord.

Local microcirculatory damage may be due to mechanical disruption of capillaries, leading to further hemorrhage, thrombosis, and loss of autoregulation.

Biochemical damage may occur due to excitotoxin release (glutamate), free radical production, arachidonic acid release, lipid peroxidation, eicosanoid production, cytokines, and electrolyte shifts.

193. Describe the three columns of Denis.

- **Anterior column**—formed by the anterior longitudinal ligament, the anterior annulus, and the anterior portion of the vertebral body.
- **Middle column**—consists of the posterior longitudinal ligament, the posterior portion of the annulus, and the posterior aspect of the vertebral body.
- **Posterior column**—includes the neural arch, facet joints and capsules, ligamentum flavum, and remaining ligamentous complex.

194. Describe the three types of instability defined by Denis.

- Mechanical (first degree)—May result in late kyphotic deformity. It requires external or operative stabilization.
- Neurologic (second degree)—Retropulsion of bone fragments predispose patients to increased risk for neurologic injury. Controversy related to operative stabilization.
- Mechanical/neurologic (third degree)—Develop after burst fractures with neurologic deficit(s) or fracture/dislocation. Highly unstable and therefore require operative decompression and stabilization.

195. What are the three types of fundamental injury pattern based on the AO classification?[104]

- Compression.
- Distraction.
- Axial torque.

196. When evaluating a patient with SCI, what are the three factors that are used in determining the most optimal treatment options based on the thoracolumbar injury classification and severity scale (TLICS)?[105]

- Injury morphology.
- Integrity of the posterior ligamentous complex.
- Neurologic status.

197. What are the three types of occipital condyle fractures?[106,107]

Occipital condyle fracture classification according to Anderson and Montesano includes the following:

- Type I injuries: comminuted fractures due to axial trauma.
- Type II injuries: extensions of linear basilar skull fractures.
- Type III injuries: avulsion fractures from varied mechanisms.

198. How are occipital condyle fractures typically treated?

Occipital condyle fractures are for the most part stable and typically treated with an external nonrigid orthosis (i.e., cervical collar such as a Miami J collar or Aspen collar) for a duration of 2 to 3 months or until the fracture is healed.

Type III fractures may present with instability; in such cases of significant displacement or in clinically symptomatic fractures, halo placement may be used. Operative interventions such as occipitocervical fusion are usually entertained when there are associated cervical fractures and/or ligamentous injuries.[106,107]

Degenerative

199. What is the most common reason for lumbar spine surgery in people older than 65 years of age?

Lumbar spinal stenosis (**Fig. 6.14**).[108]

200. What are the anatomical factors contributing to lumbar spinal stenosis?

Congenitally short pedicles, facet joint hypertrophy, disk space narrowing with upward migration of the superior articular process into the neural foramen, acute herniated disk, chronic calcified disk, disk margin osteophyte, thickening of ligamentum flavum, synovial cyst formation, and degenerative spondylolisthesis (**Fig. 6.15**).

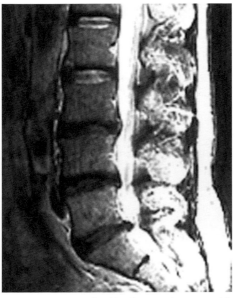

Fig. 6.14 An example of lumbar spinal stenosis with the worst level in this MRI being L5–S1.

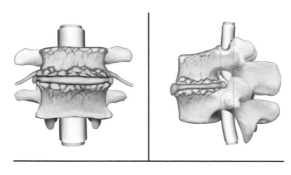

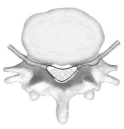

Fig. 6.15 A diagram showing how a degenerative disk can cause spinal stenosis through the shortening of disk space, osteophytes, and disk herniation.

201. What are some common immediate and delayed complications after a lumbar laminectomy?

CSF leakage, infection, hematoma, nerve injury, postlaminectomy spondylolisthesis, epidural fibrosis, and persistent pain.[109]

202. What are some of the common causes of atlantoaxial instability?

Rheumatoid arthritis, Down's syndrome, trauma, tumors, inborn errors of metabolism (e.g., mucopolysaccharidosis), infections, Morquio's syndrome, and Scott's syndrome.

203. What is the reoperation rate after initial cervical spine surgery?

2.5% per year, with ventral surgery having lower reoperation rates.[110]

204. What percentage of rheumatoid patients will experience atlantoaxial subluxation?

Approximately 25%.

205. What measurement of atlantodental interval (ADI) is considered abnormal in a normal adult, a normal child, and a patient with rheumatoid arthritis?

Three millimeters in an adult and 4 mm in a child. In a patient with rheumatoid arthritis, this distance (which is the distance from the posterior margin of the anterior ring of C1 to the anterior surface of the odontoid) can be used to monitor the patient over time. Various authors

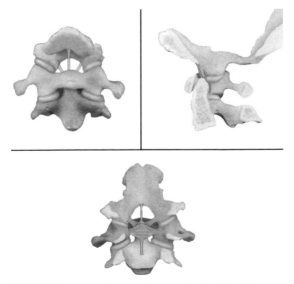

Fig. 6.16 A diagram showing the normal atlantodental interval and the normal ligaments at the C0–C1–C2 complex.

have recommended surgery when the ADI in rheumatoid patients is greater than 8 to 10 mm. In trauma, an interval of 3 to 5 mm implies rupture of the transverse ligament. An interval of 5 to 10 mm suggests additional incompetence of the alar ligaments. An interval of greater than 10 mm exists only if all other accessory odontoid ligaments are also ruptured (**Fig. 6.16**).

206. A patient with an intrathecal catheter for pain control presents with numbness and weakness in the lower extremities. What entity must be excluded and what is the best course of action?

Obtain imaging studies of the pertinent area in addition to the area where the catheter is believed to be located. Spinal catheter granuloma should be the top differential diagnosis and operative decompression and exploration may be necessary. Precipitated medication should also be in the differential diagnosis.[111,112]

207. Where do the majority of protruded thoracic disks occur?

Seventy-five percent of protruded thoracic disks occur below T8 and present most commonly with pain.[113]

208. What is happening in a dialysis patient who has an MRI and CT scan of the spine that resemble infection, but who has no laboratory markers or systemic signs of infection?

Renal destructive spondyloarthropathy.[114]

209. What diseases can result in bony softening and basilar impression?

Paget's disease, osteomalacia, hyperparathyroidism, osteogenesis imperfecta, renal rickets, and achondroplasia.

210. What are the indications for surgical intervention in rheumatoid arthritis?

Neurologic dysfunction and/or pain. If the predental space is greater than 8 mm, surgery should be considered as an option. Many patients with rheumatoid arthritis can be managed with cervical traction. If reduction has not occurred by the end of 5 days with traction, the lesion is considered irreducible. Reducible lesions are managed with a fusion stabilization procedure; irreducible lesions require decompression dictated by where impingement is occurring. Ventral decompression (if indicated) is performed before a dorsal stabilization.[115]

211. What is the mortality rate for rheumatoid arthritis?

17%.[116]

212. What is the most common inflammatory condition affecting the occipitocervical junction?

Rheumatoid arthritis.

213. What does canal elongation indicate in spondylolisthesis?

Canal elongation indicates fractures of the pars interarticularis in spondylolisthesis. Degenerative spondylolisthesis presents with spinal stenosis and an intact pars (**Fig. 6.17**).

214. What neurologic disease must always be kept in mind when making the diagnosis of cervical spondylotic myelopathy?

Amyotrophic lateral sclerosis (ALS). In ALS, sensory changes are conspicuously absent, tongue fasciculations may be seen, and atrophic weakness of the hands and forearms occurs early. With cervical spondylotic myelopathy, one may find neck and shoulder pain, sometimes intrascapular pain, and sensory changes.[117]

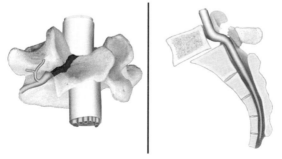

Fig. 6.17   A diagram showing a pars defect and spondylolisthesis at L5–S1. This would be a grade II spondylolisthesis.

215. What are the main clinical signs and symptoms of cervical spondylosis?

Axial pain, radiculopathy, and/or myelopathy.

216. The H-reflex is used to measure sensory conduction through nerve roots and most often to assess radiculopathy of which nerve root?

S1.

217. Diminished sensation over the medial malleolus suggests nerve root compromise at which level?

L4.

218. In acute cervical disk herniation, movement of the head in which direction accentuates the radicular pain?

In acute cervical disk herniation, lateral flexion of the head toward the side of the pain usually increases radicular pain because this motion aggravates the irritated nerve root by further decreasing the size of the intervertebral foramen.

219. What percentage of the normal adult population has some degree of straightening or reversal of cervical lordosis?

Approximately 16%.

220. What vertebral segment is most commonly affected with ossification of the posterior longitudinal ligament?

C5 is most commonly affected, followed by C4 and C6.[118]

221. How does tobacco use affect the spine?

Smoking accelerates osteoporosis, impairs blood supply to the vertebra, and impairs the metabolism of osteoblasts. These combined effects make smoking a risk factor for nonunion after attempted fusion.[119]

222. Describe osteoporosis, osteomalacia, and osteopenia.

Osteoporosis is a bone disease in which the amount of normally mineralized bone therapy unit volume decreases, which results in an increased risk of fractures. Osteomalacia is characterized by delayed or impaired mineralization of bone matrix. Rickets is osteomalacia in children. Osteopenia is a nonspecific term for decreased bone density radiologically.[120]

223. Describe the different types of osteoporosis.

Osteoporosis has been classified into primary and secondary types. Primary osteoporosis is subdivided into two types. Type 1 is seen in postmenopausal women 5 to 10 years after menopause. It predominantly affects the trabecular bone and results in fractures of the intertrochanteric hip and distal radius. Type 2 occurs due to aging and calcium deficiency in both women and men after the age of 70. It affects both cortical and trabecular bone and results in vertebral fractures, femoral neck fractures, and proximal tibia and humerus fractures. Secondary osteoporosis is a type of osteoporosis due to endocrinopathies or other disease states.

224. What are the most common causes of secondary osteoporosis?

Endocrine disorders, Cushing's disease, hyperthyroidism, hypogonadism, diabetes, hyperparathyroidism, bone marrow disorders, lymphoma, multiple myeloma, and metastatic disease.[121]

225. What are the major recommendations for physicians in relation to osteoporosis?

Counsel all women about the risk of osteoporosis; recommend bone mineral density testing for postmenopausal women with fractures. Recommend weight-bearing exercises. Counsel patients to refrain from smoking and alcohol intake.

226. What pharmacologic therapies are currently available for osteoporosis?[122,123]

Bisphosphonates. Contraindications include history of breast cancer, uterine cancer, and thromboembolism. Most common ones include the following:

- Alendronate (Fosamax).
- Risedronate (Actonel) or risedronate delayed-release (Atelvia).
- Ibandronate (Boniva).
- Zoledronic acid (Reclast).

Other agents include:

- Selective estrogen receptor modulators (SERMs): raloxifene (Evista).
- Parathyroid hormone: teriparatide (Forteo).
- Calcitonin-salmon (Fortical, Miacalcin).
- Hormone replacement therapy (HRT).
- Denosumab (Prolia) is a humanized monoclonal antibody directed against the receptor activator of the nuclear factor-kappa B ligand (RANKL), which is a key mediator of the resorptive phase of bone remodeling.

227. What are the treatment options for painful vertebral compression fractures?

A short course of a few days of bed rest, bracing, and/or pain medication. Vertebroplasty and kyphoplasty might be useful in selected patients who fail conservative treatments.[124]

228. What is the lowest accessible level for an ACDF?

Usually, T1–T2 can be reached without a manubriotomy or sternotomy. Obtaining a CT scan with sagittal reconstructions will help determine if the approach is feasible.[125]

229. After a routine ACDF at C6–C7, a patient complains of pain going down the outside of the arm. What is the phenomenon being described and how should it be managed?

C5/C6 dermatomal pain and/or palsy are not uncommon after ACDF at any level. It is thought that the palsy is caused by traction to the C5 nerve root because it is a short nerve compared with the other nerves below it. Numerous theories exist as to the underlying cause of postoperative C5 palsy, but there is no strong evidence to support any single pathomechanism. Most patients with postoperative C5 palsy experience full recovery within 6 months, although many patients continue to have some residual pain or neurologic deficit in certain cases. It is helpful to *not* use a cervical collar in the postoperative period, as the collar increases the traction on the nerve. A short course of steroids may be helpful as well. It is recommended to reimage the neck if the pain/palsy persists to rule out easily repairable causes of pain such as reherniation, missed osteophyte, or next level disease.[126]

230. In an anterior cervical diskectomy, what maneuver may decrease the incidence of right laryngeal nerve injury?

After the retractor blades are inserted, the cuff on the endotracheal tube may be deflated for a moment and then reinflated gently to produce a barely airtight seal between the cuff and the trachea. This will reduce pressure on the nerve and reduce the chances of a recurrent laryngeal nerve injury. Nerve injury probability increases with duration of procedure. Ninety minutes is acceptable for a one-level ACDF, with 45 minutes for each additional level.

231. How deep should the cadaveric bone or polyetheretherketone (PEEK) interbody cage be inserted during an ACDF?

The bone or cage should be countersunk ~1 mm; confirming this with one's index finger is sufficient. Countersinking will ensure that the graft does not extrude in the future.

232. How many weeks of conservative treatment are acceptable for patients with lumbar or cervical radiculopathy without significant motor weakness?

Six weeks of conservative therapy (physical therapy, oral pain medication, and alteration of activity) may allow the condition to resolve.

233. Describe the basic principles of the Kirkaldy-Willis three-joint complex theory for degenerative spine disease.

Each level within the spine is composed of a three-joint complex that is affected in the degenerative process. This is comprised of one intervertebral disk and two zygapophyseal joints (dorsal articulating joints). Degeneration of any one joint leads to degeneration of the other two, initiating a cascade that leads to spinal degenerative disease.[127]

234. Name the three commonly accepted stages of degenerative spine disease.

- Dysfunction stage.
- Destabilization stage.
- Restabilization stage.

235. Describe the dysfunctional stage.

This early stage is characterized by synovial reaction in the dorsal joint and small tears in the intervertebral disks. There may be some minor or absent clinical symptoms that are best treated conservatively. In more severe cases, the patients can present with a radiculopathy necessitating decompression such as diskectomy.

236. Describe the destabilization stage.

This stage is characterized by greater degeneration in the three-joint complex, manifesting as laxity and subluxation in the dorsal joints and progressive disk degeneration. There is also abnormal spinal motion. Compounded by advanced disk degeneration and disk height reduction, findings may progress to spondylolisthesis. General treatments involve core strengthening and a flexibility program to stabilize and normalize the dysfunctional motion segment. In more severe cases, the patients can present with axial mechanical back pain due to instability, which may be associated with radiculopathy as well as necessitating fusion with or without decompression of the spinal segment involved.

237. Describe the restabilization stage.

This later stage is characterized by reduced instability via osteophyte formation secondary to a prior increased joint laxity and loss of disk height. Resolution of symptoms can occur due to gradually decreased spinal motion. There may be radiculopathy from spinal nerve entrapment or claudication symptoms from central canal and lateral recess stenosis.

238. What percentage of disk herniations are far lateral versus paracentral and what is the difference in their respective presentations?

As many as 90% of herniated disks are paracentral and affect the nerve root that corresponds to the lower vertebral level; for example, a typical L4/L5 disk herniation would cause symptoms referable to the L5 nerve root. On the other hand, ~10% of herniated disks are far lateral and impinge upon the nerve root that corresponds to the upper vertebral level. A far lateral disk herniation at L4/L5 would therefore be expected to cause symptoms relative to the L4 root.

239. What is the primary goal of surgery in patients with cervical myelopathy?

The goal of surgery is to arrest the progression of myelopathy through adequate decompression of the stenosed canal. Once patients are clinically myelopathic, complete return of function or remission of symptoms almost never occurs.[7,44]

240. Describe a four-point scale of grading facet osteoarthritis.[128]

1. Normal facet joint space.
2. Narrowing of the facet joint with possible small osteophyte formation and mild hypertrophy.
3. Further narrowing of the joint space with moderate osteophyte and hypertrophy and early subarticular bony erosion.
4. Further narrowing of the joint space with large osteophyte and/or severe hypertrophy and severe subarticular bony erosion leading to subchondral cysts.

241. Describe the advantages and limitations of the direct lateral interbody fusion approach to the lumbar spine.[129,130,131]

The main advantages of this approach include:

- Minimally invasive approach with a small incision.
- Reduced length of stay.
- Reduced blood loss.
- Maintains posterior structures intact.
- Avoids risks of an anterior access surgery (anterior lumbar interbody fusion [ALIF]).
- Achieves diskectomy, graft size, and fusion surface comparable to an ALIF.

In addition to general risk factors and limitations of lumbar fusion, the following may apply specifically to this approach. The main limitations of this approach include:

- Inability to access the L5/S1 level through a traditional direct lateral route (without modification).
- Potential damage to the lumbar/sacral plexus, generally leading to a lumbar plexus neuritis postoperatively; hence, neuromonitoring is essential during this approach.

- Transient postoperative thigh weakness and/or sensory loss may be observed.
- In certain cases, the following may still occur: nonfusion, symptoms may persist or become exacerbated.

242. Describe the main advantages and disadvantages of the posterolateral (transpedicular) approach to the thoracic spine.

Main advantages include: favorable results for lateral herniated thoracic disks; this approach does not require transpleural or transmediastinal dissection; there is no violation of the rib cage or ligation of the neurovascular bundle; the technique offers a potential for less operative time and less bleeding and is familiar to most neurosurgeons.

The main disadvantage is the limited visibility of the midline of the anterior spinal canal. Another potential disadvantage is the fact that resection of the entire pedicle, the facet joint, and part of the vertebral body may lead to instability and may require fusion in certain cases.

243. What are common indications for surgical intervention (nonneuromodulative) in failed back syndrome?

Neurocompressive process such as severe spinal stenosis with intractable neurogenic claudication that cannot be effectively treated without adequate neurodecompressive surgery; for example, a disk reherniation.

Overt, intractable, and incapacitating lumbar segmental instability, such as high-grade spondylolisthesis.

The presence of epidural fibrosis alone, despite the patient's complaints, is never an indication for surgical decompressive therapy.[132]

244. What are common treatment options of failed back syndrome, postlaminectomy syndrome, or epidural fibrosis (scar formation)?[132]

Conservative treatments include:

- Patient education.
- Short-term bed rest.
- Physical and occupational therapy: intensive physical conditioning with restitution of muscle tone and full range of motion.
- Depression and anxiety management and drug abuse correction.

Medication options include gabapentin, carbamazepine, amitriptyline, NSAIDs, and steroids.

In cases of neuropathic pain, the following procedures may also be offered should the patient have failed prior conservative treatments: neuroablative procedures (i.e., dorsal rhizotomies, dorsal root ganglionectomies, anterolateral cordotomies), neuroaugmentive procedures (i.e., implanted dorsal column stimulators and deep brain stimulators), or alternatively implanted intraspinal drug infusion therapies.

245. What are the commonly accepted main advantages and disadvantages of the lateral (i.e., extracanal) approach through a paramedian incision for a far lateral or foraminal disk herniation in the lumbar spine?

Advantages: the facet joint is preserved (facet removal combined with diskectomy may lead to instability) and muscle retraction is easier.

Disadvantages: unfamiliar approach for most surgeons and the nerve roots cannot be followed medial to lateral.

246. List three mechanisms by which a patient presenting with an L4/L5 disk herniation can have an isolated L4 radiculopathy.

1. A far lateral disk herniation can impinge on the exiting nerve root (as opposed to the traversing root).
2. A migrated disk fragment can also clinically present in a similar fashion.
3. A conjoint root is an anatomical variant that can be confounding when trying to correlate the examination with the imaging findings.

247. How is sacroiliac joint (SIJ) dysfunction identified on physical examination?[133]

- Fortin's sign: tenderness when palpating the SIJ.
- Pelvic distraction: in supine position, application of posterior pressure on both anterior superior iliac spine (ASIS) points simultaneously causes pain in the SIJ area posteriorly.
- Compression test: in lateral recumbent position, application of pressure directly down on the superior hip's lateral aspect causes pain in the SIJ area posteriorly.
- FABER test: in supine position, application of flexion, abduction, and external rotation of the leg on the affected

SIJ side, while stabilizing the contralateral side, causes pain in the affected SIJ area.

- Thigh thrust: in supine position, with the contralateral hip flexed and stabilized, application of pressure down on the ASIS of the ipsilateral (affected) side causes pain in the affected SIJ area.
- Gaenslen's test: in lateral recumbent position, the contralateral hip is flexed maximally, and the ipsilateral or affected hip is extended while maintaining stability of the pelvis; this will cause pain in the affected SIJ area.

248. Describe imaging findings that suggest SIJ dysfunction requiring potential intervention.

On modalities such as X-rays, CT, or MRI, the presence of significant degenerative signs, such as evidence of sclerosis, osteophytes, subchondral cysts, or vacuum phenomenon, may be seen. Other disease processes of the SIJ may also be identified such as significant infection, SIJ disruption, and presence of neoplasm or fracture dislocation. Sacroiliac joint disruption manifests as pain in the context of asymmetric widening of SI joints on CT or X-rays, or the presence of significant contrast leakage during a diagnostic SIJ block.

Note that presence of radiographic evidence of degeneration is not required for the diagnosis of SIJ dysfunction, since most cases with hypermobility are due to extra-articular dysfunction.[133]

Neoplastic, Infectious, Vascular

249. After a minor upper respiratory illness, a patient develops acute ascending neuropathy, characterized by hyporeflexia. An MRI shows enhancement of the cauda equina nerve roots and CSF examination reveals protein elevated to over 400 mg/L. What is the diagnosis?

Guillain-Barré syndrome (GBS). MRI of the lumbosacral spine shows enhancement of the cauda equina nerve roots in 95% of patients with typical cases of GBS.[11]

250. What is the most common cause of acute flaccid paralysis in Western countries?

GBS. Seventy-five percent of patients have an antecedent event 1 to 4 weeks before the onset of weakness (most commonly this is a gastrointestinal or respiratory infection).[11]

251. What is the most common location of a spinal epidural abscess?

The thoracic spine. The majority are located posterior to the spinal cord. Spinal epidural abscess should be considered in any patient who presents with backache, fever, and spinal tenderness.[134]

252. What is the most common organism found in a spinal epidural abscess?

Staphylococcus aureus.[135]

253. What is the most common location of vertebral osteomyelitis?

The lumbar spine. Vertebral osteomyelitis is seen in IV drug abusers, patients with diabetes, and hemodialysis patients. The most common organism is *S. aureus* (**Fig. 6.18**).[134]

254. What part of the vertebra does Pott's disease have a predilection for?

Tuberculous spondylitis has a predilection for the vertebral body and spares the posterior elements.[136]

255. What is suggested when a spinal lesion is destroying the disk space?

A characteristic radiographic finding that helps distinguish infection from metastatic disease is that destruction of the disk space is highly suggestive of infection, whereas, in general, a tumor will not cross the disk space.

256. What is Grisel's syndrome?

Spontaneous subluxation of the atlantoaxial joint secondary to parapharyngeal infection. It is thought to occur through direct hematogenous spread from the inflammatory exudates to the atlantoaxial articulations. Grisel's syndrome has been associated with tonsillitis, mastoiditis, retropharyngeal abscess, otitis media, and infected tooth abscesses.[137]

257. What is the usual initial event in neurosyphilis?

Meningitis. Within 2 years of primary infection, 25% of all untreated patients develop acute symptomatic meningitis. Symptomatic meningitis responds to penicillin. Spinal syphilis presents as progressive paraplegia, radicular pain, and

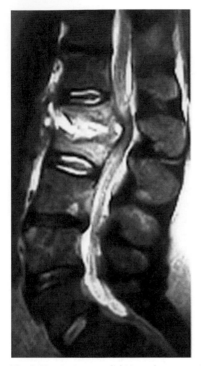

Fig. 6.18 An intense diskitis and osteomyelitis at L1–L2 causing conus compression.

upper limb atrophy. CSF shows a lymphocytosis, increased protein, increased gammaglobulin, and a positive syphilis serology.[138]

258. What is the most common intramedullary spinal cord tumor?

An ependymoma. Astrocytoma is a close second (some references put them with equal frequency).[139,140]

259. In resecting an intramedullary spinal cord tumor, what is a sure way to recognize the midline if the tumor is deforming the normal spinal cord anatomy?

The best way to recognize the posterior midline is by identifying the dorsal root entry zones bilaterally.

260. Is a dumbbell-shaped spinal cord tumor seen with neurofibromatosis type 1 (NF1) or 2 (NF2)?

It is seen with both NF1 (neurofibromas) and NF2 (schwannomas).[141]

261. What types of nerves do neurofibromas generally arise from?

The sensory nerve roots. Sometimes it is necessary to sacrifice the dorsal rootlets involved with the tumor.

262. Until proven otherwise, a mass behind the dens is what?

A chordoma must be ruled out; however, in a patient with a history of rheumatoid arthritis, a benign pannus is also in the differential diagnosis.

263. What are some characteristics of chordoma?

Chordomas are slowly growing, expansile tumors that infiltrate local bone and adjacent soft tissues, with a high chance of local recurrence or seeding after resection. Chordomas of the craniocervical junction and upper cervical spine are challenging, not only because of their rarity, but also because of their propensity to recur and their difficult location. Because they are often midline tumors, most can be approached by midline transoral and extended transoral techniques.[142]

264. What cranial nerve palsy can be present with a chordoma?

Chordomas presenting with sixth cranial nerve palsies are not uncommon.

265. What is the most common primary spinal tumor and why is the answer not multiple myeloma?

Chordoma is the most common primary malignancy found in the adult spine, placing osteosarcoma in second place.

Multiple myeloma is a systemic disease with spinal manifestation, but it is not a primary spinal tumor. Multiple myeloma is considered the most common primary malignancy of bone, appendicular and axial skeleton combined.[143,144]

266. When should you consider selective arteriography and embolization in the treatment of spinal tumors?

Selective arterial embolization is employed in the treatment of highly vascular lesions, aneurysmal bone cyst, angiosarcoma, arterial vascular malformations, renal cell carcinoma metastases, schwannoma, hemangiopericytoma, or other neural tumors requiring sacrifice of the vertebral artery.

267. Which malignant primary spine tumors have the best and worst survival rates?

Chondrosarcoma and solitary plasmocytoma have the best survival rates in primary malignant spinal tumors; osteosarcoma and lymphoma have the worst survival rates.

268. What are some features of osteosarcomas?

Most patients have local pain, and plain radiographs of the spine show osteoblastic and osteolytic activity. Tumors frequently start in the vertebral body and extend posteriorly. Ostcosarcoma has a bimodal age of onset with a peak incidence in the third decade of life for primary lesions and a second peak after 60 years old for secondary lesions due to conditions such as Paget's disease of bone, fibrous dysplasia, benign brain tumors, and retinoblastoma.[145]

269. What type of mass frequently involves the posterior elements and can present as a palpable soft tissue mass?

Chondrosarcoma.[146]

270. Where do chordomas commonly occur?

Sacrococcygeal region (50%), cranial base (35%), or vertebrae (15%).[143,147]

271. Chordomas are remnants from which embryonic tissue?

The notochord.[143,147]

272. What type of bone tumor has radiographic features of septations and fluid levels?

Aneurysmal bone cyst.[148]

273. What are some masses that grow in the sacrum?

Chordoma, giant cell tumor, metastases, myeloma, neurofibroma, aneurysmal bone cyst, chondrosarcoma, osteoblastoma, and osteosarcoma.

274. How does one determine the best surgical procedure for the treatment of sacrum tumors and how can one preserve continence postoperatively?

Surgical resection depends on the area of the sacrum invaded by the tumor. Most distal sacral tumors S3 and below will be treated with a single posterior resection. A combined anterior and posterior resection will be necessary to control sacral tumors involving the S1 and S2 segments or the entire sacrum. Preservation of all sacral nerve roots on one side can provide the patient with near-normal bowel, bladder, and sexual functions. If bilateral multiple nerve root resection is necessary for tumor control, then continence can still be preserved if the S2 nerve roots can be salvaged. Rigid spinopelvic fixation is required for postoperative stabilization and mobility.

275. During an anterior approach for complete sacrectomy, what factors should be considered?

The internal iliac vessels should be ligated during the anterior approach to control life-threatening bleeding that can occur after completion of the posterior resection as the pelvis will hinge on the pubis symphysis. The patient usually has postoperative bowel and bladder incontinence after an anterior sacral resection. A diverting colostomy and ureterostomy should be performed at the same time as the anterior resection.[149]

276. What should be considered when scoliosis presents with pain?

An osteoid osteoma may be present. Clinical symptoms include painful scoliosis, focal or radicular pain, gait disturbance, and muscle atrophy. A history of painful scoliosis is important and should point to the diagnosis of axial osteoid osteoma, particularly because idiopathic scoliosis is usually not associated with pain. Osteoid osteoma presents with intense night pain that is relieved by aspirin. This is in contrast with other tumors that produce a dull pain (like osteoblastoma).[150]

277. What bone tumors grow in the posterior elements of the spine?

Aneurysmal bone cyst, osteoid osteoma, and osteoblastoma. Aneurysmal bone cysts may display a fluid level, indicative of hemorrhage and sedimentation. Aneurysmal bone cysts are highly vascular lesions that may be cured with surgery and bone curettage.[148]

278. Most cases of osteoid osteoma present in what part of the vertebra?

In the lamina and/or pedicle.[150]

279. Where in the spine do osteochondromas seem to grow more often?

At C2. When growing from the posterior, elements may present as a palpable mass; when growing anteriorly, they may present as dysphagia and hoarseness with vascular involvement.[151]

280. What are the most common neoplasms seen at the filum terminale?

Myxopapillary ependymoma and, less commonly, paraganglioma.

281. What is the most common tumor to seed along the subarachnoid space in children?

Medulloblastoma.

282. Decompressive surgery for metastatic spine disease is usually *not* offered to which patients?

Patients with transection of the cord, more than 12 hours of paraplegia, sphincter loss of more than 24 hours, major sensory loss, or uncontrolled metastatic disease.

283. Which is the most common site for spinal meningiomas?

Thoracic (80%) and cervical (15%) (**Fig. 6.19**).[152]

284. What is the defining feature of a malignant meningioma?

Invasion of neural tissue.

285. What percentage of patients with spinal hemangioblastomas will have von Hippel–Lindau (VHL) syndrome?

25 to 40% (**Fig. 6.20**).[153]

286. What percentage of patients with VHL syndrome will have pheochromocytomas that may require excision or perioperative sympathetic blockade?

10 to 20%.[154]

287. What cranial nerve is usually the earliest one affected in a case of a glomus jugulare tumor?

The facial nerve.

288. Back pain at night should be treated as what condition until proven otherwise?

Tumor invasion of the spine.

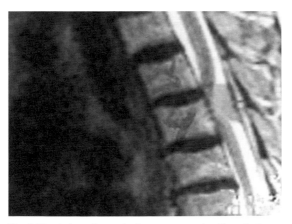

Fig. 6.19 A thoracic meningioma compressing the spinal cord. This patient presented with right-sided weakness.

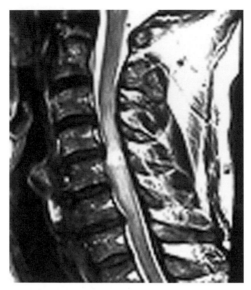

Fig. 6.20 A von Hippel–Lindau patient with a cervical spinal cord hemangioblastoma.

289. Osteoid osteoma is defined as a bone tumor less than what size in diameter?

Two centimeters. Any lesion larger than this is defined as an osteoblastoma.[150]

290. In what bone tumors may angiography be helpful?

Aneurysmal bone cyst and hemangioma. These are tumors that can be treated with embolization.[148]

291. What type of bone tumors can involve the sacrum?

Giant cell tumor, chordoma, and Ewing's sarcoma.

292. What is the most common spinal vascular malformation?

The dural arteriovenous fistula.[155]

293. Why do type I spinal arteriovenous malformations (AVMs) more commonly have lower extremity involvement as opposed to other spinal AVMs?

Intradural spinal vascular malformations (II–IV) develop during embryogenesis and present in an even distribution in the entire spine as opposed to the acquired type I lesions. Type 1 spinal AVMs are typically located in the thoracic and lumbar spine. Type I (or dural) arteriovenous fistula represent ~70% of AVMs of the spinal cord. They can present with back pain, leg weakness, and sensory deficits. To confirm the diagnosis of spinal AVM, selective spinal angiography is required.[156,157]

294. What are the differences between neurogenic and vascular claudication?

Neurogenic claudication (NC) has a dermatomal distribution of pain; vascular claudication (VC) is in the distribution of the vascular supply of the muscles. NC sensory loss is dermatomal, whereas VC is in the stocking distribution. In NC, coughing may reproduce pain and variable amounts of exercise will bring about the pain along with maintenance of a given posture for long periods. In VC, the pain is brought about with a fixed amount of exercise. More patients with NC than VC have pain on standing at rest; relief of walking symptoms with standing is typical with VC. Relief with rest is almost immediate with VC, but more gradual with NC. Discomfort on lifting is more common with NC. Foot pallor is marked with VC, peripheral pulses are decreased with VC, and skin temperature of the feet is decreased with VC. The "bicycle test" can be used to differentiate NC from VC; patients with NC can tolerate much longer periods of exercise on a bicycle than patients with VC.[158]

295. What is Cobb's syndrome?

Cobb's syndrome is a rare noninherited disorder that involves the association of spinal angiomas or AVMs with congenital, cutaneous vascular lesions in the same dermatome.[159]

296. Where is the watershed zone of the spinal cord?

The midthoracic region (T6) has a tenuous vascular supply and is described as the "watershed zone" of the spinal cord.

297. Thrombosis of which artery produces the unique syndrome of ipsilateral hypoglossal palsy and crossed hemiplegia?

Thrombosis of the anterior spinal artery.

298. Stridor and respiratory distress immediately after an ACDF should raise suspicion for what complication?

Vessel injury during the procedure and/or inadequate hemostasis during closing. Immediate evaluation and reexploration may be necessary.

299. What are the indications and contraindications for surgical intervention in patients with spinal metastasis?

Indications for surgical intervention include the following:

- Unknown primary and no tissue diagnosis (consider needle biopsy first).
- Unstable spine.
- Deficit(s) due to spinal deformity or compression by bone rather than tumor (compression fractures).
- Failure of radiation therapy (usually in radioresistant tumors such as renal cell carcinoma metastasis and melanoma).
- Recurrence after maximal radiation therapy.

Contraindications for surgery (relative) include the following:

- Very radiosensitive tumors (multiple myeloma, lymphoma) not previously irradiated.
- Total paralysis for greater than 24 hours.
- Expected survival less than 4 months.
- Multiple lesions at multiple levels.
- Patient unable to tolerate surgery due to systemic or medical causes.

Congenital and Pediatric

300. What part of the embryo develops into the dorsal root ganglia?

Neural crest cells.

301. What factors have been associated with neural tube defects?

- Geography.
- Season of conception.
- Maternal age (both older and younger).
- Socioeconomic status.
- Zinc deficiency.
- Folic acid deficiency.
- Maternal diabetes.
- Elevated maternal temperature during the first month of gestation.
- Alcohol abuse during the first month of pregnancy.
- Maternal use of valproic acid.

302. At approximately what days of gestation do the anterior and posterior neuropores close?

At 24 and 26 days, respectively.

303. How long can a myelomeningocele surgery be safely deferred?

Up to 72 hours after birth of the child. This delay may be important to stabilize a critically ill child. Myelomeningoceles repaired before 48 hours may have decreased incidence of ventriculitis and infection. It is usually routine practice to close the defect within 48 hours using antibiotics to control infection.

304. Is the exposed neural tissue of myelomeningoceles functional?

Yes. The placode may become desiccated with prolonged exposure to the air and should be covered with a wet dressing. Betadine is toxic and should be avoided.[160]

305. In a patient with a repaired myelomeningocele, the presentation of rapidly progressive scoliosis, weakness of the upper extremities, spasticity, and an ascending motor loss in the lower extremities should raise the suspicion of what?

Hydromyelia (dilation of the central canal of the spinal cord) may be a consequence of untreated or inadequately treated hydrocephalus. Most of these patients have a shunt and it is crucial to determine if the shunt is working properly in these cases.[161]

306. What is the difference between hydromyelia and syringomyelia?

Hydromyelia refers to dilations of the central canal that are at least partially lined by ependymal cells. Syringomyelia refers to all other cavities of the spinal cord outside of the central canal.[58,161]

307. What is hydrosyringomyelia?

Hydrosyringomyelia is a term to describe the pathologic findings of asymmetric cavitation of the central canal lined by both ependymal and glial tissue.

308. What other problems may go unnoticed in a newborn with an incomplete evaluation of myelomeningocele?

Diastematomyelia and/or a thickened filum terminale.[162]

309. What are the MRI criteria for spinal cord tethering?

Termination of the conus below the L3 vertebral body and a filum thicker than 2 mm. In patients with demonstrated low-lying conus, the presence of fat within the filum is suggestive of cord tethering. When the thickened filum and low-lying conus are demonstrated, surgical release of the tethered cord is justified even in the absence of neurologic impairments.

310. What diagnosis should be considered in an infant who presents with recurrent episodes of gram-negative meningitis despite successful antibiotic treatments?

Dermal sinus. The incidence of dermal sinus is ~1 in 2,500 live births. A cervical dermal sinus may accompany a posterior fossa dermoid, and MRI of the brain is crucial in working up the patient. Dermal sinuses of the sacrococcygeal region are often difficult to differentiate from pilonidal sinuses. MRI can confirm the presence of intraspinal extension.[163]

311. What is the classic triad of Klippel-Feil syndrome?

Low posterior hairline, short neck, and limitation of neck motion. The Klippel-Feil syndrome is associated with deficits in the genitourinary and cardiopulmonary systems as well as with congenital deficits of the skeletal and nervous systems. Other associated abnormalities include scoliosis, spina bifida, anomalies of the kidneys and the ribs, and cleft palate. The disorder may also be associated with abnormalities of the head and face, skeleton, muscles, brain and spinal cord, arms, legs, and fingers.[164,165]

312. All patients with Klippel-Feil syndrome should have an ultrasound examination of which system?

The renal system.[164,165]

313. In the normal adult patient, where does the conus end? Where does the thecal sac end?

L2 and S2, respectively.

314. What is the accepted diameter of a congenitally narrow cervical canal?

Any cervical canal diameter less than 12 mm.

315. What are congenital kyphosis type I and type II?

Congenital kyphosis type I involves failure of vertebral body formation, most commonly in the thoracolumbar transition area of T11–L2. Congenital kyphosis type II results from failure of vertebral segmentation. The presentation is typically in childhood with worsening kyphosis and neurologic deficits such as neurogenic bladder, lower-extremity weakness, and paresthesias. Spinal fusion is the treatment of choice.

316. What is the differential diagnosis of vertebra plana (mild flattening of the vertebral body)?

1. Eosinophilic granuloma.
2. Osteomyelitis.
3. Neoplasms such as Ewing's sarcoma, giant cell tumor, or lymphoma.
4. Aneurysmal bone cyst.
5. Advanced osteoporosis.

317. Os odontoideum can be seen in which conditions?

Down's syndrome, Morquio's syndrome, and Klippel-Feil syndrome.[166]

318. Which skeletal abnormalities can be seen with a Chiari I malformation?

Platybasia, basilar invagination, and Klippel-Feil syndrome.

319. What are some developmental and/or acquired causes of atlantoaxial instability?

Inborn errors of metabolism, Down's syndrome, infection, rheumatoid arthritis, traumatic dislocation, tumors such as neurofibromatosis, fetal warfarin syndrome, and Conradi's syndrome.

320. What is the most common site for an encephalocele?

The occipital area.

321. What determines the prognosis for encephalocele patients?

The prognosis of encephaloceles is directly proportional to the amount of brain found within the defect. Because about half of these patients have hydrocephalus, early CSF diversion is critical in preventing CSF leakage and infection.[145]

322. What are some types of occult spinal dysraphism?

Diastematomyelia, neurenteric cyst, lipomyelomeningocele, lipoma, dermoid cyst, dermal sinus tract, and tethered cord.

323. What is the ratio of incidence of myelomeningoceles compared with meningoceles?

The myelomeningocele is ~10 to 20 times more common.[160]

324. What is a type I split cord malformation (SCM) according to the Pang unified theory?

Type I SCM refers to two hemicords, each housed within its own dural tube separated by a dural, sheathed, rigid osseocartilaginous septum.[167,168]

325. What is a type II SCM?

Type II SCM refers to two hemicords housed within a single dural sheath separated only by a nonrigid fibrous sheath.[168]

326. How long should conservative therapy be instituted for a dermal sinus tract?

Dermal sinus tracts should be surgically excised once the diagnosis is made. There is no role for conservative therapy.[169]

327. What is the difference between basilar invagination and basilar impression?

Basilar invagination is a primary developmental defect that involves prolapse of the vertebral column into the base of the skull. It is often associated with developmental anomalies of the region, such as occipitalization, assimilation, and block vertebra.

Basilar impression is an acquired form of basilar invagination caused by softening of the skull. It generally manifests in diseases such as osteogenesis imperfecta, rickets, hyperparathyroidism, Paget's disease, and rheumatoid arthritis.

In contrast to basilar invagination, in basilar impression there is enfolding of the squama occipitalis; as a result, the posterior fossa floor becomes elevated and the margin of the foramen magnum curves upward. On the other hand, both could be associated with secondary hindbrain herniation and the development of syringohydromyelia.[170]

328. What are some cervical spinal abnormalities associated with Down's syndrome?

Up to 14 to 24% of patients with Down's syndrome will have atlantoaxial instability (with an atlas to dens ratio or atlantodental interval [ADI] greater than or equal to 4.5 mm). These patients, however, are symptomatic in only 1% of cases. Other abnormalities seen include os odontoideum, hypoplastic odontoid process with incomplete formation of the cruciate ligament, and rotatory atlantoaxial subluxation.[171]

329. Describe some major theories of formation of the intramedullary cyst in syringomyelia.[172,173,174,175]

1. Gardner's hydrodynamic ("water-hammer") theory postulates that the systolic pulsations are transmitted with each heartbeat from the intracranial cavity to the central canal.
2. The Williams theory is that maneuvers that raise CSF pressure (Valsalva or coughing, for example) cause "hydrodissection" through the spinal cord tissue. It is also referred to as the venous pressure gradient theory, where there is a difference between intracranial pressure and spinal pressure caused by a valvelike action at the foramen magnum. This scenario is believed to be more common in noncommunicating syringomyelia.

3. Oldfield's systolic pressure theory is also referred to as the cerebellar tonsils theory. This theory postulates that downward movement of the cerebellar tonsils during systole creates oscillations that cause a piston effect in the spinal subarachnoid space that acts on the surface of the spinal cord and forces CSF through the perivascular and interstitial spaces (Virchow-Robin spaces) into the syrinx, raising intramedullary pressure.

Cases

■ Case 1

A 67-year-old diabetic woman presents to the emergency room with increasing back pain and fever. An MRI is performed (**Fig. 6.21**). What is the diagnosis and what are the next steps in the case of this patient?

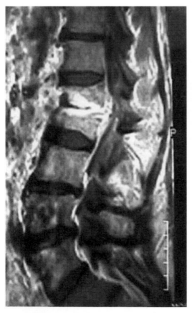

Fig. 6.21   Sagittal T1-weighted MRI with contrast.

■ Case 1 Answer

The patient is suffering from a diskitis at L1–L2. The patient should be admitted to the intensive care unit and blood cultures should be taken. Surgery should be planned quickly, and all necessary preoperative tests such as an electrocardiogram, chest X-ray, and coagulation studies should be expedited and not delay surgery. The goals of the surgery are to decompress the nerve roots in the area of L1–L2, obtain cultures, resect the infected disk, and definitively stabilize the area. An infectious disease consult should be obtained and antibiotics should be started empirically in the immediate postoperative period. The antibiotics should be tailored to the cultures taken at surgery once those results are available. A retroperitoneal approach will provide access to the disk space. A cage is used in the area of the corpectomies at L1 and L2 and screws fasten the rods from T12 to L3. The postoperative MRI and CT scans are shown in **Figs. 6.22** and **6.23**.

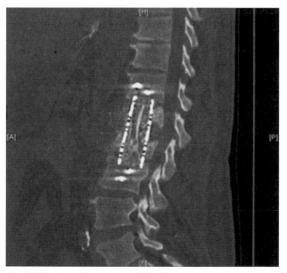

Fig. 6.22 Sagittal MRI view of lumbar spine.

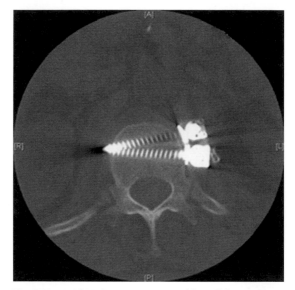

Fig. 6.23 Axial CT showing screws used for stabilization.

■ Case 2

A 50-year-old man presents with neck pain that radiates to the back of the left head and down the left arm. He had neck surgery ~5 years ago that involved an anterior fusion of the cervical spine. A CT scan is obtained (**Fig. 6.24**). He has a weak hand grip and shoulder on the left side, and reflexes are diminished. What is the diagnosis and what treatment should be instituted?

■ Case 2 Answer

The patient has a herniated disk and osteophyte at the level above the previous fusion (C3–C4), also known as "next level disease." A trial of anti-inflammatory medications and physical therapy should be conducted for 6 weeks. If the patient fails the conservative treatment, then an anterior cervical diskectomy at C3–C4 should be performed. An MRI and cervical spine X-rays will help in planning this surgery. If

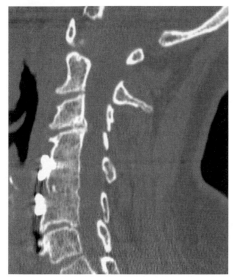

Fig. 6.24 CT scan with sagittal reconstruction.

the previous plate comes up too high on C4, then one should only place a PEEK cage or cadaver bone at C3–C4; removing the entire old plate may not be necessary. It is acceptable to place a small plate at C3–C4 if there is enough space. Currently zero-profile cages are available with diagonally angled screws to specifically treat conditions such as adjacent level disease. The postoperative CT scan is shown in **Fig. 6.25**.

■ Case 3

An 18-year-old is involved in a motorcycle accident and is thrown 20 feet from the accident. He is awake and alert and the CT of the head is negative. Cervical spine X-rays are abnormal, which prompts a CT scan of the cervical spine (**Fig. 6.26**). The patient complains of neck pain that is increasing in severity and the right arm is weak and numb. What is the diagnosis and what is the next step in the treatment of this trauma patient?

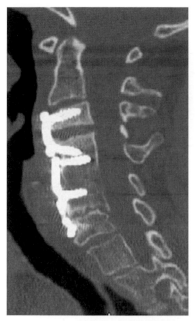

Fig. 6.25 Postoperative sagittal reconstruction of cervical spine.

■ Case 3 Answer

The patient has jumped facets at C5–C6 and should be placed in traction. An MRI of the cervical spine should be obtained provided the tongs for traction are MRI compatible. If no MRI-compatible tongs are available, the MRI should be taken first.

Traction should be placed starting at ~5 lb per level and serial X-rays and CTs should be taken to see if the subluxation corrects. If traction corrects the jumped facets, then a halo vest or cervical rigid orthosis should be worn for at least 6 weeks.

If the traction does not correct the subluxation, then surgery should be performed, first starting with a poste-

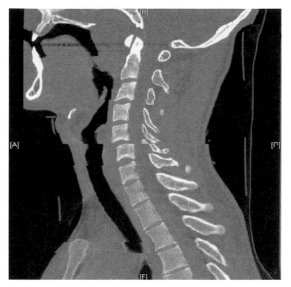

Fig. 6.26 CT scan of the cervical spine (sagittal reconstruction) postinjury.

rior approach to correct the subluxation and stabilize the area with lateral mass screws. An alternative is an anterior approach; however, the anterior approach risks not being able to correct the subluxation completely.

■ Case 4

A 44-year-old woman has been having increasing back pain and leg weakness over the past year. She has no history of trauma and she works at an office as a secretary. Her reflexes in the lower extremities are increased, and the right leg shows weakness in most muscle groups. Her gait is antalgic and mildly spastic. An MRI of the lumbar spine is performed and is shown in **Fig. 6.27**. What is the diagnosis and what is the best treatment if she has exhausted conservative measures?

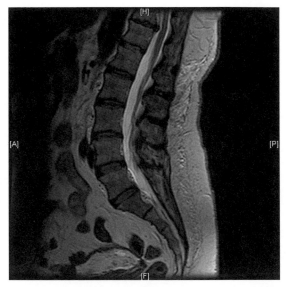

Fig. 6.27 T2-weighted sagittal MRI view of the thoracolumbar spine.

■ Case 4 Answer

The patient has a T11–T12 thoracic disk herniation. She is displaying signs of myelopathy. Thoracic disks usually present with a myelopathic rather than a radicular picture. Thoracic disk herniations are extremely uncommon and the majority occur below the T8 area. Pain may radiate to the abdominal and inguinal areas; this mimics other pathologies such as renal and gallbladder problems.

The best approach to the disk is posteriorly via a transpedicular approach. The side of approach should be on the side where the disk is herniated; however, most thoracic disks herniate centrally and the side of the approach will depend on the comfort of the surgeon. The transpedicular approach trajectory is seen in **Figs. 6.28** and **6.29**.

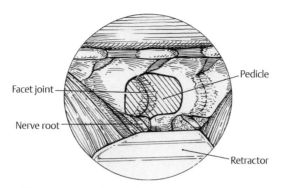

Fig. 6.28 Artist's rendering of an intraoperative view of the lumbar spine posteriorly. (Reproduced with permission from Fessler and Sekhar.[145])

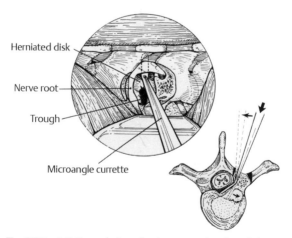

Fig. 6.29 Artist's rendering of an intraoperative view of the lumbar spine. (Reproduced with permission from Fessler and Sekhar.[145])

■ References

1. Lower Back Pain Fact Sheet. Available at: www.nih.gov. Accessed March 15, 2017

2. Joaquim AF. Initial approach to patients with acute lower back pain. Rev Assoc Med Bras (1992) 2016;62(2):186–191

3. Bogduk N. Management of chronic low back pain. Med J Aust 2004;180(2):79–83

4. van Tulder MW, Touray T, Furlan AD, Solway S, Bouter LM. Muscle relaxants for non-specific low back pain. Cochrane Database Syst Rev 2003;(2):CD004252

5. Rubinstein SM, van Tulder M. A best-evidence review of diagnostic procedures for neck and low-back pain. Best Pract Res Clin Rheumatol 2008;22(3):471–482

6. Malanga GA, Landes P, Nadler SF. Provocative tests in cervical spine examination: historical basis and scientific analyses. Pain Physician 2003;6(2):199–205

7. Cuellar J, Passias P. Cervical spondylotic myelopathy a review of clinical diagnosis and treatment. Bull Hosp Jt Dis (2013) 2017;75(1):21–29

8. Henschke N, Maher CG, Refshauge KM, et al. Prevalence of and screening for serious spinal pathology in patients presenting to primary care settings with acute low back pain. Arthritis Rheum 2009;60(10):3072–3080

9. Schober P. Lendenwirbelsäule und Kreuzschmerzen. Munch Med Wochenschr 1937;84:336–338

10. Turner MR, Talbot K. Functional vitamin B12 deficiency. Pract Neurol 2009;9(1):37–41

11. Wijdicks EF, Klein CJ. Guillain-Barré syndrome. Mayo Clin Proc 2017;92(3):467–479

12. Tubbs RS, Loukas M, Slappey JB, Shoja MM, Oakes WJ, Salter EG. Clinical anatomy of the C1 dorsal root, ganglion, and ramus: a review and anatomical study. Clin Anat 2007;20(6):624–627

13. Poncelet A. The neurologic complications of Paget's disease. J Bone Miner Res 1999;14(suppl 2):88–91

14. Gutrecht JA. Lhermitte's sign. From observation to eponym. Arch Neurol 1989;46(5):557–558

15. Brooks NP. Central cord syndrome. Neurosurg Clin N Am 2017;28(1):41–47

16. Taurog JD, Chhabra A, Colbert RA. Ankylosing spondylitis and axial spondyloarthritis. N Engl J Med 2016;374(26):2563–2574

17. Nakayama T, Ehara S. Spondylolytic spondylolisthesis: various imaging features and natural courses. Jpn J Radiol 2015;33(1):3–12

18. Ganju A. Isthmic spondylolisthesis. Neurosurg Focus 2002;13(1):E1

19. Oyinkan Marquis B, Capone PM. Myelopathy. Handb Clin Neurol 2016;136:1015–1026

20. Shaya MR. Scapular tip. J Neurosurg 2007;106(1):203, author reply 203

21. Boes CJ. The history of examination of reflexes. J Neurol 2014;261(12):2264–2274

22. Mavrogenis AF, Papagelopoulos PJ, Korres DS, Papadopoulos K, Sakas DE, Pneumaticos S. Accuracy of pedicle screw placement using intraoperative neurophysiological monitoring and computed tomography. J Long Term Eff Med Implants 2009;19(1):41-48

23. Lenke LG, Padberg AM, Russo MH, Bridwell KH, Gelb DE. Triggered electromyographic threshold for accuracy of pedicle screw placement. An animal model and clinical correlation. Spine (Phila Pa 1976). 1995 Jul 15;20(14):1585-1591

24. Allen RT, Rihn JA, Glassman SD, Currier B, Albert TJ, Phillips FM. An evidence-based approach to spine surgery. Am J Med Qual 2009;24(6, suppl):15S–24S

25. Cornett CA, Vincent SA, Crow J, Hewlett A. Bacterial spine infections in adults: evaluation and management. J Am Acad Orthop Surg 2016;24(1):11–18

26. Arutyunyan GG, Clarke MJ. Management of primary and metastatic spinal tumors. J Neurosurg Sci 2015;59(2):181–193

27. Cho KJ, Kim YT, Shin SH, Suk SI. Surgical treatment of adult degenerative scoliosis. Asian Spine J 2014;8(3):371–381

28. Rajasekaran S, Kamath V, Avadhani A. Odontoid anterior screw fixation. Eur Spine J 2010;19(2):339–340

29. Henry BM, Sanna B, Graves MJ, et al. The reliability of the tracheoesophageal groove and the ligament of Berry as landmarks for identifying the recurrent laryngeal nerve: a cadaveric study and meta-analysis. Biomed Res Int 2017;2017:4357591

30. Fountas KN, Kapsalaki EZ, Nikolakakos LG, et al. Anterior cervical discectomy and fusion associated complications. Spine 2007;32(21):2310–2317

31. Liu WJ, Hu L, Chou PH, Wang JW, Kan WS. Comparison of anterior cervical discectomy and fusion versus posterior cervical foraminotomy in the treatment of cervical radiculopathy: a systematic review. Orthop Surg 2016;8(4):425–431

32. Fringeli Y, Humm AM, Ansorge A, Maestretti G. Harlequin sign concomitant with Horner syndrome after anterior cervical discectomy: a case of intrusion into the cervical sympathetic system. J Neurosurg Spine 2017:1–4

33. Falavigna A, Piccoli Conzatti L. Minimally invasive approaches for thoracic decompression from discectomy to corpectomy. J Neurosurg Sci 2013;57(3):175–192

34. Whang PG, Vaccaro AR. Thoracolumbar fracture: posterior instrumentation using distraction and ligamentotaxis reduction. J Am Acad Orthop Surg 2007;15(11):695–701

35. Abou Al-Shaar H, Imtiaz MT, Alhalabi H, Alsubaie SM, Sabbagh AJ. Selective dorsal rhizotomy: a multidisciplinary approach to treating spastic diplegia. Asian J Neurosurg 2017

36. Daniels AH, Riew KD, Yoo JU, et al. Adverse events associated with anterior cervical spine surgery. J Am Acad Orthop Surg 2008;16(12):729–738

37. Elder BD, Ishida W, Goodwin CR, et al. Bone graft options for spinal fusion following resection of spinal column tumors: systematic review and meta-analysis. Neurosurg Focus 2017;42(1):E16

38. Leven D, Cho SK. Pseudarthrosis of the cervical spine: risk factors, diagnosis and management. Asian Spine J 2016;10(4):776–786

39. Epstein NE. Different surgical approaches to far lateral lumbar disc herniations. J Spinal Disord 1995;8(5):383–394

40. Epstein NE. Foraminal and far lateral lumbar disc herniations: surgical alternatives and outcome measures. Spinal Cord 2002;40(10):491–500

41. Abou Al-Shaar H, Alkhani A. Intrathecal baclofen therapy for spasticity: a compliance-based study to indicate effectiveness. Surg Neurol Int 2016;7(suppl 19):S539–S541

42. Shibuya N, Jupiter DC. Bone graft substitute: allograft and xenograft. Clin Podiatr Med Surg 2015;32(1):21–34

43. Farrokhi MR, Ghaffarpasand F, Khani M, Gholami M. An evidence-based stepwise surgical approach to cervical spondylotic myelopathy: a narrative review of the current literature. World Neurosurg 2016;94:97–110

44. Lebl DR, Bono CM. Update on the diagnosis and management of cervical spondylotic myelopathy. J Am Acad Orthop Surg 2015;23(11):648–660

45. Singhatanadgige W, Limthongkul W, Valone F III, Yingsakmongkol W, Riew KD. Outcomes following laminoplasty or laminectomy and fusion in patients with myelopathy caused by ossification of the posterior longitudinal ligament: a systematic review. Global Spine J 2016;6(7):702–709

46. Hanson P, Sørensen H. The lumbosacral ligament. An autopsy study of young black and white people. Cells Tissues Organs 2000;166(4):373–377

47. Almaiman M, Al-Bargi HH, Manson P. Complication of anterior iliac bone graft harvesting in 372 adult patients from May 2006 to May 2011 and a literature review. Craniomaxillofac Trauma Reconstr 2013;6(4):257–266

48. Van Royen BJ, Toussaint HM, Kingma I, et al. Accuracy of the sagittal vertical axis in a standing lateral radiograph as a measurement of balance in spinal deformities. Eur Spine J 1998;7(5):408–412

49. Berry JG, Glotzbecker M, Rodean J, Leahy I, Hall M, Ferrari L. Comorbidities and complications of spinal fusion for scoliosis. Pediatrics 2017;139(3):e20162574

50. Joaquim AF, Ghizoni E, Tedeschi H, et al. Upper cervical injuries: a rational approach to guide surgical management. J Spinal Cord Med 2014;37(2):139–151

51. Rogers WK, Todd M. Acute spinal cord injury. Best Pract Res Clin Anaesthesiol 2016;30(1):27–39

52. Fenstermaker RA. Acute neurologic management of the patient with spinal cord injury. Urol Clin North Am 1993;20(3):413–421

53. Frohna WJ. Emergency department evaluation and treatment of the neck and cervical spine injuries. Emerg Med Clin North Am 1999;17(4):739–791, v

54. Schriger DL, Larmon B, LeGassick T, Blinman T. Spinal immobilization on a flat backboard: does it result in neutral position of the cervical spine? Ann Emerg Med 1991;20(8):878–881

55. Julien TD, Frankel B, Traynelis VC, Ryken TC. Evidence-based analysis of odontoid fracture management. Neurosurg Focus 2000;8(6):e1

56. Korres DS, Chytas DG, Markatos KN, Efstathopoulos NE, Nikolaou VS. The "challenging" fractures of the odontoid process: a review of the classification schemes. Eur J Orthop Surg Traumatol 2017

57. Huybregts JG, Jacobs WC, Vleggeert-Lankamp CL. The optimal treatment of type II and III odontoid fractures in the elderly: a systematic review. Eur Spine J 2013;22(1):1–13

58. Todor DR, Mu HT, Milhorat TH. Pain and syringomyelia: a review. Neurosurg Focus 2000;8(3):E11

59. Cowan H. Autonomic dysreflexia in spinal cord injury. Nurs Times 2015;111(44):22–24

60. Mirvis SE, Young JW, Lim C, Greenberg J. Hangman's fracture: radiologic assessment in 27 cases. Radiology 1987;163(3):713–717

61. Li XF, Dai LY, Lu H, Chen XD. A systematic review of the management of hangman's fractures. Eur Spine J 2006;15(3):257–269

62. Prashant R, Franks A. Collet-Sicard syndrome—a report and review. Lancet Oncol 2003;4(6):376–377

63. Erol FS, Topsakal C, Kaplan M, Yildirim H, Ozveren MF. Collet-Sicard syndrome associated with occipital condyle fracture and epidural hematoma. Yonsei Med J 2007;48(1):120–123

64. Domenicucci M, Mancarella C, Dugoni ED, Ciappetta P, Paolo M. Post-traumatic Collet-Sicard syndrome: personal observation and review of the pertinent literature with clinical, radiologic and anatomic considerations. Eur Spine J 2015;24(4):663–670

65. Shapiro SA. Management of unilateral locked facet of the cervical spine. Neurosurgery 1993;33(5):832–837, discussion 837

66. Li G, Passias P, Kozanek M, et al. Interobserver reliability and intraobserver reproducibility of powers ratio for assessment of atlanto-occipital junction: comparison of plain radiography and computed tomography. Eur Spine J 2009;18(4):577–582

67. Hilton EL, Henderson LJ. Neurosurgical considerations in posttraumatic syringomyelia. AORN J 2003;77(1):135–139, 141–144, 146–148 passim, quiz 153–156

68. Nowak DD, Lee JK, Gelb DE, Poelstra KA, Ludwig SC. Central cord syndrome. J Am Acad Orthop Surg 2009;17(12):756–765

69. Dlouhy BJ, Dahdaleh NS, Howard MA III. Radiographic and intra-operative imaging of a hemisection of the spinal cord resulting in a pure Brown-Séquard syndrome: case report and review of the literature. J Neurosurg Sci 2013;57(1):81–86

70. Novy J. Spinal cord syndromes. Front Neurol Neurosci 2012;30:195–198

71. Radcliff KE, Kepler CK, Delasotta LA, et al. Current management review of thoracolumbar cord syndromes. Spine J 2011;11(9):884–892

72. Alvarenga MP, Thuler LC, Neto SP, et al. The clinical course of idiopathic acute transverse myelitis in patients from Rio de Janeiro. J Neurol 2010;257(6):992–998

73. Abou Al-Shaar H, AbouAl-Shaar I, Al-Kawi MZ. Acute cervical cord infarction in anterior spinal artery territory with acute swelling mimicking myelitis. Neurosciences (Riyadh) 2015;20(4):372–375

74. Herzka A, Sponseller PD, Pyeritz RE. Atlantoaxial rotatory subluxation in patients with Marfan syndrome. A report of three cases. Spine 2000;25(4):524–526

75. Kalra V, Gulati S, Kamate M, Garg A. SCIWORA-Spinal Cord Injury Without Radiological Abnormality. Indian J Pediatr 2006;73(9):829–831

76. Daniels AH, Sobel AD, Eberson CP. Pediatric thoracolumbar spine trauma. J Am Acad Orthop Surg 2013;21(12):707–716

77. Teh HS, Fadilah SA, Leong CF. Transverse myelopathy following intrathecal administration of chemotherapy. Singapore Med J 2007;48(2):e46–e49

78. Coleman WP, Benzel D, Cahill DW, et al. A critical appraisal of the reporting of the National Acute Spinal Cord Injury Studies (II and III) of methylprednisolone in acute spinal cord injury. J Spinal Disord 2000;13(3):185–199

79. Bracken MB, Shepard MJ, Collins WF, et al. A randomized, controlled trial of methylprednisolone or naloxone in the treatment of acute spinal-cord injury. Results of the Second National Acute Spinal Cord Injury Study. N Engl J Med 1990;322(20):1405–1411

80. Rasool T, Wani MA, Kirmani AR, et al. Role of methylprednisolone in acute cervical cord injuries. Indian J Surg 2004;66(3):156–159

81. Bowers CA, Kundu B, Hawryluk GW. Methylprednisolone for acute spinal cord injury: an increasingly philosophical debate. Neural Regen Res 2016;11(6):882–885

82. Fox AD. Spinal shock. Assessment & treatment of spinal cord injuries & neurogenic shock. JEMS 2014;39(11):64–67

83. American Spinal Injury Association. Standards for Neurological Classification of Spinal Injury Patients. Chicago, IL: ASIA; 1984

84. American Spinal Injury Association. Standards for Neurological Classification of Spinal Injury Patients. Chicago, IL: ASIA; 1989

85. ASIA/IMSOR Standards for Neurological and Functional Classification of Spinal Cord Injury-Revised. Chicago, IL: ASIA; 1992

86. ASIA/IMSOR International Standards for Neurological and Functional Classification of Spinal Cord Injury-Revised. Chicago, IL: ASIA; 1996

87. Kirshblum SC, Burns SP, Biering-Sorensen F, et al. International standards for neurological classification of spinal cord injury (revised 2011). J Spinal Cord Med 2011;34(6):535–546

88. Frankel HL, Hancock DO, Hyslop G, et al. The value of postural reduction in the initial management of closed injuries of the spine with paraplegia and tetraplegia. I. Paraplegia 1969;7(3):179–192

89. Casale R, Symeonidou Z, Bartolo M. Topical treatments for localized neuropathic pain. Curr Pain Headache Rep 2017;21(3):15

90. Colloca L, Ludman T, Bouhassira D, et al. Neuropathic pain. Nat Rev Dis Primers 2017;3:17002

91. Khademi H, Kamangar F, Brennan P, Malekzadeh R. Opioid therapy and its side effects: a review. Arch Iran Med 2016;19(12):870–876

92. Müller-Schwefe G, Morlion B, Ahlbeck K, et al. Treatment for chronic low back pain: the focus should change to multimodal management that reflects the underlying pain mechanisms. Curr Med Res Opin 2017:1–12

93. Menezes AH. Congenital and acquired abnormalities of the craniovertebral junction. In: Youmans J, ed. Neurological Surgery. 4th ed. Philadelphia, PA: WB Saunders; 1995:1035–1089

94. Garrett M, Consiglieri G, Kakarla UK, Chang SW, Dickman CA. Occipitoatlantal dislocation. Neurosurgery 2010;66 (3, suppl):48–55

95. Yang SY, Boniello AJ, Poorman CE, Chang AL, Wang S, Passias PG. A review of the diagnosis and treatment of atlantoaxial dislocations. Global Spine J 2014;4(3):197–210

96. Xiong M, Chen S, Yu H, Liu Z, Zeng Y, Li F. Neuroprotection of erythropoietin and methylprednisolone against spinal cord ischemia-reperfusion injury. J Huazhong Univ Sci Technolog Med Sci 2011;31(5):652–656

97. Alibai E, Zand F, Rahimi A, Rezaianzadeh A. Erythropoietin plus methylprednisolone or methylprednisolone in the treatment of acute spinal cord injury: a preliminary report. Acta Med Iran 2014;52(4):275–279

98. Kamiya K, Koda M, Furuya T, et al. Neuroprotective therapy with granulocyte colony-stimulating factor in acute spinal cord injury: a comparison with high-dose methylprednisolone as a historical control. Eur Spine J 2015;24(5):963–967

99. Takahashi H, Yamazaki M, Okawa A, et al. Neuroprotective therapy using granulocyte colony-stimulating factor for acute spinal cord injury: a phase I/IIa clinical trial. Eur Spine J 2012;21(12):2580–2587

100. Pitts LH, Ross A, Chase GA, Faden AI. Treatment with thyrotropin-releasing hormone (TRH) in patients with traumatic spinal cord injuries. J Neurotrauma 1995;12(3):235–243

101. Grossman RG, Fehlings MG, Frankowski RF, et al. A prospective, multicenter, phase I matched-comparison group trial of safety, pharmacokinetics, and preliminary efficacy of riluzole in patients with traumatic spinal cord injury. J Neurotrauma 2014;31(3):239–255

102. Shah LM, Flanders AE. Update on new imaging techniques for trauma. Neurosurg Clin N Am 2017;28(1):1–21

103. Oh JJ, Asha SE. Utility of flexion-extension radiography for the detection of ligamentous cervical spine injury and its current role in the clearance of the cervical spine. Emerg Med Australas 2016;28(2):216–223

104. Reinhold M, Audigé L, Schnake KJ, Bellabarba C, Dai LY, Oner FC. AO spine injury classification system: a revision proposal for the thoracic and lumbar spine. Eur Spine J 2013;22(10):2184–2201

105. Lee JY, Vaccaro AR, Lim MR, et al. Thoracolumbar injury classification and severity score: a new paradigm for the treatment of thoracolumbar spine trauma. J Orthop Sci 2005;10(6):671–675

106. Anderson PA, Montesano PX. Morphology and treatment of occipital condyle fractures. Spine 1988;13(7):731–736

107. Theodore N, Aarabi B, Dhall SS, et al. Occipital condyle fractures. Neurosurgery 2013;72(suppl 2):106–113

108. Weinstein JN, Tosteson TD, Lurie JD, et al; SPORT Investigators. Surgical versus nonsurgical therapy for lumbar spinal stenosis. N Engl J Med 2008;358(8):794–810

109. Stadler JA III, Wong AP, Graham RB, Liu JC. Complications associated with posterior approaches in minimally invasive spine decompression. Neurosurg Clin N Am 2014;25(2):233–245

110. King JT Jr, Abbed KM, Gould GC, Benzel EC, Ghogawala Z. Cervical spine reoperation rates and hospital resource utilization after initial surgery for degenerative cervical spine disease in 12,338 patients in Washington state. Neurosurgery 2009;65(6):1011–1022, discussion 1022–1023

111. Zacest AC, Carlson JD, Nemecek A, Burchiel KJ. Surgical management of spinal catheter granulomas: operative nuances and review of the surgical literature. Neurosurgery 2009;65(6):1161–1164, discussion 1164–1165

112. Wadhwa RK, Shaya MR, Nanda A. Spinal cord compression in a patient with a pain pump for failed back syndrome: a chalk-like precipitate mimicking a spinal cord neoplasm: case report. Neurosurgery 2006;58(2):E387

113. Vanichkachorn JS, Vaccaro AR. Thoracic disk disease: diagnosis and treatment. J Am Acad Orthop Surg 2000;8(3):159–169

114. Bindi P, Chanard J. Destructive spondyloarthropathy in dialysis patients: an overview. Nephron 1990;55(2):104–109

115. Gillick JL, Wainwright J, Das K. Rheumatoid arthritis and the cervical spine: a review on the role of surgery. Int J Rheumatol 2015;2015:252456

116. Pellicci PM, Ranawat CS, Tsairis P, Bryan WJ. A prospective study of the progression of rheumatoid arthritis of the cervical spine. J Bone Joint Surg Am 1981;63(3):342–350

117. Hardiman O, Chalabi AA, Brayne C, et al. The changing picture of amyotrophic lateral sclerosis: lessons from European registers. J Neurol Neurosurg Psychiatry 2017:2016-314495

118. Saetia K, Cho D, Lee S, Kim DH, Kim SD. Ossification of the posterior longitudinal ligament: a review. Neurosurg Focus 2011;30(3):E1

119. Hadley MN, Reddy SV. Smoking and the human vertebral column: a review of the impact of cigarette use on vertebral bone metabolism and spinal fusion. Neurosurgery 1997;41(1):116–124

120. Wintermeyer E, Ihle C, Ehnert S, et al. Crucial role of vitamin D in the musculoskeletal system. Nutrients 2016;8(6):E319

121. Sheu A, Diamond T. Secondary osteoporosis. Aust Prescr 2016;39(3):85–87

122. Sözen T, Özışık L, Başaran NÇ. An overview and management of osteoporosis. Eur J Rheumatol 2017;4(1):46–56

123. Langdahl B, Ferrari S, Dempster DW. Bone modeling and remodeling: potential as therapeutic targets for the treatment of osteoporosis. Ther Adv Musculoskelet Dis 2016;8(6):225–235

124. Yuan WH, Hsu HC, Lai KL. Vertebroplasty and balloon kyphoplasty versus conservative treatment for osteoporotic vertebral compression fractures: a meta-analysis. Medicine (Baltimore) 2016;95(31):e4491

125. Karikari IO, Powers CJ, Isaacs RE. Simple method for determining the need for sternotomy/manubriotomy with the anterior approach to the cervicothoracic junction. Neurosurgery 2009;65(6, suppl):E165–E166, discussion E166

126. Nassr A, Eck JC, Ponnappan RK, Zanoun RR, Donaldson WF III, Kang JD. The incidence of C5 palsy after multilevel cervical decompression procedures: a review of 750 consecutive cases. Spine 2012;37(3):174–178

127. Yong-Hing K, Kirkaldy-Willis WH. The pathophysiology of degenerative disease of the lumbar spine. Orthop Clin North Am 1983;14(3):491–504

128. Feydy A, Pluot E, Guerini H, Drapé JL. Osteoarthritis of the wrist and hand, and spine. Radiol Clin North Am 2009;47(4):723–759

129. Shirzadi A, Birch K, Drazin D, Liu JC, Acosta F Jr. Direct lateral interbody fusion (DLIF) at the lumbosacral junction L5-S1. J Clin Neurosci 2012;19(7):1022–1025

130. Nasca RJ. Newer lumbar interbody fusion techniques. J Surg Orthop Adv 2013;22(2):113–117

131. Pawar A, Hughes A, Girardi F, Sama A, Lebl D, Cammisa F. Lateral lumbar interbody fusion. Asian Spine J 2015;9(6):978–983

132. Baber Z, Erdek MA. Failed back surgery syndrome: current perspectives. J Pain Res 2016;9:979–987

133. Zelle BA, Gruen GS, Brown S, George S. Sacroiliac joint dysfunction: evaluation and management. Clin J Pain 2005;21(5):446–455

134. Boody BS, Jenkins TJ, Maslak J, Hsu WK, Patel AA. Vertebral osteomyelitis and spinal epidural abscess: an evidence-based review. J Spinal Disord Tech 2015;28(6):E316–E327

135. DeFroda SF, DePasse JM, Eltorai AE, Daniels AH, Palumbo MA. Evaluation and management of spinal epidural abscess. J Hosp Med 2016;11(2):130–135

136. Kumar K. Spinal tuberculosis, natural history of disease, classifications and principles of management with historical perspective. Eur J Orthop Surg Traumatol 2016;26(6):551–558

137. Youssef K, Daniel S. Grisel syndrome in adult patients. Report of two cases and review of the literature. Can J Neurol Sci 2009;36(1):109–113

138. Marra CM. Neurosyphilis. Continuum (Minneap Minn) 2015;21(6 Neuroinfectious Disease):1714–1728

139. Cristante L, Herrmann HD. Surgical management of intramedullary spinal cord tumors: functional outcome and sources of morbidity. Neurosurgery 1994;35(1):69–74, discussion 74–76

140. Nakamura M, Ishii K, Watanabe K, et al. Surgical treatment of intramedullary spinal cord tumors: prognosis and complications. Spinal Cord 2008;46(4):282–286

141. Kivrak AS, Koc O, Emlik D, Kiresi D, Odev K, Kalkan E. Differential diagnosis of dumbbell lesions associated with spinal neural foraminal widening: imaging features. Eur J Radiol 2009;71(1):29–41

142. Choi D, Melcher R, Harms J, Crockard A. Outcome of 132 operations in 97 patients with chordomas of the craniocervical junction and upper cervical spine. Neurosurgery 2010;66(1):59–65, discussion 65

143. Heery CR. Chordoma: the quest for better treatment options. Oncol Ther 2016;4(1):35–51

144. Bingham N, Reale A, Spencer A. An Evidence-Based Approach to Myeloma Bone Disease. Curr Hematol Malig Rep 2017

145. Fessler RG, Sekhar L. Atlas of Neurosurgical Techniques: Spine and Peripheral Nerves. Stuttgart: Georg Thieme Verlag; 2006

146. Strike SA, McCarthy EF. Chondrosarcoma of the spine: a series of 16 cases and a review of the literature. Iowa Orthop J 2011;31:154–159

147. Koutourousiou M, Snyderman CH, Fernandez-Miranda J, Gardner PA. Skull base chordomas. Otolaryngol Clin North Am 2011;44(5):1155–1171

148. Rapp TB, Ward JP, Alaia MJ. Aneurysmal bone cyst. J Am Acad Orthop Surg 2012;20(4):233–241

149. Zhang HY, Thongtrangan I, Balabhadra RS, Murovic JA, Kim DH. Surgical techniques for total sacrectomy and spinopelvic reconstruction. Neurosurg Focus 2003;15(2):E5

150. Atesok KI, Alman BA, Schemitsch EH, Peyser A, Mankin H. Osteoid osteoma and osteoblastoma. J Am Acad Orthop Surg 2011;19(11):678–689

151. Sinelnikov A, Kale H. Osteochondromas of the spine. Clin Radiol 2014;69(12):e584–e590

152. Solero CL, Fornari M, Giombini S, et al. Spinal meningiomas: review of 174 operated cases. Neurosurgery 1989;25(2):153–160

153. Conway JE, Chou D, Clatterbuck RE, Brem H, Long DM, Rigamonti D. Hemangioblastomas of the central nervous system in von Hippel-Lindau syndrome and sporadic disease. Neurosurgery 2001;48(1):55–62, discussion 62–63

154. Lonser RR, Oldfield EH. Microsurgical resection of spinal cord hemangioblastomas. Neurosurgery 2005;57(4, suppl):372–376, discussion 372–376

155. Maimon S, Luckman Y, Strauss I. Spinal dural arteriovenous fistula: a review. Adv Tech Stand Neurosurg 2016;(43):111–137

156. Rosenblum B, Oldfield EH, Doppman JL, Di Chiro G. Spinal arteriovenous malformations: a comparison of dural arteriovenous fistulas and intradural AVM's in 81 patients. J Neurosurg 1987;67(6):795–802

157. Ferch RD, Morgan MK, Sears WR. Spinal arteriovenous malformations: a review with case illustrations. J Clin Neurosci 2001;8(4):299–304

158. Varcoe RL, Taylor CF, Annett P, Jacobsen EE, McMullin G. The conundrum of claudication. ANZ J Surg 2006;76(10):916–927

159. Johnson WD, Petrie MM. Variety of spinal vascular pathology seen in adult Cobb syndrome. J Neurosurg Spine 2009;10(5):430–435

160. Song RB, Glass EN, Kent M. Spina bifida, meningomyelocele, and meningocele. Vet Clin North Am Small Anim Pract 2016;46(2):327–345

161. Wisoff JH. Hydromyelia: a critical review. Childs Nerv Syst 1988;4(1):1–8

162. Bedru A, Mune T, Assefa G, Meseret S. Diastematomyelia: a case report with review of litratures. Ethiop Med J 2006;44(2):195–200

163. Kanev PM, Park TS. Dermoids and dermal sinus tracts of the spine. Neurosurg Clin N Am 1995;6(2):359–366

164. Tracy MR, Dormans JP, Kusumi K. Klippel-Feil syndrome: clinical features and current understanding of etiology. Clin Orthop Relat Res 2004;(424):183–190

165. Boos N. Surgery of a Klippel-Feil malformation of the cervicothoracic junction. Eur Spine J 2009;18(8):1237–1238

166. Rozzelle CJ, Aarabi B, Dhall SS, et al. Os odontoideum. Neurosurgery 2013;72(suppl 2):159–169

167. Tubbs RS, Salter EG, Oakes WJ. Split spinal cord malformation. Clin Anat 2007;20(1):15–18

168. Lao L, Zhong G, Li X, Liu Z. Split spinal cord malformation: report of 5 cases in a single Chinese center and review of the literature. Pediatr Neurosurg 2013;49(2):69–74

169. Alexiou GA, Prodromou N. Spinal dermal sinus tract. Childs Nerv Syst 2010;26(5):597

170. Pinter NK, McVige J, Mechtler L. Basilar invagination, basilar impression, and platybasia: clinical and imaging aspects. Curr Pain Headache Rep 2016;20(8):49

171. McKay SD, Al-Omari A, Tomlinson LA, Dormans JP. Review of cervical spine anomalies in genetic syndromes. Spine 2012;37(5):E269–E277

172. Pillay PK, Awad IA, Hahn JF. Gardner's hydrodynamic theory of syringomyelia revisited. Cleve Clin J Med 1992;59(4):373–380

173. Williams B. Cerebrospinal fluid pressure changes in response to coughing. Brain 1976;99(2):331–346

174. Oldfield EH, Muraszko K, Shawker TH, Patronas NJ. Pathophysiology of syringomyelia associated with Chiari I malformation of the cerebellar tonsils. Implications for diagnosis and treatment. J Neurosurg 1994;80(1):3–15

175. Rusbridge C, Greitz D, Iskandar BJ. Syringomyelia: current concepts in pathogenesis, diagnosis, and treatment. J Vet Intern Med 2006;20(3):469–479

7 Peripheral Nerves

General

■ History and Physical

1. What types of sensation are affected in amyotrophic lateral sclerosis (ALS)?

None, sensation is intact.[1]

2. What muscle group should be examined in the lower extremities to differentiate a foot drop from radiculopathy versus a foot drop from peroneal nerve palsy?

Test foot inversion, which is controlled by the tibialis posterior and anterior. In a pure peroneal neuropathy, foot inversion is intact. Also, note that gluteus medius (internal rotation of a flexed hip) is spared in peroneal nerve palsy.[2]

3. What is the usual presentation of anterior interosseous nerve entrapment?

Pain located in the proximal forearm that increases with exercise and decreases with rest; up to 85% of patients will present in this way.[3]

4. What muscles are involved in anterior interosseous nerve entrapment?

Flexor digitorum profundus 1 and 2, flexor pollicis longus, and the pronator quadratus.[4]

5. What symptoms may be present with the rare T1 radiculopathy caused by a Pancoast tumor in the apical pleura of the lung?

Irritation in the medial upper arm and a Horner syndrome.[5]

6. What are the standard laboratory tests in a peripheral neuropathy work-up?

Thyroid panel, rheumatology profiles, vitamin B_{12}, folic acid, hemoglobin A1C, erythrocyte sedimentation rate, rapid protein reagent, heavy metals, and immunoelectrophoresis of serum protein.[2]

7. What is a Froment sign?

Paralysis of the adductor pollicis produces a Froment sign; when grasping a piece of paper between the thumb and index finger, the flexor pollicis longus is used (resulting in interphalangeal [IP] joint flexion) because the adductor pollicis does not work.[6]

8. What is the pinch or "O" sign?

To test for anterior interosseous nerve palsy, the thumb and index finger are unable to make a circle ("O"); instead, the pulps of the thumb and index finger touch each other. This is the result of weakness of flexion of the distal phalanges (**Fig. 7.1**).[4,6]

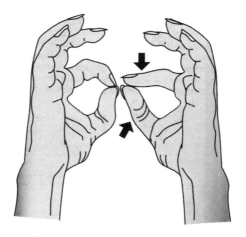

Fig. 7.1 Pinch or "O" sign. (Reproduced with permission from Alberstone et al.[7])

9. How can one differentiate an ulnar nerve injury below the midforearm and an ulnar nerve injury above the midforearm if there are no external signs of injury to the arm?

If the ulnar nerve is divided below the midforearm, an ulnar claw hand is produced. The fourth and fifth digits are hyperextended at the metacarpophalangeal (MP) joints by the long extensors, but are flexed at the IP joints. This posture is sometimes called the "hand of benediction." If an ulnar nerve lesion is above the midforearm, the clawing of the ulnar side two fingers may not occur if the extrinsic muscles producing IP joint flexion are also denervated.[6]

10. How does a lower plexus lesion result in a claw hand?

Lower brachial plexus lesions are usually injuries caused by excessive abduction of the arm as a result of someone clutching for an object when falling from a height. The first thoracic nerve (T1) is usually torn. The fibers from this segment of the spinal cord help form the ulnar and median nerves; the small muscles of the hand (interossei and lumbricals) are affected and the hand has a clawed appearance due to hyperextension of the MP joints and flexion of the IP joints. The extensor digitorum is unopposed by the lumbricals and extends the MP joints. Because the flexor digitorum superficialis and profundus are unopposed by the lumbricals and interossei, the claw hand results. There is also sensory loss along the medial side of the forearm, hand, and medial two fingers. Lower brachial plexus lesions may also be the result of malignant metastases from the lungs in the lower deep cervical lymph nodes and an aberrant cervical rib.[7,8]

11. A golfer complains of palmar pain on the ulnar side of the hand that is aggravated by grasping his club; what is the primary diagnosis?

Hook of hamate fracture. The hook of the hamate forms the lateral (radial) border of tunnel of the Guyon, which transports the ulnar nerve and artery to the hand.[9]

12. What branch of the ulnar nerve takes an abrupt turn around the hook of the hamate?

The deep branch.[9]

13. In neuropathies, which muscles most commonly first show wasting in the upper extremities and in the lower extremities?

The first dorsal interosseus muscle in the upper limbs and extensor digitorum brevis in the lower limbs.

14. What is the rate of axonal regeneration in a peripheral nerve lesion?

In a peripheral nerve injury, the axon progresses down the distal stump at a rate of 1 mm per day. The rate is greater if the lesion is close to the central nervous system and lesser if the injury is more distal. Thus, proximal lesions may grow as rapidly as 2 to 3 mm per day, whereas distal lesions may progress as slowly as 0.5 mm per day.[2,6]

15. What is the significance of a positive Tinel sign in the setting of peripheral nerve regeneration?

A Tinel sign signifies that fine fibers have reached the area of stimulation. If the nerve is indeed regenerating, then the patient will report paresthesias in the distribution of the nerve that is stimulated. The absence of a Tinel sign many months after injury may be an indication for operative exploration.[6]

16. How can one radiologically differentiate ganglia from other masses such as schwannomas?

Ganglia exhibit lack of contrast enhancement and display a connection with the joint space. For example, in peroneal nerve compression, a para-articular ganglion is connected to the superior tibiofibular joint capsule.[10]

17. What type of neuropathy can a patient with acquired immunodeficiency syndrome (AIDS) have?

AIDS patients can present with a distal sensory neuropathy or an antiretroviral toxic neuropathy caused by exposure to specific nucleoside reverse transcriptase inhibitors. The conditions can coexist as well, resulting in burning dysesthesias and debilitating paresthesias. Symptoms are typically limited to the feet, but often extend to the lower extremities.[2,11]

18. Describe the Sunderland classification of a seventh cranial nerve injury.[12]

- First degree:
  - Neurapraxia.
  - Nerve fiber and covering are intact.
  - No wallerian degeneration.
  - Full recovery.
  - Nerve stimulation across the nerve is not present initially.
- Second degree:
  - Axonotmesis.
  - Endoneurium is intact.
  - Wallerian degeneration in 24 hours.
  - Axon regeneration.
  - Potential full recovery.
- Third degree:
  - Neurotmesis.
  - Endoneurium is damaged.
  - Wallerian degeneration.
  - Synkinesis.
  - Incomplete recovery.
- Fourth degree:
  - Neurotmesis.
  - Perineurium is damaged.
  - Wallerian degeneration.
  - Worse synkinesis.
  - Less recovery.
- Fifth degree:
  - Epineurium also is damaged.
  - No recovery unless repaired.

19. The middle trunk of the brachial plexus is formed by anterior rami of which cord segments?

C7.

■ Emergencies

20. What is the most common neuropathy in a patient on anticoagulation medication?

Femoral neuropathy from a hematoma near the psoas muscle.[2]

21. What is the diagnosis of progressive paralysis, an expanding mass in a limb, and/or a bruit detected in that limb?

An aneurysm or fistula may be present and urgent decompression may be required.

■ Technique

22. Where is the approximate location of the sural nerve?

Halfway between the lateral malleolus and Achilles tendon.[4]

23. What are the steps in performing a sural nerve biopsy?

The patient is supine with the leg elevated. A 3-cm incision is made proximal to the lateral malleolus at the groove formed by the lateral malleolus and the Achilles tendon. A 2- to 3-cm piece of whole nerve is sectioned and given to the pathologist. Make sure that on closing the proximal stump of nerve does not retract beyond the incision line and become entrapped within the healing skin.[4]

24. How is a sural nerve block performed?

The needle is introduced just lateral to the Achilles tendon ~1 to 2 cm proximal to the level of the distal tip of lateral malleolus. The needle is directed to the posteromedial aspect of the fibula, and 5 mL of anesthetic is injected after aspiration of the syringe to ensure that a vessel was not breached.[13]

25. How does one administer a Tensilon test?

One milliliter of 1% edrophonium chloride (10 mg/mL, Tensilon) is prepared. The patient is given an initial dose of 0.1 mL and observed for a response. If the patient's symptoms do not change, the remaining 0.9 mL is administered and the response observed again. Administration of an acetylcholinesterase inhibitor, such as edrophonium, causes transient improvement in symptoms of myasthenia gravis.[11]

26. Where is the location of an incision in tarsal tunnel surgery?

Start 2 cm proximal to the medial malleolus, about halfway between the medial malleolus and the Achilles tendon. The incision is extended distally, directly superficial to the course of the posterior tibial nerve.[4]

27. Where is the greater saphenous vein located?

Immediately posterior to the medial malleolus and superficial to the medial malleolar ligament. It is important to identify the distal portion of the vein during dissection so that the proper orientation of the valves is made when grafting the vein to another location.[14]

28. How is a tibial nerve block performed?

The posterior tibial artery is palpated as a landmark. The needle is passed adjacent to the Achilles tendon toward the posterior tibial artery behind the medial malleolus. To block the posterior tibial nerve, direct the needle just medial to the Achilles tendon. Proceed with the needle through the deep fascia until it impinges on the bone behind the medial malleolus. After aspiration, 5 mL of anesthetic is injected.[15]

29. Where is the location for harvesting the medial antebrachial cutaneous nerve for a graft?

The medial antebrachial cutaneous nerve can be used for nerve cable grafts. The anterior branch of this nerve is harvested two fingerbreadths anterior and distal to the medial epicondyle.[16]

30. How does one perform a suprascapular nerve block?

A suprascapular nerve block is performed by needle insertion behind the lateral end of the clavicle at its junction with the insertion of the trapezius muscle; the needle is directed downward and backward.[17]

31. Where is the palmar cutaneous branch of the median nerve and in what common surgery is it at risk?

The palmar cutaneous branch of the median nerve arises from the radial border of the median nerve ~5 to 6 cm proximal to distal transverse flexion crease of the wrist. It runs along the median nerve for 2 to 3 cm, and then runs along the ulnar border of the flexor carpi radialis tendon. An anatomical cadaver study showed that in no case did the palmar cutaneous branch extend ulnar to the axial line of the ring finger. It is at risk in carpal tunnel surgery. That is why it is important to err on the ulnar side when performing carpal tunnel surgery.[4,9]

32. What are the attachments of the flexor retinaculum?

Medial attachments are the pisiform and the hook of the hamate. Lateral attachments are the scaphoid tuberosity and the crest of the trapezium.[18]

33. What are the complications of carpal tunnel operations?[9]

- Inadequate release of the ligament resulting in persistence of symptoms.
- Postoperative fibrosis.
- Tender neuroma of the palmar cutaneous branch of the median nerve.
- Hypertrophic scars.
- Section of the motor branch, resulting in complete denervation and atrophy of the thenar muscle mass.
- Reflex sympathetic dystrophy.
- Bowstringing of the flexor tendons.
- Wound infection and hematoma.

34. What is pillar pain?

Pillar pain is a deep wrist pain after carpal tunnel release thought to result from a redistribution of forces between the carpal bones after the surgery. It usually subsides spontaneously after carpal tunnel surgery in ~6 months.[19]

35. What is the significance of nerve action potential recordings across a lesion in determining what type of surgery is to be done?

If no potential is recorded distal to the lesion, it is resected and a repair is done. When a nerve action potential is recorded, then only a neurolysis is performed. Neurolysis is usually the initial technical step in the surgical management of any lesion in continuity.[4]

36. What are the most common causes of failure of nerve repair?

The leading causes of failure of nerve repair back to healthy tissue are inadequate resection and distraction of the repair site. Use of grafts can help with this problem, as the surgeon is encouraged to resect back to healthy nerves and using grafts permits repair with minimal tension. The use of grafts is not advisable for making up small gaps that can be readily closed with proper mobilization and end-to-end repair.[4]

37. When harvesting iliac crest bone for a fusion procedure, what nerve is at risk if the bone is harvested too far laterally?

The surgeon may use the medial 6 to 8 cm of the iliac crest to avoid injuring the superior cluneal nerves (**Fig. 7.2**).[20]

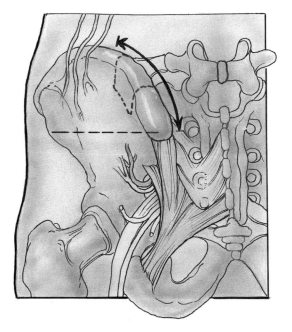

Fig. 7.2   Illustration of posterior iliac crest bone graft harvesting. Note the location of the superior cluneal nerves lateral to the incision site. (Reproduced with permission from Fessler and Sekhar.[21])

38. After a brachial plexus avulsion injury of nerve roots C5 though C7, what type of nerve repair procedures are available?[22]

- Spinal accessory nerve (XI) to suprascapular nerve.
- Spinal accessory nerve (XI) to musculocutaneous nerve.
- Phrenic nerve to suprascapular nerve.
- Pectoralis branches or intercostals to musculocutaneous nerve.
- Contralateral C7 root neurotization to median nerve.

39. List general options for secondary nerve repair.[23,24]

- Placement of interposed nerve graft (need to harvest another site, e.g., sural).
- Nerve transposition.
- Joint casting—flexing the joint to shorten the distance of nerves, then gradually extending the joint (not very effective, may tear nerve graft in the process).
- Synthetic polymer bridging.
- Biologic conduits (vein filler with muscle, for example).

40. Which nerve is most likely to be injured in a fracture of the medial epicondyle?

The ulnar nerve.[25]

41. Name the main advantages and disadvantages of a primary nerve repair.

Advantages:

- Anatomy is relatively easy to assess.
- Associated injuries usually can be treated at the same time.
- Retraction is minimal.
- Grafts are not necessary, which may increase distal reinnervation rates in certain cases.

Disadvantages:

- Tension may need to be applied on the nerve if a gap is present.
- Dissection of the nerve that may be necessary for mobilization may cause undue devascularization.

42. List indications for a secondary nerve repair.

- Initial injury site dirty or infected.
- Late presentation of nerve injury.
- Gunshot wounds to an extremity.
- Traction injuries.
- Blunt injuries.

■ Electrophysiology

43. What are three crucial phases one needs to record when performing electromyography (EMG)?

1. Recording of insertional activity.
2. Determination of the presence or absence of spontaneous discharges at rest.
3. Assessment of the presence and type of muscle action potential.[6]

44. What are some findings on EMG that one sees with nerve compression?

- Sharp positive waves.
- Insertional activity.
- Fibrillations.
- Spontaneous rest activity.
- Decreased recruitment.[26]

45. What is the electrophysiologic equivalent of the tendon jerk?

An H reflex.[26]

46. What electrophysiologic reflex occurs with supramaximal stimulus to the nerve?

An F reflex.[26]

47. What is the only muscle from which an H reflex can be readily elicited?

Soleus (in response to stimulation of the posterior tibial nerve).[26]

48. Compare and contrast a neurogenic motor unit potential and a myogenic motor unit potential.

Both are polyphasic; however, neurogenic motor unit potentials have increased amplitude and long duration compared with myogenic (reduced amplitude and short duration).[26]

49. What else must be present in an EMG examination for an observed fasciculation to be considered abnormal?

Fibrillations and/or positive sharp waves.[26]

50. What is the most common disorder of neuromuscular transmission?

Myasthenia gravis.[27]

51. Is electrodiagnostic testing useful in the acute setting?

A frequent misconception is that electrodiagnostic testing is not useful in an acute injury. EMG changes take 1 to 3 weeks to become recordable in the muscles. Nerve conduction abnormalities, however, are present immediately and can be helpful in the immediate determination of the extent of injury.[2]

52. What study, if positive, increases the diagnostic yield of a sural nerve biopsy?

Nerve conduction velocities. Decreased nerve conduction velocities in the lower extremities increase the diagnostic yield of a sural nerve biopsy.

53. What is the Erb point?

The point on the side of the neck 2 to 3 cm above the clavicle and in front of the transverse process of the sixth cervical vertebra. Pressure over this point elicits Duchenne-Erb paralysis, and electrical stimulation over this area causes various arm muscles to contract.[2]

54. Fibrillations, fasciculations, and atrophy are all manifestations of what type of nerve injury?

Lower motor neuron paralysis.[26]

55. What is the resting membrane potential of a peripheral nerve?

–90 to –70 mV.

56. What is the effect of cooling an extremity on nerve conduction?

Increase in amplitudes, prolonged distal latencies, and slowing of conduction velocities.[28]

■ Pain

57. What are common causes of neuropathic pain?[2]

- Diabetic neuropathy.
- Alcoholic neuropathy.
- Acute inflammatory demyelinating polyradiculopathy.
- Human immunodeficiency virus (HIV)–related neuropathy.
- Postherpetic neuralgia.
- Trigeminal neuralgia.
- Posttraumatic neuralgia.
- Postradiation plexopathy.
- Thalamic stroke.
- Radiculopathy caused by spinal osteoarthritis or discopathy, compressive myelopathy.

58. What is causalgia and what are features of the skin in this condition?

Causalgia is an intense, continuous, burning pain produced by an incomplete peripheral nerve injury. Touching the limb brings about the pain, and the skin is red, warm, and swollen. Causalgia and reflex sympathetic dystrophy are now termed complex regional pain syndrome (CRPS).[2]

59. What are the different types of CRPS?

CRPS may follow a simple soft tissue injury (CRPS-I) or injury to a large peripheral nerve (CRPS-II). Allodynia and hyperalgesia are noted and there may be changes in skin appearance and temperature.[2]

60. What is phantom limb pain?

It is a continuous burning pain following amputation of a limb. It occurs in 60 to 80% of amputees, and is severe in up to 10% of cases. It is caused by a neuroma formation in the stump.[29]

61. What is the most likely cause of a rheumatoid arthritis patient's complaining of occipital pain in the distribution of the greater occipital nerve?

Patients with rheumatoid arthritis are at risk for atlantoaxial subluxation. This subluxation can compress nervous structures between the C1 and C2 lamina and can entrap the C2 dorsal ramus, giving occipital neuralgia. Surgical fixation of the unstable joint (such as C1–C2 wiring) can help with this occipital pain and provide stabilization to the C1–C2 area in these patients.[30]

62. What is allodynia?

Pain evoked by normally nonnoxious stimuli. This may be due to hyperexcitability of nociceptors and/or abnormal cross-talk between axons, termed ephaptic transmission.[31]

63. What differentiates typical from atypical trigeminal neuralgia?

In typical trigeminal neuralgia, the patient is pain-free between paroxysms, whereas in atypical trigeminal neuralgia, aching or burning background pain occurs between attacks. It has been suggested that atypical trigeminal neuralgia is an evolution of the typical variety.[32]

64. What is hyperpathia?

Increased sensitivity with increasing threshold to repetitive stimulation.

65. What is Prinzmetal's angina and what type of neurosurgical procedure is known to help with this problem?

Prinzmetal's angina is a form of angina that is often refractory to medications or coronary bypass grafting. It is believed to be due to coronary artery spasm. Thoracic sympathectomy is helpful in medically refractory angina of this type.[33]

66. List treatments for deafferentation pain syndrome.[34,35]

- Medication management initially, such as gabapentin, amitriptyline, and pregabalin.
- Spinal cord stimulator.
- Pain pump placement.
- Dorsal root entry zone ablation surgically.
- Thalamotomy.
- Motor cortex stimulation.

Upper Extremity

67. What are the common entrapment syndromes in the upper extremities?

- Median nerve entrapment at the carpal tunnel.
- Ulnar nerve entrapment at the cubital and Guyon's tunnel.
- Radial nerve entrapment at the spiral groove of the humerus.
- Posterior interosseous syndrome from radial nerve entrapment at the fibrous arch of the supinator muscle (arcade of Fröhse).[36]

68. List and classify some causes of hand and arm pain.

- Congenital: muscular dystrophies, osteogenesis imperfecta.
- Infection: herpes zoster, cellulites.
- Trauma: fractures, muscle contusion, muscle sprain.
- Tumor: Pancoast's tumor, metastases, neurofibroma (NF1), schwannoma, pathologic fracture, bone tumor, sarcoma.
- Inflammatory/autoimmune: Raynaud's phenomenon, vasculitis, brachial plexitis.
- Endocrine: hypo- or hyperthyroidism.
- Metabolic: potassium, calcium, or magnesium disturbances.
- Neuropathic: cervical spondylosis, referred pain, peripheral neuropathy.
- Medications.
- Vascular: myocardial infarction, peripheral vascular disease.

69. What is meant by a prefixed brachial plexus? What is a postfixed brachial plexus?

Occasionally, the brachial plexus is prefixed where C4 contributes to the upper trunk or is postfixed where T2 contributes to the lower trunk (**Fig. 7.3**). The brachial plexus normally includes C5–T1 nerves.[6]

70. What are the most common types of injuries to the brachial plexus?

Stretch and contusion injuries from motorcycles, falls, sports injuries, and blows to the shoulders.[6]

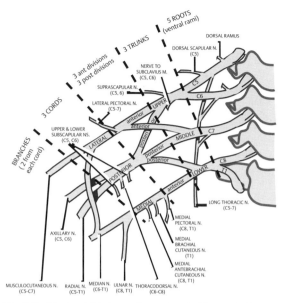

Fig. 7.3 The brachial plexus. (Reproduced with permission from Alberstone et al.[7])

71. What is the Martin-Gruber anastomosis?

An anatomical variation occurring 10 to 15% of the time where there is median to ulnar crossover of motor fibers in the forearm, which can be mistaken for a conduction block in the ulnar nerve during EMG. In half of these cases, the nerve communication arises from the anterior interosseous branch (**Fig. 7.4**).[26]

72. What is a Riche-Cannieu anastomosis?

An anatomical variation whereby there is a connection between the deep branch of the ulnar nerve and the recurrent motor branch of the median nerve. In this variant, the median and ulnar nerves are connected in the palm. Even with an ulnar nerve injury at the wrist, some intrinsic function still persists.[37]

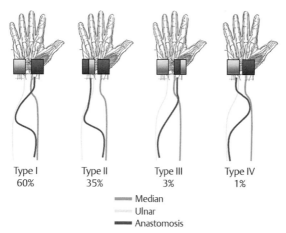

Type I   Type II   Type III   Type IV
60%   35%   3%   1%

━━━ Median
━━━ Ulnar
━━━ Anastomosis

Fig. 7.4   Variations in Martin-Gruber anastomosis.

73. Which syndrome affects the flexor digitorum profundus I and II, pronator quadratus, and flexor pollicis longus, but retains normal sensation?

Anterior interosseous nerve palsy.[36]

74. How can a palsy of the anterior interosseous branch of the median nerve lead to loss of hand intrinsics?

In cases of Martin-Gruber anastomosis.[38]

75. In a hand with normal anatomy, which muscles are controlled by the median nerve?

The lumbricals 1 and 2, the opponens pollicis, the abductor pollicis brevis, and the flexor pollicis brevis; all other hand intrinsics are controlled by the ulnar nerve.[2]

76. How can hand intrinsics be maintained from a low ulnar nerve injury?

A Martin-Gruber anastomosis between the anterior interosseous nerve and the ulnar nerve.[38]

77. What is the Gantzer muscle?

An aberrant accessory head to the flexor pollicis longus that may be a point of compression of the anterior interosseous nerve.[39]

78. What is the most common site of a radial nerve injury?

The spiral groove of the humerus.[36]

79. What diseases can cause carpal tunnel syndrome by connective tissue thickening?

- Rheumatoid arthritis.
- Acromegaly.
- Hypothyroidism or hyperthyroidism.
- Amyloid disease.
- Fluid retention.
- Weight gain.
- Pregnancy (self-limiting after birth).
- Multiple myeloma from amyloid deposition.

A malaligned carpal fracture, ganglion or synovial cyst, and other benign masses can also compromise the carpal tunnel without connective tissue thickening.[24]

80. What item in the patient history can best differentiate pronator syndrome from carpal tunnel syndrome?

Nocturnal exacerbation with carpal tunnel syndrome (with shaking of the hands to get relief) is not seen with pronator syndrome.[36]

81. What is the most common cause of failure of carpal tunnel surgery?

Incomplete transection of the transverse carpal ligament.[36]

82. What radial nerve–innervated muscle is usually spared in a radial nerve lesion involving the spiral groove?

The triceps.

83. Which ulnar nerve–innervated muscle is spared in a cubital tunnel lesion?

The flexor carpi ulnaris.

84. What types of arm abduction are affected in a C5 root injury compared with an axillary nerve injury?

A C5 root injury affects 180 degrees of shoulder abduction; an axillary nerve injury affects only the second 90 degrees of movement.[40]

85. How can one differentiate a C6 root lesion from a lesion of the musculocutaneous nerve?

A C6 root lesion affects the biceps, brachioradialis, and brachialis muscles; a musculocutaneous nerve lesion spares the brachioradialis.[2,7]

86. What muscle does the musculocutaneous nerve pass through?

The coracobrachialis. The nerve enters the muscle from the medial side 5 cm distal to the coracoid process. The musculocutaneous nerve has only motor innervation above the elbow and sensory innervation below the elbow.[4]

87. What are some C7 muscle movements that are not involved with the radial nerve?

Shoulder adduction and wrist flexion.[2]

88. What are the nerves involved with the control of thumb movement?

The median nerve controls abduction, flexion, and opposition; the ulnar controls adduction; and the radial nerve (by way of the posterior interosseous nerve) controls extension and abduction.

89. What is the common root of the suprascapular nerve and the radial nerve?

C6.

90. How does paralysis of the nerve to the rhomboids and long thoracic nerve help to localize an upper plexus lesion?

When these nerves are involved, it localizes the plexus lesion to a proximal rather than distal location.[7]

91. What findings would indicate that a brachial plexus lesion is very proximal?

- Rhomboid paralysis and winging of the scapula due to loss of serratus anterior muscle function.
- Phrenic nerve paralysis.
- Cervical spine fracture with or without myelopathy.
- Extensive paraspinal denervation.
- Presence of meningoceles at multiple levels as shown on myelography.
- Presence of a Horner syndrome.
- Peripheral sensory potentials or positive results for multiple nerves on histamine injection tests.[41]

92. What are the characteristics that differentiate an infraganglionic brachial plexus lesion (as opposed to supraganglionic or proximal lesion)?

- There is a positive Tinel sign.
- On nerve conduction studies, both motor conduction and sensory conduction are absent below the lesion.
- Absence of positive signs described in the question above.

93. What are some general contraindications to peripheral nerve surgery on a proximal brachial plexus lesion?

- Joint contractures.
- Severe edema.
- Advanced patient age.
- Lack of patient motivation or lack of patient understanding of surgical goals.

94. What are the types of entrapment that result in weakness specific to the supraspinatus and/or infraspinatus muscles?

Compression at the scapular notch by the suprascapular ligament (or a cyst) results in weakness of the supraspinatus and infraspinatus muscles. If compression occurs at the spinoglenoid notch (after branches have left for the supraspinatus), then only the infraspinatus muscle is affected. The supraspinatus is involved with glenohumeral joint stability and abduction of the humerus. The infraspinatus is mainly involved with external rotation of the upper arm.[36,42]

95. How can one demonstrate supraspinatus weakness and infraspinatus weakness on physical examination?

Supraspinatus weakness is best demonstrated by weakness in the first 15 degrees of abduction of the arm. Infraspinatus weakness is demonstrated with weakness of external rotation of the arm with the elbow held in 90 degrees of flexion.

96. What nerve innervates the angle of the mandible?

C2 via the greater auricular nerve.

97. How can one differentiate ulnar palsy from T1 root lesion?

The abductor pollicis brevis (invariably median nerve innervated) is spared in ulnar neuropathy, but is involved in a T1 lesion.[2,7]

98. How can one test for weakness of the abductor pollicis brevis?

Weakness of the abductor pollicis brevis may be demonstrated by having the patient abduct the thumb from the plane of the palm against resistance.[36]

99. What nerve entrapment can occur with hypertrophic scalene musculature from occupations where people lift things over their heads or after anterior cervical decompression resulting in postoperative subluxation?

Dorsal scapular nerve.

100. Which first branch from the posterior cord supplies the "cough muscle"?

The thoracodorsal nerve supplying the latissimus dorsi, which contracts when one coughs.

101. Which thoracic ganglia control palmar hyperhidrosis, axillary hyperhidrosis, and facial hyperhidrosis?

The second and third thoracic ganglia control palmar hyperhidrosis, the fourth controls axillary hyperhidrosis, and the first controls facial hyperhidrosis.[43]

102. What cardiac condition presents like a left C6 radiculopathy?

An acute myocardial infarction.

103. A medial cord brachial plexus injury and a C7–C8 root injury both affect median-innervated and ulnar-innervated muscles. How can one differentiate between them electrophysiologically?

The paraspinal muscles are involved in a root injury.

104. What nerve gives sensation to the "snuff box"?

The radial nerve.

105. The posterior interosseous branch of the radial nerve can be compressed at its point of entry into which muscle?

The supinator muscle.

106. What is the arcade of Fröhse?

The most proximal portion of the superficial head of the supinator muscle. It is a location of entrapment of the posterior interosseous nerve.[36]

107. How can one differentiate PIN (posterior interosseous nerve) palsy from a C7 nerve root syndrome?

In C7 nerve root syndrome, the triceps muscle is involved, unlike in PIN. Also, in a C7 nerve root injury, the wrist extensor muscles are usually spared, whereas in PIN palsy there is a weakness of the wrist extensors with a radial drift.[2,36]

108. How does one differentiate a PIN palsy from a more proximal radial nerve injury?

A radial nerve injury typically produces a complete wrist drop because the extensor carpi radialis longus is involved.[2,36]

109. What is Parsonage-Turner syndrome?

Parsonage-Turner syndrome, also known as brachial plexus neuritis or neuralgic amyotrophy, is a condition characterized by inflammation of a network of nerves that control the muscles of the chest, shoulders, and arms (brachial plexus). Individuals with the condition first experience a sudden onset of severe pain across the shoulder and upper arm. Within a few hours or days, the muscles of the affected shoulder may be affected by weakness, wasting, and paralysis. Although individuals with the condition may experience paralysis of the affected areas for months or, in some cases, years, recovery is usually complete.

The exact cause of Parsonage-Turner syndrome is not known.[2]

110. What muscles does the brachial plexus pass between?

The anterior and middle scalene.[4]

111. The C5 root is usually adherent to the lateral border of what muscle?

The anterior scalene muscle.

112. What can cause a lower root injury, and why are these roots more susceptible to injury?

A lower root injury (C8 and T1) may be caused by forceful abduction of the shoulder. A lower root injury produces weakness in intrinsics of the hand as well as long flexors and extensors of the fingers. Sensory deficit is along the medial aspect of the arm, forearm, and hand. There may be an associated Horner's syndrome if there is a T1-associated preganglionic injury due to disruption of the first sympathetic ganglion. The reason why the lower roots are more susceptible is because the upper roots are secured in their respective vertebrae; the lower roots are not as well secured.[7]

113. What anatomical space does the axillary nerve traverse between the teres minor and teres major muscles?

The quadrangular space in association with the posterior circumflex humeral artery.[4]

114. How can one diagnose quadrangular space syndrome?

By injecting lidocaine into the quadrangular space, also known as the quadrilateral space or the foramen of Velpeau. Alleviation of pain is diagnostic and therapeutic.[44,45]

115. How can the axillary nerve be injured?

Because of its relatively fixed position at the posterior cord and at the deltoid, any downward subluxation of the proximal humerus can result in traction and injury to the axillary nerve. It is also susceptible to injury with anterior shoulder dislocations because of its close relationship to the inferior capsule. In patients with axillary nerve injuries following anterior dislocation, a sensory examination over the lateral shoulder will be normal. An axillary nerve injury causes loss of shoulder abduction and external rotation. Occasionally, shoulder pain can be caused by entrapment of the axillary nerve.[39]

116. What is the thoracic outlet?

A space bounded by the clavicle, first rib, subclavius muscle, costoclavicular ligament, and anterior scalene muscle (**Fig. 7.5**).[7]

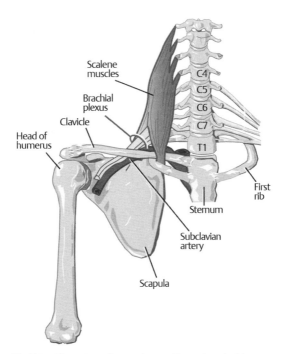

Fig. 7.5 Thoracic outlet syndrome. (Reproduced with permission from Alberstone et al.[7])

117. What is the culprit in thoracic outlet syndrome?

The most obvious structure that is occasionally present in this area is a cervical rib or an anomalous transverse process of C7. An anomalous fibrous band connecting the end of the cervical rib to the first rib may also be present. The supraclavicular approach provides the best visualization of the anatomy of the scalenus muscles and their relationship to the components of the brachial plexus in thoracic outlet surgery.[40]

118. Name other conditions that can mimic thoracic outlet syndrome.[46]

- Herniated disk disease (C7–C8 or C8–T1).
- Cervical spondylitis.
- Mediastinal venous obstruction (e.g., Pancoast's tumor).
- Brachial plexitis.
- Fibromyalgia.
- Raynaud's disease.
- Trauma.
- Ulnar nerve compression at the elbow.
- Vasculitis.
- Vasospastic disorder.

119. What is the Wartenberg sign? What is Wartenberg's syndrome?

The Wartenberg sign is the abducted posture of the small finger from ulnar nerve compromise from weakness of a palmar interosseous muscle. Wartenberg's syndrome is entrapment of the sensory branch of the radial nerve resulting in altered sensation over the dorsum of the hand. Tight casts, watch bands, and handcuffs are usually causes of Wartenberg's syndrome.[2,47]

120. What are signs and symptoms of first-order neuron Horner's syndrome?[48]

- Hemisensory loss.
- Dysarthria.
- Dysphagia.
- Ataxia.
- Vertigo.
- Nystagmus.
- Anhydrosis affects the ipsilateral side of the body.

121. What are signs and symptoms of second-order neuron Horner's syndrome?[48]

- Facial, neck, axillary, shoulder, or arm pain.
- Cough, hemoptysis.
- Anhydrosis of the ipsilateral face.

122. What are signs and symptoms of third-order neuron Horner's syndrome?[48]

- Diplopia from sixth nerve palsy.
- Numbness and pain in the distribution of the first or second division of the trigeminal nerve.
- Anhydrosis is either absent or limited to an area above the ipsilateral brow.

123. Name some common causes of Horner's syndrome.

- Brainstem stroke.
- Syringomyelia.
- Brachial plexus trauma.
- Pancoast tumors.
- Upper lobe pneumonia.
- Carotid dissecting aneurysm.
- Carotid artery ischemia.
- Migraine.
- Intracavernous or middle cranial fossa tumor.
- Iatrogenic post-ACDF (post–anterior cervical diskectomy and fusion) procedure.

Lower Extremity

124. What are the common entrapment syndromes of the lower extremities?

- Sciatic nerve entrapment at the piriformis muscle.
- Peroneal nerve entrapment at the fibular head.
- Plantar nerve entrapment at the tarsal tunnel.[36]

125. What reflex may help to differentiate intraspinal from peroneal causes of foot drop?

Internal hamstring reflex.[49]

126. Which set of muscles evert the foot?

Peroneus longus and brevis.[2]

127. Which muscle function may differentiate a femoral lesion from an L4 lesion?

The iliopsoas muscles are involved in a femoral lesion, not in an L4 lesion. The quadriceps muscle is weak in both femoral neuropathy and L4 radiculopathy. Thigh adduction may be weak in L4 radiculopathy, but normal in femoral neuropathy.

128. What sensation finding may help to distinguish a femoral lesion from an L4 lesion?

In femoral neuropathy, the anterior thigh may have a sensation loss; in L4 radiculopathy, the sensation loss is from the knee to the medial malleolus.

129. What is the femoral stretch test?

With the patient prone, lifting the leg to test for irritation of the nerve roots at L4 and above. This is also called the reverse leg raising test. Recall that the straight leg raise is performed with the patient supine and raising the leg stretches the L5 and S1 nerve roots.[50]

130. If injured exclusively, which nerve in the lower extremity will result in a foot drop and minimal sensory loss?

The deep peroneal nerve.[40]

131. Which nerve innervates the web space between the first and second toes?

The deep peroneal nerve.[40]

132. What are two common sites of stretch injury to the peroneal nerve?

1. The peroneal nerve can be stretched in association with fibular head trauma.
2. The peroneal division of the sciatic nerve can be stretched secondary to hip dislocation.

This reinforces the fact that damage may be located more proximal than the examiner suspects.[51]

133. How can one differentiate a common peroneal nerve injury from a superficial peroneal nerve injury?

Both have weak foot eversion; however, there is no foot drop with superficial peroneal nerve injury.[2]

134. What are some causes of a painless foot drop?

- ALS.
- Parasagittal brain tumor.
- Some cases of peroneal neuropathy.[2]

135. Which nerve is compressed in anterior tarsal tunnel syndrome (pain in the dorsum of the foot and atrophy of the extensor digitorum brevis)?

The deep peroneal nerve.[9]

136. How can one differentiate an L3 root lesion from a femoral lesion?

Adductors are involved in a root lesion.

137. How is pain and weakness elicited in piriformis syndrome?

With external rotation and abduction of the hip. The Freiberg test (forced internal rotation of the hip with thigh extension) can exacerbate the symptoms.[52]

138. What nerve is most likely injured in a patient with an externally rotated foot on walking and weakness in internal rotation and adduction?

The obturator nerve.[2]

139. In any peroneal nerve injury, what muscle above the knee is important to evaluate by physical examination and EMG?

Short head of biceps femoris. If this muscle demonstrates membrane instability on EMG (positive sharp waves and fibrillations), then the lesion is most likely proximal to the fibular head.[40]

140. What is the first sensory branch of the lumbar plexus?

The iliohypogastric nerve (**Fig. 7.6**).[7]

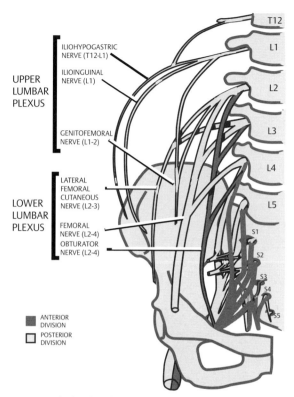

Fig. 7.6 The lumbar plexus. (Reproduced with permission from Alberstone et al.[7])

141. What is the only thigh muscle supplied by the peroneal division of the sciatic nerve?

Short head of the biceps femoris (**Fig. 7.7**).[2,4]

142. Forced internal rotation of the hip is a provocative test to elicit pain from what syndrome?

Piriformis syndrome.[52]

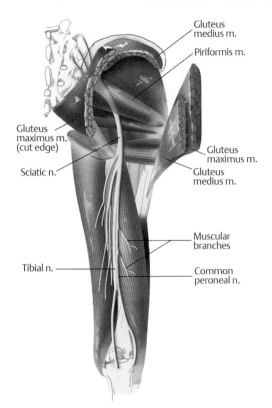

Fig. 7.7 Course of the sciatic nerve. (Reproduced with permission from Midha and Zager.[39])

143. What nerve innervates the main medial rotators of the thigh?

The superior gluteal nerve (L4, L5) (**Fig. 7.8**).[2]

144. Dysfunction of the superior gluteal nerve results in what type of gait?

A Trendelenburg gait.[53]

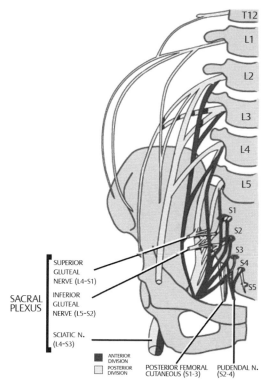

Fig. 7.8 The sacral plexus. (Reproduced with permission from Alberstone et al.[7])

145. What alternative innervation can the extensor digitorum brevis have?

Accessory deep peroneal nerve (a branch of the superficial peroneal nerve).[54]

146. What is the most common location of an intraneural ganglion cyst?

The peroneal nerve behind the fibula head.[40]

147. What is the most frequently injured nerve in the lower extremities?

The peroneal nerve and peroneal division of the sciatic nerve are the most frequently injured nerves in the lower extremities because of their exposed position and susceptibility to trauma.[36,40]

148. What is the best L5-innervated muscle to test clinically?

The extensor hallucis longus. Sometimes an S1 radiculopathy can weaken this muscle.

149. What is the differential diagnosis of a sacral nerve root mass?

- Schwannoma.
- Neurofibroma.
- Traumatic neuroma, perineuroma.
- Malignant peripheral nerve sheath tumor.
- Neurogenic sarcoma (malignant schwannoma).
- Ganglion cyst.
- Glomus.
- AVM.

Cases

■ Case 1

A patient presents with numbness and paresthesias of his pinky and half of the ring finger, with some weakness of his hand. His hand has the deformity pictured in **Fig. 7.9**. What is the likely diagnosis?

■ Case 1 Answer

This is a case of ulnar nerve entrapment. The figure demonstrates a claw hand. Symptoms tend to be weakness of fourth and fifth digit finger flexion and interosseous muscles seen with finger abduction. There may be hypothenar and interosseous wasting. The claw deformity forms by weakness of the lumbricals 3 and 4. Sensory loss is in the pinky and ulnar half of the ring finger. The thumb, index and middle fingers, and medial side of the ring finger are innervated by the median nerve. The Tinel sign may be

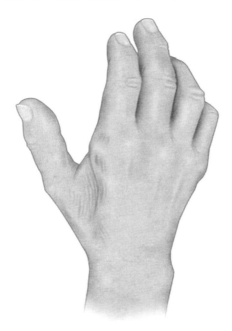

Fig. 7.9 Illustration showing hand position. (Reproduced with permission from Rohkamm.[55])

positive at the elbow. Ulnar nerve neurolysis with or without transposition is the standard treatment.[40]

■ Case 2

A patient fractures his forearm and develops an inability to dorsiflex the wrist. What is the likely injury?

■ Case 2 Answer

This is a radial nerve injury. A problem in the midupper arm would likely cause wrist drop without triceps weakness, as the branch innervating the triceps will have left the nerve proximal to the injured site. Treatment is exploration if there

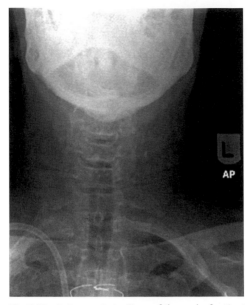

Fig. 7.10 Anteroposterior X-ray of the neck of patient with cervical rib.

is no improvement in 8 weeks. A nerve conduction study would be used for evaluation.[7,40]

■ Case 3

A patient presents with right shoulder and arm pain with numbness and weakness of the hand. An X-ray (**Fig. 7.10**) shows this abnormality. What is the diagnosis?

■ Case 3 Answer

This is a C7 cervical rib causing thoracic outlet syndrome. The subclavian artery, vein, and brachial plexus pass between the anterior and medial scalene muscles, which insert into the first rib. Arterial compression may cause Raynaud-type symptoms. Nerve compression may mimic ulnar nerve compression.[7]

■ Case 4

A patient presents with weakness of his arms and legs. There are no sensory deficits noted. He has no autonomic dysfunction. There is no cognitive dysfunction. He has tongue fasciculations noted on examination. He is hyperreflexic in some muscle groups and hyporeflexic in others. His magnetic resonance imaging (MRI) scan is normal. What is the diagnosis?

■ Case 4 Answer

ALS. This is caused by degeneration of motor neurons in the spinal cord and brainstem as well as the corticospinal tract. It tends to present with lower and upper motor neuron problems. There is no cognitive or sensory dysfunction. Extraocular muscles and urinary sphincter are usually spared. Tongue fasciculations are common.[11]

■ Case 5

A patient presents with significant weakness in dorsiflexion at the ankle as well as the big toe with numbness of the lateral foot but normal sensation of the medial foot. What is the likely cause?

■ Case 5 Answer

Foot drop may be caused by an L5 radiculopathy or also a peroneal nerve entrapment just below the fibular head. In this case, there is numbness of the lateral foot. This is more consistent with peroneal nerve dysfunction, as the L5-mediated dorsiflexion weakness would cause numbness of the medial foot. Also, L5 innervates the hip abductors and on examination one will notice that the patient has difficulty abducting the leg. This would not be present with a peroneal nerve problem. Foot drop may also be caused by a parasagittal brain tumor.[7]

■ References

1. Morgan S, Orrell RW. Pathogenesis of amyotrophic lateral sclerosis. Br Med Bull 2016;119(1):87–98
2. Greenberg MS. Handbook of Neurosurgery. 8th ed. New York, NY: Thieme Medical Publishers; 2016

3. Kim DH, Murovic JA, Kim YY, Kline DG. Surgical treatment and outcomes in 15 patients with anterior interosseous nerve entrapments and injuries. J Neurosurg 2006;104(5):757–765

4. Kline DJ, Hudson AR, Kim DH. Atlas of Peripheral Nerve Surgery. Philadelphia, PA: WB Saunders; 2001

5. Davis GA, Knight S. Pancoast tumor resection with preservation of brachial plexus and hand function. Neurosurg Focus 2007;22(6):E15

6. Kline DG, Hudson AR. Acute injuries of peripheral nerves. In: Youmans JR, ed. Neurological Surgery. 4th ed. Philadelphia, PA: WB Saunders; 1996:2103–2181

7. Alberstone CD, Steinmetz MP, Najm IM, Benzel EC. Anatomic Basis of Neurologic Diagnosis. New York, NY: Thieme Medical Publishers; 2007

8. Drake JM, Siddiqi SN. Birth trauma. In: Youmans JR, ed. Neurological Surgery. 4th ed. Philadelphia, PA: WB Saunders; 1996:1767–1777

9. Tindall SC. Chronic injuries of peripheral nerves by entrapment. In: Youmans JR, ed. Neurological Surgery. 4th ed. Philadelphia, PA: WB Saunders; 1996:2182–2208

10. Pavlus JD, Carter BW, Tolley MD, Keung ES, Khorashadi L, Lichtenberger JP III. Imaging of thoracic neurogenic tumors. AJR Am J Roentgenol 2016;207(3):552–561

11. Mumenthaler M, Mattle H. Neurology. Stuttgart: Georg Thieme Verlag; 2005

12. Peitersen E. Bell's palsy: the spontaneous course of 2,500 peripheral facial nerve palsies of different etiologies. Acta Otolaryngol Suppl 2002;(549):4–30

13. Schabort D, Boon JM, Becker PJ, Meiring JH. Easily identifiable bony landmarks as an aid in targeted regional ankle blockade. Clin Anat 2005;18(7):518–526

14. Diaz FG, Johnson RR. Extracranial occlusive disease of the vertebral artery. In: Youmans JR, ed. Neurological Surgery. 4th ed. Philadelphia, PA: WB Saunders; 1996

15. Lévecque JP, Borne M, Saïssy JM. Analgesia with continuous lateral posterior tibial nerve block. Reg Anesth Pain Med 1999;24(2):191–192

16. Masear VR, Meyer RD, Pichora DR. Surgical anatomy of the medial antebrachial cutaneous nerve. J Hand Surg Am 1989;14(2, pt 1):267–271

17. Barber FA. Suprascapular nerve block for shoulder arthroscopy. Arthroscopy 2005;21(8):1015

18. Hohenberger GM, Maier MJ, Grechenig C, Schwarz AM, Matzi V, Weiglein AH. Carpal tunnel release: safe and simple identification of the flexor retinaculum based on superficial anatomical landmarks. Clin Anat 2017;30(4):512–516

19. Boya H, Ozcan O, Oztekin HH. Long-term complications of open carpal tunnel release. Muscle Nerve 2008;38(5):1443–1446

20. Connolly ES, McKhann GM, Huang J, Choudhri TF. Fundamentals of Operative Techniques in Neurosurgery. New York, NY: Thieme Medical Publishers; 2002

21. Fessler RG, Sekhar L. Atlas of Neurosurgical Techniques—Spine & Peripheral Nerve. New York, NY: Thieme Medical Publishers; 2006

22. Venkatramani H, Bhardwaj P, Faruquee SR, Sabapathy SR. Functional outcome of nerve transfer for restoration of shoulder and elbow function in upper brachial plexus injury. J Brachial Plex Peripher Nerve Inj 2008;3:15

23. Trehan SK, Model Z, Lee SK. Nerve repair and nerve grafting. Hand Clin 2016;32(2):119–125

24. Perretta D, Green S. Bridging the gap in peripheral nerve repair. Bull Hosp Jt Dis (2013) 2017;75(1):57–63

25. Pathy R, Dodwell ER. Medial epicondyle fractures in children. Curr Opin Pediatr 2015;27(1):58–66

26. Subramony SH, Carpenter DE. Electromyography. In: Youmans JR, ed. Neurological Surgery. 4th ed. Philadelphia, PA: WB Saunders; 1996:223–246

27. Phillips WD, Vincent A. Pathogenesis of myasthenia gravis: update on disease types, models, and mechanisms. F1000Res 2016;5. pii: F1000 Faculty Rev-1513

28. Olney RK. Clinical trials for polyneuropathy: the role of nerve conduction studies, quantitative sensory testing, and autonomic function testing. J Clin Neurophysiol 1998;15(2):129–137

29. Nikolajsen L, Staehelin Jensen T. Phantom limb pain. Curr Rev Pain 2000;4(2):166–170

30. Hartlev LB, Gudmundsdottir G, Mosdal C, Stengaard-Pedersen K. Rheumatoid arthritis with atlanto-axial subluxation. Pre- and postoperative symptoms, radiological findings and operative complications [in Danish]. Ugeskr Laeger 2008;170(8):647–650

31. Jensen TS, Finnerup NB. Allodynia and hyperalgesia in neuropathic pain: clinical manifestations and mechanisms. Lancet Neurol 2014;13(9):924–935

32. Jacob RP, Rhoton AL Jr. Diagnosis and non-operative management of trigeminal neuralgia. In: Youmans JR, ed. Neurological Surgery. 4th ed. Philadelphia, PA: WB Saunders; 1996:3376–3385

33. Henrard L, Pierard L, Limet R. Treatment of Prinzmetal's angina with normal coronary vessels by thoracic sympathectomy [in French]. Arch Mal Coeur Vaiss 1982;75(11):1317–1320

34. Chang Chien GC, Candido KD, Saeed K, Knezevic NN. Cervical spinal cord stimulation treatment of deafferentation pain from brachial plexus avulsion injury complicated by complex regional pain syndrome. A A Case Rep 2014;3(3):29–34

35. Carvalho GA, Nikkhah G, Samii M. Pain management after post-traumatic brachial plexus lesions. Conservative and surgical therapy possibilities [in German]. Orthopade 1997;26(7):621–625

36. Rengashary S. Entrapment neuropathies. In: Rengashary SS, Wilkins RH, eds. Neurosurgery. 2nd ed. New York, NY: McGraw-Hill; 1996:3073–3098

37. Ahadi T, Raissi GR, Yavari M, Majidi L. Prevalence of ulnar-to-median nerve motor fiber anastomosis (Riché-Cannieu communicating branch) in hand: an electrophysiological study. Med J Islam Repub Iran 2016; 30:324

38. Piagkou M, Tasigiorgos S, Lappas D, et al. Median to ulnar nerve anastomosis: a review of the literature. Chirurgia (Bucur) 2012;107(4):442–446

39. al-Qattan MM. Gantzer's muscle. An anatomical study of the accessory head of the flexor pollicis longus muscle. J Hand Surg [Br] 1996;21(2):269–270

40. Midha R, Zager E. Surgery of Peripheral Nerves: A Case-Based Approach. New York, NY: Thieme Medical Publishers; 2007

41. Guha A, Graham B, Kline DG, Hudson AR. Brachial plexus injuries. In: Rengachary SS, Wilkins RH, eds. Neurosurgery. 2nd ed. New York, NY: McGraw-Hill; 1996:3121–3134

42. Maniker A. Operative Exposures in Peripheral Nerve Surgery. New York, NY: Thieme Medical Publishers; 2005

43. Cameron AE. Selecting the right patient for surgical treatment of hyperhidrosis. Thorac Surg Clin 2016;26(4):403–406

44. Lester B, Jeong GK, Weiland AJ, Wickiewicz TL. Quadrilateral space syndrome: diagnosis, pathology, and treatment. Am J Orthop (Belle Mead NJ) 1999;28(12):718–722, 725

45. Cahill BR, Palmer RE. Quadrilateral space syndrome. J Hand Surg Am 1983;8(1):65–69

46. Laulan J, Fouquet B, Rodaix C, Jauffret P, Roquelaure Y, Descatha A. Thoracic outlet syndrome: definition, aetiological factors, diagnosis, management and occupational impact. J Occup Rehabil 2011;21(3):366–373

47. Zöch G, Aigner N. Wartenberg syndrome: a rare or rarely diagnosed compression syndrome of the radial nerve? [in German]. Handchir Mikrochir Plast Chir 1997;29(3):139–143

48. Reede DL, Garcon E, Smoker WR, Kardon R. Horner's syndrome: clinical and radiographic evaluation. Neuroimaging Clin N Am 2008;18(2):369–385, xi

49. Miller DW, Hahn JF. General methods of clinical examination. In: Youmans JR, ed. Neurological Surgery. 4th ed. Philadelphia, PA: WB Saunders; 1996:31–40

50. Nadler SF, Malanga GA, Stitik TP, Keswani R, Foye PM. The crossed femoral nerve stretch test to improve diagnostic sensitivity for the high lumbar radiculopathy: 2 case reports. Arch Phys Med Rehabil 2001;82(4):522–523

51. Kim DH, Murovic JA, Tiel RL, Kline DG. Management and outcomes in 318 operative common peroneal nerve lesions at the Louisiana State University Health Sciences Center. Neurosurgery 2004;54(6):1421–1428, discussion 1428–1429

52. Niu CC, Lai PL, Fu TS, Chen LH, Chen WJ. Ruling out piriformis syndrome before diagnosing lumbar radiculopathy. Chang Gung Med J 2009;32(2):182–187

53. Petrofsky JS. The use of electromyogram biofeedback to reduce Trendelenburg gait. Eur J Appl Physiol 2001;85(5):491–495

54. Kayal R, Katirji B. Atypical deep peroneal neuropathy in the setting of an accessory deep peroneal nerve. Muscle Nerve 2009;40(2):313–315

55. Rohkamm R. Color Atlas of Neurology. Stuttgart: Georg Thieme Verlag; 2004

8 Neurology

General

1. What is the Dandy maneuver?

To assess for a possible cerebrospinal fluid (CSF) leak, the patient's head is held below the waist for several minutes while in a sitting position.[1] Walter Dandy (1886–1946) was one of the founding fathers of neurosurgery. He described CSF circulation, was the first neurosurgeon to clip an aneurysm, and established the first intensive care unit.

2. What is the name of the syndrome that comprises quadriplegia, anarthria, and preserved consciousness?

Locked-in syndrome. It is most commonly seen with upper brainstem infarction and can also involve the third nerve nucleus.[2]

3. What are the common features of normal pressure hydrocephalus?

Gait apraxia, urinary incontinence, and dementia.[3]

4. What is the Adam triad?

The Adam triad of symptoms of normal pressure hydrocephalus includes gait apraxia, incontinence, and dementia.

5. Failure of ventriculoperitoneal shunting in patients with idiopathic normal pressure hydrocephalus may be attributed to what other causes of dementia?

Vascular dementia or Alzheimer's disease.

6. What are the top three causes of dementia?

Alzheimer's disease, Lewy's body dementia, and multiinfarct dementia.[4] Other disorders linked to dementia are Huntington's disease, traumatic brain injury, and Parkinson's disease.

7. What are the main differentiating factors between Alzheimer's disease and Lewy's body dementia?

In Alzheimer's disease, cortical neuritic plaques and neurofibrillary tangles are seen; early impairment in short-term memory is evident. It is more prevalent in women. In Lewy's body dementia, there is relatively preserved memory with impairments in executive functions; parkinsonian and autonomic features are present. It is more prevalent in men.[5]

8. What is pseudobulbar affect?

Pseudobulbar affect (also known as intermittent emotional expression disorder) is characterized by involuntary displays of crying or laughing, typically without any associated feelings of sadness, depression, or euphoria. Pseudobulbar affect is associated with a variety of neurologic illnesses including multiple sclerosis (MS), amyotrophic lateral sclerosis, Alzheimer's disease, Huntington's disease, Parkinson's disease, stroke, and traumatic brain injury.[6]

9. How is the hearing loss from Ménière's disease different from the hearing loss caused by an acoustic tumor?

The hearing loss from Ménière's disease fluctuates, whereas the hearing loss from a tumor is usually progressive. Also, the brainstem auditory evoked potentials are normal in Ménière's disease.[7,8]

10. What is the most common cause of Cushing syndrome?

Iatrogenic administration of exogenous steroids.[9] Harvey Cushing (1869–1939) is considered the "father of neurosurgery." He developed local anesthetic, the tourniquet, and heart pressure and oxygen level monitoring. He received a Pulitzer Prize for the biography of Sir William Osler. The rivalry and antagonism between Cushing and Dandy is a subject of interest among neurosurgical historians.

11. What are the classic symptoms of Parkinson's disease?

Resting tremor, cogwheel rigidity, and bradykinesia.[10]

12. What is the abduction relief sign?

The abduction relief sign is performed by the patient abducting the shoulder and placing the hand ipsilateral to the radiculopathy on the top of his head. Relief of radicular symptoms is a positive sign. A worsening of symptoms may point to thoracic outlet syndrome.[11]

Emergencies and Epilepsy

13. What are the features of baclofen withdrawal?

Rebound spasticity, hemodynamic lability, severe hyperthermia, altered mental status, pruritus, diaphoresis, diffuse intravascular coagulopathy, rhabdomyolysis, and multiorgan system failure.[12]

14. What is the difference between an early and a late posttraumatic seizure?

Early implies less than or equal to 7 days, whereas late is more than 7 days.[13]

15. What is the definition of status epilepticus?

An epileptic seizure of greater than 5 minutes or more than one seizure within a 5-minute period without the person returning to normal between them.[14]

16. What is the most common cause of status epilepticus in an adult?

Subtherapeutic antiepileptic drug levels in a patient with known seizure disorder.

17. What is the pharmacologic treatment of status epilepticus?

Intravenous (IV) glucose 50% 50 mL, IV thiamine 100 mg (folate/multivitamin).

Treatment is according to the following, in order:

- Lorazepam 1 to 2 mg every 5 minutes, up to 9 mg (0.1 mg/kg) or diazepam 5 mg every 5 minutes, up to 20 mg (0.2 mg/kg).
- Phenytoin—loading dose 20 mg/kg.
- Phenobarbital drip—loading dose 20 mg/kg.
- Pentobarbital drip—20 mg/kg if seizure does not arrest in 30 minutes.[15,16]

18. What are some common causes of changes in mental status or coma?

The mnemonic "AEIOU TIPS" is a help in identifying common causes:

- *A*lcohol (drugs and toxins).
- *E*ndocrine, *e*xocrine, *e*lectrolyte.
- *I*nsulin.
- *O*piates, *o*verdose.
- *U*remia.
- *T*rauma, *t*emperature (abnormal).
- *I*nfection.
- *P*sychiatric disorder.
- *S*eizure, *s*troke, *s*hock, *s*pace-occupying lesion.[17]

19. What is sudden unexpected death in an epileptic patient typically attributed to?

Seizure-related cardiac arrhythmia.[18]

20. What is the long-term outcome of patients who suffer from prolonged refractory status epilepticus?

Approximately 50% mortality. Of the patients surviving, only about half to two-thirds will have functional cognitive status.[19]

21. What are some indications for a hemispherectomy?

Intractable epilepsy in the setting of unilateral hemisphere damage, congenital hemiplegia, chronic encephalitis, hemimegalencephaly, and Sturge-Weber syndrome.[20,21]

22. Sturge-Weber syndrome is associated with intracranial calcifications, seizures, glaucoma, and port-wine stains in the distribution of which cranial nerve?

The trigeminal nerve. The intracranial findings in Sturge-Weber syndrome are only seen in patients in whom the port-wine lesions involve the first division of the trigeminal nerve.

23. What does the electroencephalogram (EEG) show in an absence seizure?

Spike-and-wave pattern at exactly three per second.[22]

24. What is the most common type of seizure?

Febrile convulsions.[23]

25. Which type of seizure is associated with West syndrome?

Infantile spasms, also known as epileptic spasms. West syndrome produces seizures in early childhood and consists of the classic triad of mental retardation, infantile spasms, and hypsarrhythmia on EEG (completely chaotic and disorganized background pattern).[24]

26. What is the treatment of infantile spasms?

Adrenocorticotropic hormone (ACTH) rather than antiepileptics.[25]

27. What is Aicardi syndrome?

A triad of callosal agenesis, ocular abnormalities, and infantile spasm.[26] Aicardi syndrome is a rare neurologic disorder first described by French neurologist Jean Aicardi in 1965. It occurs most commonly in females, but it can also occur in males with Klinefelter's syndrome.

28. What is the most common cause of complex partial seizures?

Mesial temporal lobe epilepsy is the most common cause of complex partial seizures. About 70 to 80% of these seizures arise from the temporal lobe, and more than 65% of these originate in the mesial temporal lobe structures, especially the hippocampus, amygdala, and parahippocampal gyrus.

29. Which region of the hippocampus is spared in mesial temporal lobe epilepsy?

The CA2 subregion and the dentate granule cells are relatively spared, as cell loss is more pronounced in the CA1, CA3, and CA4 subregions.

Infectious and Inflammatory

■ Infectious Diseases

30. What are the most common agents that cause transplacental infections?

Use the mnemonic "TORCHES":

- *T*oxoplasma.
- *O*ther agents such as human immunodeficiency virus (HIV).

- *R*ubella.
- Cytomegalovirus (CMV).
- *H*erpes virus.
- *S*yphilis.[27]

31. Discuss the CSF profile in the different types of meningitis.

Refer to **Table 8.1** for details.

32. What is the most common cause of viral meningitis?

Enterovirus in ~80% of cases.[28] Coxsackie or echovirus groups of enteroviruses are the most common enterovirus. Most infections produce no symptoms, or mild symptoms such as sore throats, colds, and flulike illnesses.

33. Which histologic stain is used to diagnose cryptococcosis?

An India ink stain is utilized to identify cryptococcosis, which is shown as single budding yeasts with a thick capsule.[29]

Table 8.1   Cerebrospinal fluid profile in infectious meningitis

Infectious agent	Opening pressure (mm H_2O)	Glucose (mg/dL)	Protein (mg/dL)	White blood cell (type)
Bacteria	High (< 200)	Low (< 40)	High (> 100)	Elevated (neutrophilic)
Viral/aseptic	Normal/mildly elevated (< 200)	Normal (50–70)	Normal/mildly elevated (15–40)	Elevated (lymphocytic)
Tuberculosis	Normal/mildly elevated (180–300)	Very low (< 40)	High (> 100)	Elevated (pleocytosis)
Fungal	Normal/mildly elevated (180–300)	Low (< 40)	Mildly elevated (50–200)	Elevated (lymphocytic)

34. What is the most common central nervous system (CNS) fungal infection?

Candidiasis, which is caused by *Candida albicans*.

35. What is the causative agent of neurocysticercosis?

The larval stage of the pork tapeworm *Taenia solium*. It is the most common parasitic infection involving the CNS.[30]

36. What antihelmintics are used to treat neurocysticercosis?

Praziquantel and albendazole. Steroids are also given concurrently to reduce the edema that tends to occur initially during treatment with antihelmintics.[31]

37. What is Gradenigo syndrome?

Petrous apex osteomyelitis with sixth cranial nerve palsy and retro-orbital pain. It occurs in children from extension of severe otitis.[32]

38. What are Negri bodies?

Intracytoplasmic eosinophilic collections in neurons seen with rabies.[33]

39. How does the rabies virus reach the CNS?

The virus travels in a retrograde fashion through the peripheral nerves to reach the CNS.[34]

40. What is the treatment of rabies?

Passive immunization for 10 to 20 days with rabies immunoglobulin.[35]

41. What is the causative agent of Lyme disease?

Borrelia burgdorferi.[36]

42. What antibiotic is most commonly used to treat Lyme disease?

Antibiotics commonly used for oral treatment include doxycycline, amoxicillin, or cefuroxime.[37]

43. Which organism is associated with Sydenham's chorea?

Group A β-hemolytic streptococcus. Sydenham's chorea is one of the main criteria of rheumatic fever. Other features include arthritis, erythema marginatum, and endocarditis.[38]

44. What are the major symptoms and signs of tabes dorsalis?

The major symptoms are ataxia, lightning pains, and urinary incontinence; the chief signs are absent tendon reflexes at the knee and ankle, impaired vibratory and position sense in the legs and feet, and a positive Romberg's sign. An Argyll Robertson pupil is found in 90% of cases.[39]

45. What is Hutchinson's triad (congenital syphilis)?

Notched teeth, deafness, and interstitial keratitis.[40]

46. The presence of an "owl's eye" intranuclear inclusion is suggestive of what kind of infection?

CMV encephalitis. Cowdry type A intranuclear inclusions are characteristic of CMV, but these are also found with other infections.

47. What does *Aspergillus* look like with silver stain?

It has branching septate hyphae.

48. What does *Mucor* look like histologically?

It has nonseptate right-angle branching hyphae.

49. What patients are at risk of suffering from mucormycosis?

Diabetic patients. This disease is fatal within a few days unless treated aggressively.[41]

50. What is the most common pathogen that causes brain abscess?

Streptococcus. These abscesses occur most commonly at the gray–white matter junction and are multiple in ~30% of cases.

51. How is a brain abscess acquired?

An abscess can form from local spread of an adjacent ear or sinus infection, from hematogenous spread from another infected site (most commonly lung), or from trauma, or it can rarely be iatrogenic.[42]

52. In what U.S. states can histoplasmosis be found?

In Ohio and Mississippi.

53. Where is blastomycosis found in the United States?

In the eastern United States.

54. Where is coccidioidomycosis found in the United States?

In the Southwest, especially in California and Arizona.

55. What is the intermediate host in hydatid disease?

Sheep. Hydatid disease is caused by *Echinococcus granulosus*, a dog tapeworm. Cysts form in the liver, lung, and brain.[43]

56. What is the intermediate host in schistosomiasis?

The snail. Schistosomiasis is caused by *Schinia masoni*, *Schistosoma haematobium*, and *Schistosoma japonicum*. These trematodes live in blood vessels.

57. What are the cells of origin that are found in primary CNS lymphoma in a patient with HIV?

B cell origin.[44]

58. What is the most common cause of myelopathy in HIV?

Vacuolar myelopathy. It is prudent to obtain a magnetic resonance imaging (MRI) scan to exclude a mass lesion before giving this diagnosis because vacuolar myelopathy is a diagnosis of exclusion.[45]

59. Which parts of the spinal cord does acquired immunodeficiency syndrome (AIDS)–associated vacuolar myelopathy involve?

It mainly involves the posterior and lateral columns of the thoracic spinal cord.[46]

60. Subacute sclerosing panencephalitis is a postinfectious process of which viral infection?

Measles. It occurs several years after a measles infection, usually before 2 years of age. Death occurs within 1 to 3 years.[47]

61. What is the causative agent of cat-scratch disease?

Bartonella henselae. Most people acquire this bacterial infection following a scratch or a bite by a cat. Local inflammation and regional adenitis develop. In immunocompromised people, this disease can progress to produce virulent encephalitis associated with status epilepticus. A brain MRI scan may show a characteristic hyperintensity in the pulvinar region.[48]

62. What types of treatments are given for ADEM (acute disseminated encephalomyelitis)?

High-dose steroids, plasmapheresis, and IV immunoglobulin.[49]

63. What viruses have been associated with ADEM?

Paramyxovirus, varicella, rubella, and Epstein-Barr virus.[50]

64. What do CSF studies typically show with ADEM?

Protein slightly elevated with a lymphocytic pleocytosis.[51]

65. What is the clinical triad of neurologic manifestations in Lyme disease?[52]

1. Cranial neuritis (mimicking Bell's palsy).
2. Meningitis.
3. Radiculopathy.

66. What is the causative agent of PML (progressive multifocal leukoencephalopathy)?

PML is the result of infection of the brain with the JC virus (a papovavirus). PML is usually associated with impaired immunity, specifically altered cell-mediated immunity.[53]

67. What is the drug of choice for the treatment of herpes simplex encephalitis?

Acyclovir. Because it is a relatively safe drug, it is acceptable to start this drug empirically in presumptive cases of herpes encephalitis.[54]

68. What is the most common organism found in hematogenous pyogenic vertebral osteomyelitis?

Staphylococcus aureus.[55]

69. What are the most common ganglia involved in herpes zoster?

The trigeminal and thoracic ganglia are the most common neuronal sites in herpes zoster; these dermatomes are also the most common sites of cutaneous eruption.[56]

■ Inflammatory

70. What is the most common human prion disease?

Creutzfeldt-Jakob disease accounts for ~85% of all human prion disease.[57]

71. What type of inflammatory response is seen in Creutzfeldt-Jakob disease histologically?

None.

72. Positive immunoassay for what protein in the CSF supports the diagnosis of Creutzfeldt-Jakob disease?

14–3–3-brain protein.[58] Instruments used for a procedure on a patient with Creutzfeldt-Jakob disease should be discarded. Sterilization protocols from the World Health Organization (WHO), the Centers for Disease Control and Prevention (CDC), and the Association for the Advancement of Medical Instrumentation (AAMI) conflict with one another.

73. What is the most frequent chronic neurologic disease of young adults?

MS.[59]

74. Describe the revised McDonald's criteria for diagnosis of MS.

Revised McDonald's criteria were initiated in 2005. They are as follows[60,61]:

• Two or more acute attacks with clinical evidence of two or more lesions

or

- Two or more attacks with clinical evidence of at least one lesion and two or more lesions found on MRI, or CSF findings suggestive of MS

or

- One or more attacks with clinical evidence of two or more lesions with dissemination in time (DIT) evidence

or

- One attack and clinical evidence of a lesion with either dissemination in space with more than two lesions found on MRI with CSF findings or at least DIT by another attack.

75. Describe the criteria for an acute MS attack.

- Symptoms lasting > 24 hours.
- Each attack should be separated from another one by at least 1 month.

Congenital and Pediatric

76. Below what spinal level does one make the diagnosis of tethered cord?

Tethered cord is defined as a conus medullaris below the level of L2. The diagnosis of tethered cord syndrome is made clinically with presenting symptoms of bladder dysfunction, deficits in the lower extremities, abnormal gait, and/or pain in the back or lower extremities.[62]

77. What is the most common condition associated with syringomyelia?

Chiari I malformation.[63] Depending on the symptomatology of the Chiari, one can observe or operate if the symptoms are daily. Eliminating the Chiari will usually resolve the syrinx.

78. Supplementation with which vitamin can reduce the incidence of open neural tube defects (NTDs)?

Folate. Taking 400 mg of synthetic folic acid daily from fortified foods and/or supplements has been suggested. The Recommended Dietary Allowance (RDA) for folate equivalents for pregnant women is 600 mg.[64]

79. What is the most common malignant brain tumor in children?

Medulloblastoma.[65]

80. What is the lifetime risk of cancer when a patient in early childhood gets a computed tomography (CT) scan of the head? What is ALARA?

A 0.5% lifetime risk of fatal cancer in addition to reduced cognitive abilities. As low as reasonably achievable (ALARA) refers to radiation dose and children.[66]

81. What is the most common pediatric CNS tumor?

Pilocytic astrocytoma.[67]

82. What is the most common cause of shunt failure?

Mechanical obstruction. About half of implanted CSF shunts fail within 2 years.[68]

83. What are the types of cerebral lesions encountered in tuberous sclerosis patients?

There are three types of cerebral lesions encountered in tuberous sclerosis patients: cortical tubers, subependymal nodules, and subependymal giant cell astrocytoma. Cortical tubers and subependymal nodules are hamartomatous lesions; a subependymal giant cell astrocytoma is a benign neoplastic lesion.[69]

84. When does the anterior neuropore close?

At 24 days of gestation. During development, the neural folds fuse at 22 days to form the neural tube. This tube closes like a zipper starting at the hindbrain.

85. When does the posterior neuropore close?

At 26 days of gestation.

86. When should folic acid supplementation begin?

Before conception. It is recommended that women planning on conceiving start taking folate a few months before conception.[70]

87. What is the developmental pathology that causes NTDs?

Failure of disjunction of the neural and cutaneous ectoderm during neurulation causes failure of fusion of the neural tube, resulting in NTDs (dysraphism).[71]

88. Myelomeningocele, which results from a failure of primary neurulation, is associated with what developmental syndrome?

Chiari II malformation. Almost all patients with myelomeningocele also have the Chiari II hindbrain malformation. Brainstem-associated defects include medullary kinking, tectal beaking, and intrinsic nuclei abnormalities. Supratentorial abnormalities include dysgenesis of the corpus callosum, gray matter heterotopias, polymicrogyria, and large massa intermedia.[71]

89. How are open NTDs diagnosed *in utero*?

Maternal serum α fetoprotein (MSAFP) is the initial screening test best performed at 16 to 18 weeks. In the amniotic fluid, the AFP concentration is 100-fold less than in the fetal CSF. The diagnostic accuracy of a single MSAFP level is 60 to 70%. High-resolution fetal ultrasonography can also be used to visualize the abnormalities. Amniocentesis is indicated if the MSAFP and ultrasound study suggest the presence of an open NTD. If an NTD is present, neural acetylcholinesterase (AChE) from the CSF leaks into the amniotic fluid and can also be measured. The amniotic AFP and AChE level have an accuracy of ~99%, and a false-positive rate of ~0.35%.[72]

90. What is the most common chromosomal cause of mental retardation?

Fragile X syndrome. It has a male predominance. These patients tend to exhibit autistic behaviors. They have a dysmorphic appearance with long face, enlarged ears, and macro-orchidism.[73]

91. What is the chromosomal abnormality seen in fragile X syndrome?

It is caused by a mutation of the *FMR1* gene on the X chromosome. Normally, the *FMR1* gene contains between 6 and 55 repeats of the CGG codon. Affected individuals have over 230 repeats and carriers have 60 to 230 repeats. Expansion of the CGG repeating codon to such a degree causes methylation of the *FMR1* locus, which results in constriction and fragility of the X chromosome.[73,74]

92. What is the chromosomal defect of cri-du-chat syndrome?

The defect is 5 p monosomy (deletion in the short arm of chromosome 5). Cri-du-chat is a French phrase meaning "scream of the cat."[75,76]

93. What is the chromosomal disorder in Patau syndrome?

Trisomy 13.[77]

94. What is the chromosomal disorder in Edwards syndrome?

Trisomy 18.[78]

95. What is colpocephaly?

A rare malformation of the brain that consists of marked dilatation of the occipital horns, thickening of the gray matter, and thinning of the white matter. Clinically, these patients have mental retardation, spasticity, and seizures. This disorder has been associated with trisomy 8.[79]

96. What is hydranencephaly?

This occurs when most of or the entire cortex is replaced by CSF. This may result from cerebral ischemia or infection (CMV or toxoplasma).[80]

97. What is holoprosencephaly?

This is a form of neuronal migratory defect that results from failure of the telencephalic vesicle to cleave into two cerebral hemispheres. The degree of cleavage ranges from severe (alobar) to less severe (semilobar and lobar). It is often accompanied by failure of fetal facial midline structures to form properly, and midline facial defects such as cleft lip, cleft palate, and cyclopia are seen.[81]

98. What is lissencephaly?

Lissencephaly, which literally means "smooth brain," is the most severe neuronal migration abnormality. This disorder is characterized by the lack of normal convolutions (folds) in the brain and an abnormally small head (microcephaly).[82]

99. What is schizencephaly?

Schizencephaly is a rare developmental disorder characterized by abnormal slits, or clefts, in the brain's cerebral hemispheres. The cleft can communicate with the ventricle, and is lined with cortical gray matter.[83]

100. What is the most common craniosynostosis?

Sagittal synostosis. Premature closure of the sagittal suture causes scaphocephaly (boat-shaped head).[84]

101. What head shape is associated with bilateral coronal synostosis?

Brachycephaly—the head is excessively wide and short.[85]

102. What are the two most common congenital craniofacial syndromes?

Crouzon's syndrome is the most frequent, followed by Apert's syndrome. Both of these syndromes have autosomal dominant or sporadic inheritance.

103. What is the enzyme deficiency in Tay-Sachs disease?

Hexosaminidase A. This is the most common of all gangliosidoses. This enzyme deficiency results in the accumulation of GM_2 ganglioside, principally in the brain.[86]

104. What is the enzyme deficiency in Niemann-Pick disease?

Sphingomyelinase. This results in the accumulation of sphingomyelin.[87]

105. What is the enzyme deficiency in Gaucher's disease?

Glucocerebrosidase. This results in the accumulation of glucocerebroside.[88]

106. What is the mode of inheritance of Hunter's syndrome?

X-linked recessive, unlike its counterpart, Hurler's syndrome, which is autosomal recessive.[89]

107. What substance(s) can be found in the urine of patients with Hurler's disease?

Heparin and dermatan sulfate. These are also found in the urine of patients with Hunter's syndrome (see **Table 8.2** for a summary).[89]

108. What is the mode of inheritance of Duchenne's muscular dystrophy (DMD)?

X-linked recessive.[90]

Table 8.2 Inborn errors of metabolism and genetic defects

Disease/ syndrome	Type of genetic disorder	Genetic defect	Accumulation
Fragile X	CGG triplet repeat in X chromosome	FMR1 gene	N/A
Cri-du-chat	Chromosomal deletion in the short (p) arm	Chromosome 5	N/A
Patau	Trisomy	Chromosome 13	N/A
Edwards	Trisomy	Chromosome 18	N/A
Tay-Sachs	Autosomal recessive	Hexosaminidase A gene	GM2 ganglioside
Niemann-Pick	Autosomal recessive	Sphingomyelinase gene	Sphingomyelin
Gaucher	Autosomal recessive	Glucocerebrosidase gene	Glucocerebroside
Hurler	Autosomal recessive	α-L-iduronidase gene	Heparan sulfate/ dermatan sulfate
Hunter	X-linked recessive	L-Iduronate sulfatase gene	Heparan sulfate/ dermatan sulfate

109. What is the gene responsible for DMD?

The dystrophin gene. Its product, dystrophin, is a protein that is normally expressed in skeletal, cardiac, and smooth muscle. The dystrophin gene is one of the largest known genes, spanning more than 2 Mb of genomic DNA.[91]

110. What is the difference between DMD and Becker's muscular dystrophy?

Whereas dystrophin is absent in patients with the Duchenne phenotype, it is present but structurally abnormal in the Becker type. The symptoms in the Becker phenotype begin later in life and tend to be milder.[92]

111. What is the etiology of kernicterus?

It is caused by an increased level of unconjugated bilirubin that stains the gray matter and causes neuronal necrosis.[93]

112. What is the treatment of an elevated bilirubin level in infants?

Phototherapy using ultraviolet light. If the bilirubin level is very high (> 20), treatment with an exchange transfusion is warranted.[94]

113. What is CADASIL?

Cerebral autosomal dominant arteriopathy with subcortical infarcts and leukoencephalopathy. CADASIL is the most common form of hereditary stroke disorder, and is thought to be caused by mutations of the Notch 3 gene on chromosome 19. The disease belongs to a family of disorders called the leukodystrophies.

114. Which part of the CNS is specifically involved in CADASIL?

On MRI, increased T2-weighted signal intensity and a corresponding decreased T1-weighted signal intensity are seen in anterior temporal, frontal, and periventricular white matter as well as in the pons and basal ganglia.

115. Which gene is associated with CADASIL?

Chromosome 19 (Notch 3 gene).

Functional and Pain

116. What is hyperpathia?

Normally painful stimuli eliciting disproportional severe pain.[95]

117. What is allodynia?

Normally nonpainful stimuli eliciting pain.[96]

118. What is the most common adult muscular dystrophy involving multiple organs?

Myotonic dystrophy.[97]

119. What type of muscle manifestations are seen with Creutzfeldt-Jakob disease?

Myoclonic jerks are seen in ~90% of cases. These jerks often persist during sleep.[98]

120. What is the most common pattern of facial involvement in trigeminal neuralgia?

The most common pattern of involvement is pain in the second and third divisions of the nerve simultaneously.

121. What neurologic deficits are associated with classic trigeminal neuralgia?

None.[99]

122. What is the most common point of neurovascular conflict in trigeminal neuralgia?

Superior cerebellar artery is the most common point of vascular contact with the trigeminal root entry zone from anatomical studies.[100] Radiosurgery is now the standard of care for trigeminal neuralgia.

123. What is the first-line drug for trigeminal neuralgia?

Carbamazepine.[99]

124. What is the most common seizure type in epileptic adults?

Complex partial seizures.[101]

125. What is the treatment of choice in patients with intractable pain from brachial plexus avulsion once medical therapy has been exhausted?

Dorsal root entry zone lesioning.[102]

126. What is the most common form of atypical parkinsonism?

Multisystem atrophy is the most common form of atypical parkinsonism and is characterized by autonomic failure.[103]

127. What is the most common cervical radiculopathy?

C6.

128. What cervical radiculopathy is difficult to distinguish from a primary shoulder disorder?

C5.

129. What is the most likely cervical radiculopathy that can present with unilateral axial neck pain without muscle weakness?

C4.

130. What is a cervicogenic headache?

A cervicogenic headache is a suboccipital headache often present with pressure behind the eyes and tinnitus. It is caused by cervical stenosis or herniated disk in the cervical spine. It is often misdiagnosed as a migraine headache. The pain is thought to be caused by irritation of the trigeminal nerve fibers that dip down into the upper cervical spinal cord. The headache is often resolved with cervical traction or, in refractory cases, anterior cervical diskectomy or cervical laminectomy.

Cases

■ Case 1

A child presents with lateral gaze palsy and retro-orbital pain after an ear injection. What is the likely diagnosis?

■ Case 1 Answer

Gradenigo's syndrome is petrous apex osteomyelitis with sixth cranial nerve palsy and retro-orbital pain that may occur from an extension of otitis.

■ Case 2

A patient with a distant history of a penile rash develops balance deterioration and blurry vision with a small pupil that reacts to accommodation, but not light. What is the diagnosis?

■ Case 2 Answer

This patient has neurosyphilis. The eye abnormality is Argyll Robertson pupils. The posterior column dysfunction is due to tabes dorsalis.

■ Case 3

A patient presents with pain in the eye and difficulty moving the eye with double vision. What is in the differential diagnosis?

■ Case 3 Answer

This appears to be a diabetic third nerve lesion. Compressive third nerve lesions usually are painless and tend to affect the pupil's ability to constrict before it would affect extraocular movements. Diabetic mononeuropathy tends to cause pain and first affects the inside fibers that are involved with moving the eye. The fibers involved with pupillary constriction are mainly on the outside of the nerve. Pituitary apoplexy also may cause headache and ophthalmoplegia.

■ Case 4

A young toddler presents with frequent jack-knife flexion and extension of the trunk and limbs with myoclonic head jerk, and an EEG with continuous large bilateral slow waves (hypsarrhythmia). He is also developmentally delayed. What is the diagnosis?

■ Case 4 Answer

He has West's syndrome. Seizures usually disappear by 5 years; treatment is with ACTH.

■ Case 5

A patient presents with unilateral lancinating electric-type pain in the V2 and V3 distributions. What is the likely diagnosis?

■ Case 5 Answer

This appears to be trigeminal neuralgia. Usually, it is caused from pressure from the superior cerebellar artery onto the trigeminal nerve at the junction of central and peripheral myelin implant. Occasionally, a vein or another artery may be involved. A tumor may sometimes be found pressing the nerve; thus a preoperative MRI is warranted. About 70% of patients respond to carbamazepine. Opiates tend not to be successful. If symptoms do not respond to carbamazepine or other antiepileptics, the diagnosis should be in question. Treatments can be classified into destructive procedures such as balloon gangliolysis, radiosurgery, and alcohol injection versus nondestructive procedures such as microvascular decompression. The latter option has a lower likelihood of postoperative numbness. Damage to the trigeminal nerve may cause anesthesia dolorosa, which may cause even worse pain than the trigeminal neuralgia itself, as it is a deafferentation syndrome.

■ References

1. Robertson J, Brodkey J. Glomus jugulare tumors. In: Youmans JR, ed. Neurological Surgery. 4th ed. Philadelphia, PA: WB Saunders; 1996

2. Doble JE, Haig AJ, Anderson C, Katz R. Impairment, activity, participation, life satisfaction, and survival in persons with locked-in syndrome for over a decade: follow-up on a previously reported cohort. J Head Trauma Rehabil 2003;18(5):435–444

3. Woodworth GF, McGirt MJ, Williams MA, Rigamonti D. Cerebro-spinal fluid drainage and dynamics in the diagnosis of normal pressure hydrocephalus. Neurosurgery 2009;64(5):919–925, discussion 925–926

4. Lautenschlager NT, Martins RN. Common versus uncommon causes of dementia. Int Psychogeriatr 2005;17(suppl 1):S27–S34

5. Preobrazhenskaya IS, Mkhitaryan EA, Yakhno NN. Comparative analysis of cognitive impairments in Lewy body dementia and Alzheimer's disease. Neurosci Behav Physiol 2006;36(1):1–6

6. Schiffer R, Pope LE. Review of pseudobulbar affect including a novel and potential therapy. J Neuropsychiatry Clin Neurosci 2005;17(4):447–454

7. Cacace AT, Parnes SM, Lovely TJ, Kalathia A. The disconnected ear: phenomenological effects of a large acoustic tumor. Ear Hear 1994;15(4):287–298

8. Coelho DH, Lalwani AK. Medical management of Ménière's disease. Laryngoscope 2008;118(6):1099–1108

9. Carroll TB, Findling JW. Cushing's syndrome of nonpituitary causes. Curr Opin Endocrinol Diabetes Obes 2009;16(4):308–315

10. Kalenka A, Schwarz A. Anaesthesia and Parkinson's disease: how to manage with new therapies? Curr Opin Anaesthesiol 2009;22(3):419–424

11. Fast A, Parikh S, Marin EL. The shoulder abduction relief sign in cervical radiculopathy. Arch Phys Med Rehabil 1989;70(5):402–403

12. Fernandes P, Dolan L, Weinstein SL. Intrathecal baclofen withdrawal syndrome following posterior spinal fusion for neuromuscular scoliosis: a case report. Iowa Orthop J 2008;28:77–80

13. Teasell R, Bayona N, Lippert C, Villamere J, Hellings C. Post-traumatic seizure disorder following acquired brain injury. Brain Inj 2007;21(2):201–214

14. Al-Mufti F, Claassen J. Neurocritical care: status epilepticus review. Crit Care Clin 2014;30(4):751–764

15. Treiman DM. Treatment of convulsive status epilepticus. Int Rev Neurobiol 2007;81:273–285

16. Nandhagopal R. Generalised convulsive status epilepticus: an overview. Postgrad Med J 2006;82(973):723–732

17. Greenberg MS. Handbook of Neurosurgery. 6th ed. New York, NY: Thieme Medical Publishers; 2006

18. Mumenthaler M, Mattle H. Neurology. Stuttgart: Georg Thieme Verlag; 2005

19. Cooper AD, Britton JW, Rabinstein AA. Functional and cognitive outcome in prolonged refractory status epilepticus. Arch Neurol 2009;66(12):1505–1509

20. McClelland S III, Maxwell RE. Hemispherectomy for intractable epilepsy in adults: the first reported series. Ann Neurol 2007;61(4):372–376

21. Morino M, Shimizu H, Uda T, et al. Transventricular hemispherotomy for surgical treatment of intractable epilepsy. J Clin Neurosci 2007;14(2):171–175

22. Durá Travé T, Yoldi Petri ME. Typical absence seizure: epidemiological and clinical characteristics and outcome [in Spanish]. An Pediatr (Barc) 2006;64(1):28–33

23. Vestergaard M, Basso O, Henriksen TB, Østergaard JR, Olsen J. Risk factors for febrile convulsions. Epidemiology 2002;13(3):282–287

24. Hrachovy RA. West's syndrome (infantile spasms). Clinical description and diagnosis. Adv Exp Med Biol 2002;497:33–50

25. Mackay MT, Weiss SK, Adams-Webber T, et al; American Academy of Neurology; Child Neurology Society. Practice parameter: medical treatment of infantile spasms: report of the American Academy of Neurology and the Child Neurology Society. Neurology 2004;62(10):1668–1681

26. Steffensen TS, Gilbert-Barness E, Lacson A, Margo CE. Cerebellar migration defects in Aicardi syndrome: an extension of the neuropathological spectrum. Fetal Pediatr Pathol 2009;28(1):24–38

27. Ford-Jones EL, Kellner JD. "Cheap torches": an acronym for congenital and perinatal infections. Pediatr Infect Dis J 1995;14(7):638–640

28. Ihekwaba UK, Kudesia G, McKendrick MW. Clinical features of viral meningitis in adults: significant differences in cerebrospinal fluid findings among herpes simplex virus, varicella zoster virus, and enterovirus infections. Clin Infect Dis 2008;47(6):783–789

29. Gazzoni AF, Pegas KL, Severo LC. Histopathological techniques for diagnosing cryptococcosis due to capsule-deficient Cryptococcus: case report [in Portuguese]. Rev Soc Bras Med Trop 2008;41(1):76–78

30. Rajshekhar V, Raghava MV, Prabhakaran V, Oommen A, Muliyil J. Active epilepsy as an index of burden of neurocysticercosis in Vellore district, India. Neurology 2006;67(12):2135–2139

31. Mehta SS, Hatfield S, Jessen L, Vogel D. Albendazole versus praziquantel for neurocysticercosis. Am J Health Syst Pharm 1998;55(6):598–600

32. Motamed M, Kalan A. Gradenigo's syndrome. Postgrad Med J 2000;76(899):559–560

33. González-Angulo A, Márquez-Monter H, Feria-Velasco A, Zavala BJ. The ultrastructure of Negri bodies in Purkinje neurons in human rabies. Neurology 1970;20(4):323–328

34. Jackson AC. Rabies virus infection: an update. J Neurovirol 2003;9(2):253–258

35. Champion JM, Kean RB, Rupprecht CE, et al. The development of monoclonal human rabies virus-neutralizing antibodies as a substitute for pooled human immune globulin in the prophylactic treatment of rabies virus exposure. J Immunol Methods 2000;235(1–2):81–90

36. Ohlenbusch A, Matuschka FR, Richter D, et al. Etiology of the acrodermatitis chronica atrophicans lesion in Lyme disease. J Infect Dis 1996;174(2):421–423

37. CDC Guidelines, 2015. Diagnosing and Testing Lyme Disease.

38. Cairney S, Maruff P, Currie J, Currie BJ. Increased anti-saccade latency is an isolated lingering abnormality in Sydenham chorea. J Neuroophthalmol 2009;29(2):143–145

39. Nitrini R. The history of tabes dorsalis and the impact of observational studies in neurology. Arch Neurol 2000;57(4):605–606

40. Williams J, Kanniappan VK, Manickavasagan T. Hutchinson's triad in a 9-year-old girl. Int J STD AIDS 1992;3(4):295–296

41. Rashid M, Bari Au, Majeed S, Tariq KM, Haq Iu, Niwaz A. Mucormycosis: a devastating fungal infection in diabetics. J Coll Physicians Surg Pak 2005;15(1):43–45

42. Ni YH, Yeh KM, Peng MY, Chou YY, Chang FY. Community-acquired brain abscess in Taiwan: etiology and probable source of infection. J Microbiol Immunol Infect 2004;37(4):231–235

43. Bortoletti G, Gabriele F, Seu V, Palmas C. Epidemiology of hydatid disease in Sardinia: a study of fertility of cysts in sheep. J Helminthol 1990;64(3):212–216

44. Gasser O, Bihl FK, Wolbers M, et al; Swiss HIV Cohort Study. HIV patients developing primary CNS lymphoma lack EBV-specific CD4+ T cell function irrespective of absolute CD4+ T cell counts. PLoS Med 2007;4(3):e96

45. Anneken K, Fischera M, Evers S, Kloska S, Husstedt IW. Recurrent vacuolar myelopathy in HIV infection. J Infect 2006;52(6):e181–e183

46. Di Rocco A, Simpson DM. AIDS-associated vacuolar myelopathy. AIDS Patient Care STDS 1998;12(6):457–461

47. Otaki M, Sada K, Kadoya H, Nagano-Fujii M, Hotta H. Inhibition of measles virus and subacute sclerosing panencephalitis virus by RNA interference. Antiviral Res 2006;70(3):105–111

48. Herremans M, Bakker J, Vermeulen MJ, Schellekens JF, Koopmans MP. Evaluation of an in-house cat scratch disease IgM ELISA to detect Bartonella henselae in a routine laboratory setting. Eur J Clin Microbiol Infect Dis 2009;28(2):147–152

49. Lu RP, Keilson G. Combination regimen of methylprednisolone, IV immunoglobulin, and plasmapheresis early in the treatment of acute disseminated encephalomyelitis. J Clin Apher 2006;21(4):260–265

50. Ranasuriya DG, Feld RJ, Nairn SJ. A case of acute disseminated encephalomyelitis in a 12-year-old boy. Pediatr Emerg Care 2008;24(10):697–699

51. Höllinger P, Sturzenegger M, Mathis J, Schroth G, Hess CW. Acute disseminated encephalomyelitis in adults: a reappraisal of clinical, CSF, EEG, and MRI findings. J Neurol 2002;249(3):320–329

52. Pachner AR, Steere AC. The triad of neurologic manifestations of Lyme disease: meningitis, cranial neuritis, and radiculoneuritis. Neurology 1985;35(1):47–53

53. Muñoz-Mármol AM, Mola G, Fernández-Vasalo A, Vela E, Mate JL, Ariza A. JC virus early protein detection by immunohistochemistry in progressive multifocal leukoencephalopathy: a comparative study with in situ hybridization and polymerase chain reaction. J Neuropathol Exp Neurol 2004;63(11):1124–1130

54. Bell JB, Davies RA, Thompson EJ. Herpes simplex encephalitis. A study of seven patients and their immunological response prior to routine acyclovir treatment. J Infect 2003;47(2):161–163

55. Adatepe MH, Powell OM, Isaacs GH, Nichols K, Cefola R. Hematogenous pyogenic vertebral osteomyelitis: diagnostic value of radionuclide bone imaging. J Nucl Med 1986;27(11):1680–1685

56. Muraki R, Iwasaki T, Sata T, Sato Y, Kurata T. Hair follicle involvement in herpes zoster: pathway of viral spread from ganglia to skin. Virchows Arch 1996;428(4–5):275–280

57. Stewart LA, Rydzewska LH, Keogh GF, Knight RS. Systematic review of therapeutic interventions in human prion disease. Neurology 2008;70(15):1272–1281

58. Saiz A, Graus F, Dalmau J, Pifarre A, Marin C, Tolosa E. Detection of 14-3-3 brain protein in the cerebrospinal fluid of patients with paraneoplastic neurological disorders. Ann Neurol 1999;46(5):774–777

59. Franklin GM, Tremlett H. Multiple sclerosis and pregnancy: what should we be telling our patients? Neurology 2009;73(22):1820–1822

60. Dalton CM, Brex PA, Miszkiel KA, et al. Application of the new McDonald criteria to patients with clinically isolated syndromes suggestive of multiple sclerosis. Ann Neurol 2002;52(1):47–53

61. Lo CP, Kao HW, Chen SY, et al. Prediction of conversion from clinically isolated syndrome to clinically definite multiple sclerosis according to baseline MRI findings: comparison of revised McDonald criteria and Swanton modified criteria. J Neurol Neurosurg Psychiatry 2009;80(10):1107–1109

62. Khealani B, Husain AM. Neurophysiologic intraoperative monitoring during surgery for tethered cord syndrome. J Clin Neurophysiol 2009;26(2):76–81

63. Attenello FJ, McGirt MJ, Gathinji M, et al. Outcome of Chiari-associated syringomyelia after hindbrain decompression in children: analysis of 49 consecutive cases. Neurosurgery 2008;62(6):1307–1313, discussion 1313

64. Mosley BS, Cleves MA, Siega-Riz AM, et al; National Birth Defects Prevention Study. Neural tube defects and maternal folate intake among pregnancies conceived after folic acid fortification in the United States. Am J Epidemiol 2009;169(1):9–17

65. Gulino A, Arcella A, Giangaspero F. Pathological and molecular heterogeneity of medulloblastoma. Curr Opin Oncol 2008;20(6):668–675

66. Slovis TL. Children, computed tomography radiation dose, and the As Low As Reasonably Achievable (ALARA) concept. Pediatrics 2003;112(4):971–972

67. Rodriguez FJ, Giannini C, Asmann YW, et al. Gene expression profiling of NF-1-associated and sporadic pilocytic astrocytoma identifies aldehyde dehydrogenase 1 family member L1 (ALDH1L1) as an underexpressed candidate biomarker in aggressive subtypes. J Neuropathol Exp Neurol 2008;67(12):1194–1204

68. Piatt JH Jr, Garton HJ. Clinical diagnosis of ventriculoperitoneal shunt failure among children with hydrocephalus. Pediatr Emerg Care 2008;24(4):201–210

69. Au KS, Ward CH, Northrup H. Tuberous sclerosis complex: disease modifiers and treatments. Curr Opin Pediatr 2008;20(6):628–633

70. Lee JI, Lee JA, Lim HS. Effect of time of initiation and dose of prenatal iron and folic acid supplementation on iron and folate nutriture of Korean women during pregnancy. Am J Clin Nutr 2005;82(4):843–849

71. Brand MC. Examining the newborn with an open spinal dysraphism. Adv Neonatal Care 2006;6(4):181–196

72. Ennever FK, Lave LB. Parent preferences and prenatal testing for neural tube defects. Epidemiology 1995;6(1):8–16

73. Saul RA, Friez M, Eaves K, et al. Fragile X syndrome detection in newborns-pilot study. Genet Med 2008;10(10):714–719

74. Schneider A, Hagerman RJ, Hessl D. Fragile X syndrome — from genes to cognition. Dev Disabil Res Rev 2009;15(4):333–342

75. Saito N, Ebara S, Fukushima Y, Wakui K, Takaoka K. Progressive scoliosis in cri-du-chat syndrome over a 20-year follow-up period: a case report. Spine 2001;26(7):835–837

76. Vera-Carbonell A, Bafalliu JA, Guillén-Navarro E, et al. Characterization of a de novo complex chromosomal rearrangement in a patient with cri-du-chat and trisomy 5p syndromes. Am J Med Genet A 2009;149A(11):2513–2521

77. Fukushima H, Harada T, Morita N, Paparella MM. Trisomy 13 syndrome. Otol Neurotol 2008;29(8):1209–1210

78. Bhat BV, Usha TS, Pourany A, Puri RK, Srinvasan S, Mitra SC. Edward syndrome with multiple chromosomal defects. Indian J Pediatr 1989;56(1):137–139

79. Herskowitz J, Rosman NP, Wheeler CB. Colpocephaly: clinical, radiologic, and pathogenetic aspects. Neurology 1985;35(11):1594–1598

80. Tsai JD, Kuo HT, Chou IC. Hydranencephaly in neonates. Pediatr Neonatol 2008;49(4):154–157

81. Guion-Almeida ML, Richieri-Costa A, Zechi-Ceide RM. Holoprosencephaly spectrum, ano/microphthalmia, and first branchial arch defects: evidence for a new disorder. Clin Dysmorphol 2008;17(1):41–46

82. Gleeson JG. Classical lissencephaly and double cortex (subcortical band heterotopia): LIS1 and doublecortin. Curr Opin Neurol 2000;13(2):121–125

83. Oh KY, Kennedy AM, Frias AE Jr, Byrne JL. Fetal schizencephaly: pre- and postnatal imaging with a review of the clinical manifestations. Radiographics 2005;25(3):647–657

84. Butzelaar L, Breugem CC, Hanlo P, Mink van der Molen AB. Is isolated sagittal synostosis an isolated condition? J Craniofac Surg 2009;20(2):399–401

85. Koh KS, Kang MH, Yu SC, Park SH, Ra YS. Treatment of nonsyndromic bilateral coronal synostosis using a multiple bone flap rotation-reposition technique. J Craniofac Surg 2004;15(4):603–608

86. Martin DC, Mark BL, Triggs-Raine BL, Natowicz MR. Evaluation of the risk for Tay-Sachs disease in individuals of French Canadian ancestry living in New England. Clin Chem 2007;53(3):392–398

87. van Diggelen OP, Voznyi YV, Keulemans JL, et al. A new fluorimetric enzyme assay for the diagnosis of Niemann-Pick A/B, with specificity of natural sphingomyelinase substrate. J Inherit Metab Dis 2005;28(5):733–741

88. Charrow J. Enzyme replacement therapy for Gaucher disease. Expert Opin Biol Ther 2009;9(1):121–131

89. Martin R, Beck M, Eng C, et al. Recognition and diagnosis of mucopolysaccharidosis II (Hunter syndrome). Pediatrics 2008;121(2):e377–e386

90. Davidson ZE, Truby H. A review of nutrition in Duchenne muscular dystrophy. J Hum Nutr Diet 2009;22(5):383–393

91. Evans NP, Misyak SA, Robertson JL, Bassaganya-Riera J, Grange RW. Dysregulated intracellular signaling and inflammatory gene expression during initial disease onset in Duchenne muscular dystrophy. Am J Phys Med Rehabil 2009;88(6):502–522

92. Bradley WG, Jones MZ, Mussini JM, Fawcett PR. Becker-type muscular dystrophy. Muscle Nerve 1978;1(2):111–132

93. Rice AC, Shapiro SM. A new animal model of hemolytic hyperbilirubinemia-induced bilirubin encephalopathy (kernicterus). Pediatr Res 2008;64(3):265–269

94. Kuzniewicz MW, Escobar GJ, Newman TB. Impact of universal bilirubin screening on severe hyperbilirubinemia and phototherapy use. Pediatrics 2009;124(4):1031–1039

95. Parkes A. Post-trumatic hyperpathia in the limbs. Proc R Soc Med 1970;63(1):71–72

96. Keizer D, Fael D, Wierda JM, van Wijhe M. Quantitative sensory testing with Von Frey monofilaments in patients with allodynia: what are we quantifying? Clin J Pain 2008;24(5):463–466

97. Prior TW; American College of Medical Genetics (ACMG) Laboratory Quality Assurance Committee. Technical standards and guidelines for myotonic dystrophy type 1 testing. Genet Med 2009;11(7):552–555

98. Cyngiser TA. Creutzfeldt-Jakob disease: a disease overview. Am J Electroneurodiagn Technol 2008;48(3):199–208

99. Gronseth G, Cruccu G, Alksne J, et al. Practice parameter: the diagnostic evaluation and treatment of trigeminal neuralgia (an evidence-based review): report of the Quality Standards Subcommittee of the American Academy of Neurology and the European Federation of Neurological Societies. Neurology 2008;71(15):1183–1190

100. Lorenzoni JG, Massager N, David P, et al. Neurovascular compression anatomy and pain outcome in patients with classic trigeminal neuralgia treated by radiosurgery. Neurosurgery 2008;62(2):368–375, discussion 375–376

101. Cascino GD. Complex partial seizures. Clinical features and differential diagnosis. Psychiatr Clin North Am 1992;15(2):373–382

102. Samii M, Bear-Henney S, Lüdemann W, Tatagiba M, Blömer U. Treatment of refractory pain after brachial plexus avulsion with dorsal root entry zone lesions. Neurosurgery 2001;48(6):1269–1275, discussion 1275–1277

103. Nicholl DJ, Bennett P, Hiller L, et al; European Study Group on Atypical Parkinsonism. A study of five candidate genes in Parkinson's disease and related neurodegenerative disorders. Neurology 1999;53(7):1415–1421

9 Neuroradiology

Cranial

1. What is the characteristic angiographic appearance of vessels in fibromuscular dysplasia (FMD)?

FMD is an angiopathy that affects medium-sized arteries predominantly in young women of childbearing age. FMD most commonly affects the renal arteries and can cause refractory renovascular hypertension. Of patients with identified FMD, renal involvement occurs in 60 to 75%, cerebrovascular involvement occurs in 25 to 30%, visceral involvement occurs in 9%, and arteries of the limbs are affected in approximately 5%. The classic "beads on a string" appearance is typical of medial fibroplasia, the most common type of FMD (**Fig. 9.1**).[1,2]

2. What are the three anatomical appearances of a normal pineal gland on contrast-enhanced imaging?

A normal pineal gland could appear as a nodule (52%), or have a crescent (26%) or ringlike (22%) shape.[3]

3. What is the common computed tomography (CT) finding both in pseudotumor cerebri and in ventriculoperitoneal (VP) shunt overdrainage?

Slitlike ventricles. These are small ventricles, sometimes so small that they are barely visible on CT or magnetic resonance imaging (MRI) scans. Slit ventricles can occur after severe head injury or viral infection of the brain. In the case of a VP shunt, the ventricles become completely decompressed due to very low draining pressure. Pseudotumor cerebri is characterized by increased intracranial pressure without hydrocephalus, mass or meningitis, or hypertensive encephalitis. The problem is cerebrospinal fluid malabsorption causing cerebral edema.[4]

4. What is the angiographic finding of mass effect due to a brain tumor on an anteroposterior (AP) view?

The pericallosal arteries are seen as a bayonet- or stair-step-shaped bend under the falx cerebri. This phenomenon is called square shift. The same type of shift is observed in the displacement of callosomarginal artery under the anterior falx.

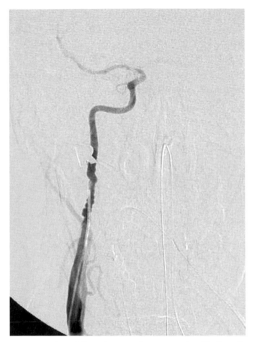

Fig. 9.1 Carotid angiogram demonstrating findings in fibromuscular dysplasia.

5. What is the most common nontumoral MRI finding in patients with complex partial epilepsy?

Chronic temporal lobe seizures are typically associated with atrophy of the hippocampus and, less commonly, the para-hippocampal gyrus. This type of atrophy is associated with sclerosis most of the time.[5]

6. In what forms can hemangioblastomas appear on CT or MRI?

Vascular nodule on the side of the cyst, vascular nodule encompassing the cyst, and solid vascular mass are the types encountered on contrast-enhanced CT or MRI. However, a cyst with a nodule on the side is most commonly seen (60%).[6]

7. What can be seen in the anterior vascular MRI/magnetic resonance angiography in relation to a presellar versus a postsellar tumor?

A presellar localization causes elevation of A1 segments of anterior cerebral arteries, whereas a postsellar tumor does not generally displace them.

8. What is the normal expected range of the diameter of an internal acoustic opening to assess any abnormal widening due to acoustic neuroma on a CT scan?

Most acoustic neurinomas enlarge the ostium of the internal acoustic canal; only 3 to 5% of these tumors do not cause enlargement. An internal acoustic opening more than 5 to 8 mm in diameter should raise a question whether this is caused by an intracanalicular neuroma.[7]

9. What is the differential diagnosis for a spherical hypointense mass in the suprasellar region in the MRI?

The most important two are Rathke's cleft cyst and aneurysm due to the flow void. If a vascular lesion is suspected, a formal angiogram must be performed. Cystic microadenoma and epidermoid cysts are also considered among the differential diagnosis.[8]

10. What is the enhancement pattern of a pituitary adenoma with contrast relative to a normal gland?

Normal gland will enhance immediately after the contrast injection as opposed to adenoma that remains unchanged; however, 30 minutes postinjection, the normal gland loses its enhancement and tumor enhances.[9]

11. What are the MRI signs of acute intracranial hypotension?

Diffuse pachymeningeal (dural) enhancement, bilateral subdural effusion/hematomas, downward displacement of brain, enlargement of the pituitary gland, engorgement of the dural venous sinuses, prominence of spinal epidural venous plexus, venous sinus thrombosis, and isolated cortical vein thrombosis.[10]

12. What type of imaging is most helpful to detect diffuse axonal (shearing) injury?

Diffuse axonal injury is notorious for poor visualization on CT. When it is nonhemorrhagic, it is best demonstrated with T2-weighted (T2W) MRI. When it is hemorrhagic, long echo time gradient-echo (GRE) MRI shows the injury best.[11]

13. What are the findings of Dandy-Walker malformation on a coronal T2W MRI?

Dandy-Walker malformation is characterized by cystic dilatation of the fourth ventricle, complete or partial agenesis of the cerebellar vermis, and an enlarged posterior fossa. Keyhole formation in the large fourth ventricle and inverted Y due to elevated tentorium and torcula are highly suggestive of the disease.[12]

14. What are the best diagnostic clues for Sturge-Weber syndrome in MRI?

Cortical calcification, atrophy, and enlarged ipsilateral choroid plexus are the typical MRI findings. In skull radiography, tram-track calcification is also considered a typical sign.[13]

15. What are the best diagnostic tools and the findings they provide to confirm the diagnosis of traumatic extracranial arterial dissection?

MRI and CT angiography (CTA) are the modalities of choice. MRI reveals a crescentic hyperintensity. On CTA, a tapered narrowing with or without a block is highly suggestive of dissection. Vertebral arteries are the most common location.[14]

16. What are the diagnostic clues on CT and MRI in a patient with suspected traumatic carotid-cavernous fistula?

Enlarged superior ophthalmic vein on contrast CT and dilated cavernous sinus as flow voids on T1W MRI, along with marked proptosis and swelling of eyelids.[15]

17. What are the components of an infundibulum seen on cerebral angiography?

The most common location is the posterior communicating artery; it arises directly from its apex. It is conical in shape and less than 3 mm in size.[16]

18. What are the image characteristics of multiple sclerosis (MS) on MRI?

Multiple perpendicular callososeptal hyperintensities along the penetrating venules (Dawson's fingers), bilateral asymmetric ovoid FLAIR (fluid-attenuated inversion recovery) hyperintensities, and transient enhancement during active demyelination.[17]

19. How is cerebellopontine angle (CPA) arachnoid cyst differentiated from an epidermoid cyst?

Epidermoid cysts present restricted diffusion in diffusion-weighted image (DWI) sequence, whereas arachnoid cysts do not. An arachnoid cyst is the closest differential diagnosis that carries similar MRI features, except for the restricted diffusion on DWI.[18,19]

20. What is the term "Medusa head" used to describe on MRI or angiogram?

A developmental venous anomaly that is characterized by dilated medullary veins that course in the white matter, resembling "caput medusae" or "Medusa head." These anomalous venous structures tend to coincide with cavernomas (**Fig. 9.2**). The risk of bleeding is lower than for the other vascular malformations such as arteriovenous malformations (AVMs) and cavernous malformations.[20]

21. What are the MRI findings of Wilson's disease?

Wilson's disease is suggested mainly in T2W images by brain atrophy (focal/diffuse), high signal intensity at the lentiform nuclei (with bilateral symmetric and concentric lamellar putaminal pattern), thalamic and caudate nuclei, substantia nigra, periaqueductal gray matter, pontine tegmentum, cerebellum, and cortical and subcortical areas with frontal lobe predilection.[21]

22. What is the best imaging tool for cavernous malformations and what are the most common findings?

T2W GRE MRI is the best tool for cavernous malformations. Hypointense "blooming" and numerous punctate hypointense foci ("black dots") if the lesion is greater than 3 cm are the most common findings on T2W GRE, giving them a characteristic popcorn appearance.[22]

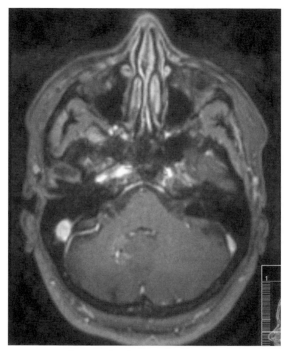

Fig. 9.2 Axial T1-weighted magnetic resonance image demonstrating cavernous angioma (or cavernoma) of the cerebellar hemisphere with associated venous angioma.

23. What are the commonly accepted angiographic criteria for AVMs with a relatively higher risk of bleeding?

Stenotic venous drainage, single draining vein, intranidal aneurysm, smaller nidus, and deep location are the features seen in the AVMs that are more prone to bleed.[22]

24. What is the chronologic order of angiographic findings in moyamoya disease?

A narrowing in the circle of Willis and the internal carotid artery (ICA) is the earliest finding. After that, the lenticulostriate and thalamoperforator collaterals develop in the intermediate phase. Transdural external carotid–internal carotid collaterals emerge in the late phases of the disease (**Fig. 9.3**).[23]

25. What are the imaging findings of intracranial artery dissection?

Hyperintense crescent within the vessel wall on axial T1W MRIs, and tapered stenosis, string sign (long-segment stenosis), and abrupt occlusion or intimal flap/double lumen on angiography.[24]

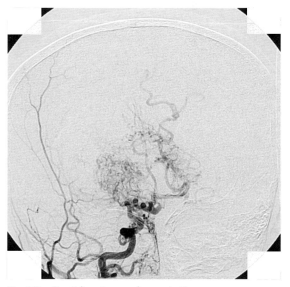

Fig. 9.3 Carotid angiogram demonstrating moyamoya disease with formation of moyamoya vessels after occlusion of the anterior and middle cerebral arteries.

26. What is the differential diagnosis for false-positive empty delta sign?

An empty delta sign is typical contrast CT or MRI evidence for a superior sagittal sinus thrombosis. This is caused by enhancing dura surrounding a clot in a thrombosed sinus. Subdural hematoma, subdural empyema, or arachnoid granulations can commonly mimic this appearance with a false-positive empty delta sign.[25,26]

27. What is the differential diagnosis for an atherosclerotic fusiform aneurysm in the vertebrobasilar system?

A long-segment focal irregular fusiform or ovoid arterial dilatation is characteristic for an atherosclerotic fusiform aneurysm. Atherosclerotic dolichoectasia (nonfocal fusiform or saccular dilatation), giant serpentine aneurysm (partially thrombosed mass), or nonatherosclerotic fusiform vasculopathy (younger patient with inherited vasculopathy) may be indistinguishable from atherosclerotic fusiform aneurysms.[27]

28. What are the central nervous system (CNS) manifestations of Lhermitte-Duclos disease?

Lhermitte-Duclos disease is recently considered to be part of a multiple hamartoma–neoplasia syndrome (Cowden's disease). It is a rare pathologic entity with progrediating, diffuse hypertrophy chiefly of the stratum granulosum of the cerebellum. The CNS involvement always occurs in cerebellum characterized by a relatively well-defined mass containing a gyriform pattern. In T1W images, hypointense mass with striations ("corduroy" or "tiger-striped" pattern) is characteristic.[28]

29. What is the angiographic finding associated with high risk of hemorrhage in the Cognard grading system for dural AV fistula?

Reflux (retrograde drainage) into cortical veins is associated with higher hemorrhage risk compared with those that do not have this type of drainage. In the grading system, type IIB, III, IV, and V involve this angiographic feature.[29]

30. Fluid–fluid level on a radiologic study is seen in which conditions?

- Aneurysmal bone cyst.
- Giant cell tumor.
- Telangiectatic osteosarcoma.
- Chondroblastoma.
- Nonneoplastic cyst with fracture.

31. Describe dissemination in space lesions on MRI for MS.

Three out of four conditions are needed:

- One enhancing lesion or nine nonenhancing lesions on T2W MRI.
- Three or more periventricular lesions.
- One or more juxtacortical lesions.
- One or more infratentorial lesions (or a spinal cord lesion).[17]

32. Describe dissemination in time lesions on MRI for MS.

- One enhancing lesion on T2W MRI at a different site in 3 months.
- One enhancing lesion on T2W MRI after another 3 months *or* a new lesion on T2W MRI.[17]

33. What are the characteristic MR spectroscopy findings for brain tumors?

Tumors exhibit elevated choline (Cho) and decreased *N*-acetyl aspartate (NAA). On the contrary, strokes and focal cortical dysplasias exhibit elevated Cho.[30]

34. How do you differentiate recurrent tumor from radiation necrosis?

Positron emission tomography (PET) is useful to distinguish between them, as radiation necrosis is hypometabolic on PET in contrast to tumors. In addition, perfusion MRI may also be useful for distinguishing recurrent tumor from radiation necrosis, as higher cerebral blood volume is evident in the former.[31]

35. What are the segments of Bouthillier's angiographic classification of the ICA?[32]

- Cervical segment.
- Petrous segment.
- Lacerum segment.
- Cavernous segment.
- Clinoid segment.
- Ophthalmic (supraclinoid) segment.
- Communicating (terminal) segment.

36. How do you differentiate brain tumor from a tumefactive demyelinating lesion?

The presence of a T2-hypointense rim and peculiar diffusion findings in the form of increased diffusion with a restriction at periphery on DWI along with the absence of elevated cerebral blood volume on perfusion studies suggest a tumefactive demyelinating lesion.[33]

37. What are the imaging findings of ICA dissection?

On CT scan, arterial wall hematoma in the upper portion of the ICA (crescent-shaped) hyperdense area may be seen.

CTA demonstrates enlargement of the dissected artery along with narrowed eccentric lumen surrounded by a crescent-shaped mural thrombus and thin annular enhancement.

On MRI, ICA dissection is depicted as hyperintense crescent sign within the wall of the vessel on T2W images along with absent flow-void.

Angiography is considered the gold standard imaging modality in the diagnosis of ICA dissection. Angiography commonly demonstrates vessel wall irregularities, string sign (thin string of contrast distal to a stenotic ICA area), string and pearl sign (focal narrowing with a distal site of dilatation), and pseudoaneurysm formation.[34]

38. What is the differential diagnosis of ring-enhancing lesion in the brain?[35]

- High-grade glioma.
- Lymphoma.
- Brain abscess.
- Tuberculoma.
- Toxoplasmosis.
- Metastasis.
- Tumefactive demyelinating lesion.

39. What is the differential diagnosis of dural enhancement?[36]

- Tumor.
- Infection.
- Metastasis.
- Postoperative states.
- Intracranial hypotension.
- Cerebral venous thrombosis.
- Neurosarcoidosis.
- Idiopathic pachymeningitis.

40. What are the radiologic clues to diagnose different dementias radiologically?[37,38,39]

On MRI, Alzheimer's disease demonstrates medial temporal and parietal lobe atrophy. There might be severe global atrophy in end-stage disease.

Vascular dementia appears on MRI as global atrophy, diffuse white matter lesions, lacunes, and strategic infarcts, which are infarcts in regions that are involved in cognitive function.

On T2W MRI, cerebral amyloid angiopathy is depicted as multiple microhemorrhages, typically in a peripheral location. FLAIR usually reveals moderate-to-severe white matter hyperintensities.

Frontotemporal lobar degeneration (Pick's disease) has pronounced atrophy of frontal and/or temporal lobes.

The role of imaging is very limited in Lewy's body dementia. Brain MRI is usually normal.

Creutzfeldt-Jakob disease spongiform changes can sometimes be detected on FLAIR, but are most visible on DWI, affecting either the striatum or the neocortex, or a combination of both.

Spinal

41. What are the characteristic MRI findings of infectious spondylitis?

The destruction of two adjacent end plates and the intervening disk associated with large paraspinal masses are the characteristic MRI findings of infectious spondylitis. The paraspinal masses are the abscess formations and are usually present with calcifications.[40]

42. What is the neuroradiologic assessment for the integrity of atlantoaxial (transverse) ligament?

Atlantodental distance > 3 mm on lateral C-spine or the sum overhang distance of both C1 lateral masses on C2 ≥ 7 mm on an open-mouth odontoid X-ray indicates transverse ligament disruption.[41]

43. What is the appropriate evaluation in a patient with rheumatoid arthritis, where cervical stability is concerned?

On neutral lateral views, the atlantodental interval, measured from the posteroinferior margin of the anterior arch of the atlas to the anterior surface of the odontoid process, should not exceed 3 mm in adults, or 5 mm in very young children. If the distance is above these limits, it suggests a possible transverse ligament laxity and atlantoaxial instability or subluxation. This instability can be better appreciated on a sagittal reconstructed CT of the cervical spine (**Fig. 9.4**).[42]

44. What specific radiographic view is important to obtain when planning a C1–C2 transarticular screw fixation?

A sagittal reconstructed paramedian CT scan through the pars interarticularis (preferably CTA) to visualize the course of the vertebral artery and determine whether there is enough room to place a screw without violating the vertebral canal (**Fig. 9.5**).[43]

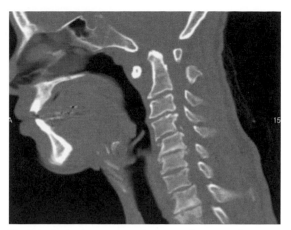

Fig. 9.4 Sagittal reconstructed computed tomography scan of the cervical spine demonstrating atlantoaxial instability with increased atlantodental interval (ADI).

45. What are Modic changes?

Vertebral body marrow changes at the end plates. They are typically associated with degenerative or inflammatory conditions. There are three types. Type 1 shows increased signal only on T2W MRI and is associated with bone edema or acute inflammation. Type 2 shows increased signal on both T1W and T2W MRIs and signifies replacement of marrow by fat. Type 3 shows decreased signal on both T1W and T2W MRIs and suggests osteosclerosis. Both types 2 and 3 are chronic changes.[44]

46. What are the five types of spondylolisthesis?

Isthmic (pars interarticularis defect), degenerative, dysplastic (congenital), traumatic, and pathologic.[45]

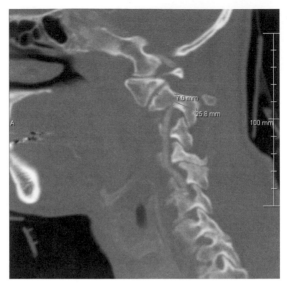

Fig. 9.5 Sagittal reconstructed computed tomography angiogram scan with contrast of the cervical spine, demonstrating trajectory of the vertebral artery and width of the pars interarticularis of C2 in relation to the vertebral artery and projected tract of a transarticular screw.

47. How do you differentiate scar tissue from a recurrent disk herniation radiographically?

The best study to differentiate the two conditions is an MRI with contrast. In cases of scar tissue or epidural fibrosis, there will be uptake of contrast throughout the fragment, whereas in disk reherniation, contrast enhancement will only be seen circumferentially around the lesion/fragment (**Fig. 9.6**).[46]

48. What are the radiographic indications for surgical fusion/instrumentation of the lumbar spine in a patient with an L2 burst fracture?

Canal compromise of greater than 50%, loss of height of greater than 50%, and/or kyphosis of greater than 30 degrees.[47]

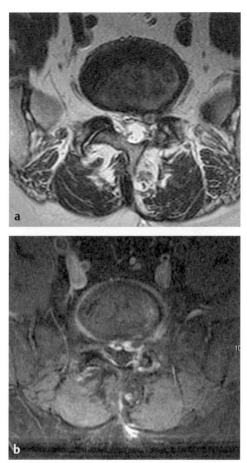

Fig. 9.6 Axial T2-weighted **(a)** and T1-weighted magnetic resonance images with contrast **(b)** of the lumbar spine, demonstrating recurrent disk herniation with circumferential enhancement from epidural fibrosis (the central nonenhancing portion seen amid the scar tissue is the recurrent disk).

49. What is the Spence rule?

When looking at an AP odontoid view of a C-spine X-ray, the sum of the lateral overhang of the C1 lateral masses from the C2 vertebra should not exceed 7 mm. If the distance of excursion of lateral masses is 7 mm or more, there is a transverse ligament rupture.[45]

50. What is the Steele rule of thirds?

The dens, subarachnoid space, and spinal cord each occupy one-third of the area of the canal at the level of the atlas.

51. What is the normal thickness of the prevertebral soft tissue anterior to the cervical spine on plain X-ray lateral images?

At C2, it is 6 mm; at C6, it is ~22 mm.[48]

52. What is the McGregor line? What is it used for?

The McGregor line is an imaginary line drawn from the posterior edge of the hard palate to the most inferior point of the occiput on a sagittal view of the cervical spine. It is used in conditions such as rheumatoid arthritis to determine the vertical settling of the odontoid process. There should not be more than 4.5 mm of protrusion of the odontoid process above this line (**Fig. 9.7**).[49]

53. What is the most common cause of spinal cord compression in patients with cancer?

Metastatic tumor in the epidural space.[51]

54. What is usually the earliest indication of spinal cord compression in a cancer patient?

Central back pain.[52]

55. What are the two most common intramedullary spinal cord tumors?

Ependymomas and astrocytomas.[53,54]

56. What are the two most common intradural extramedullary spinal tumors?

Meningiomas and schwannomas.[55]

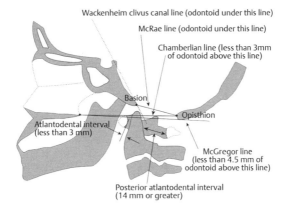

Fig. 9.7 Craniometric lines in lateral view of the cervical spine. (Reproduced with permission from Nader and Sabbagh.[50])

57. What are the two most common extradural spinal tumors?

Metastatic and bone tumors.[56,57]

58. Where do myxopapillary ependymomas occur?

At the conus or filum terminale.[58,59]

59. Which intramedullary tumors most commonly present with a cyst?

Hemangioblastomas followed by ependymomas, astrocytomas, and arachnoid cysts.

60. What is the rule of imaging in multiple myeloma?

To diagnose and monitor the response to treatment. On X-rays, multiple myeloma will appear as punched-out osteolytic lesions. CT scan is more sensitive than X-rays in detecting bone lesions. Lesions with less than 5% of trabecular bone destruction can be detected on CT. PET-CT can detect active disease. MRI is the gold standard imaging modality in multiple myeloma. MRI detects the replacement of normal bone marrow with neoplastic cells, made evident by the progressive increase in T1W signal intensity in the marrow. Both PET-CT and MRI can be used to monitor response to therapy.[60]

61. What is the radiologic definition of osteoporosis?

Osteoporosis is defined as a T-score ≤ 2.5 and osteopenia as a T-score ≤ 1.0 at any skeletal site on dual-energy X-ray absorptiometry scan.[61]

62. How do you identify the artery of Adamkiewicz radiologically?

The artery can be identified based on the presence of a branching artery from the radiculomedullary artery running obliquely along the anterior surface of the spinal cord with a hairpin turn connection to the anterior spinal artery at the allocated level of the spinal cord (lumbar or lower thoracic).[62]

63. What is the most common radiologic appearance of transverse myelitis on MRI?

Transverse myelitis appears as medullary cord swelling at the level of the lesion with hyperintensity on T2W MRI.[63]

64. What is the differential diagnosis of dumbbell-shaped tumors?[64]

- Neurofibroma.
- Malignant peripheral nerve sheath tumor.
- Solitary bone plasmacytoma.
- Chordoma.
- Superior sulcus tumor.
- Spine metastasis.
- Tuberculous spondylitis.
- Vertebral hydatid disease.
- Aneurysmal bone cyst.
- Intraforaminal synovial cyst.
- Traumatic pseudomeningocele.
- Extradural arachnoid cyst.

65. What is Cobb's angle? What is it used for? How do you measure it?

It is a measurement used in spinal deformities, particularly scoliosis, to quantify the magnitude of the deformity on plain radiographs. It is measured by drawing lines from the upper and lower ends of the deformity end plates, and then measuring the angle between the two lines, where they intersect. Scoliosis is defined as a lateral spinal curvature with a Cobb angle of 10 degrees or more.[65,66]

■ References

1. Escalona AO, Pradel ZG, Pisón JL, et al. Pediatric cerebrovascular accident secondary to fibromuscular dysplasia [in Spanish]. An Pediatr (Barc) 2009;71(4):339–342

2. Al-Katib S, Shetty M, Jafri SM, Jafri SZ. Radiologic assessment of native renal vasculature: a multimodality review. Radiographics 2017;37(1):136–156

3. Sener RN. The pineal gland: a comparative MR imaging study in children and adults with respect to normal anatomical variations and pineal cysts. Pediatr Radiol 1995;25(4):245–248

4. Rekate HL. Shunt-related headaches: the slit ventricle syndromes. Childs Nerv Syst 2008;24(4):423–430

5. Zijlmans M, de Kort GA, Witkamp TD, et al. 3T versus 1.5T phased-array MRI in the presurgical work-up of patients with partial epilepsy of uncertain focus. J Magn Reson Imaging 2009;30(2):256–262

6. Torreggiani WC, Keogh C, Al-Ismail K, Munk PL, Nicolaou S. Von Hippel-Lindau disease: a radiological essay. Clin Radiol 2002;57(8):670–680

7. Yamakami I, Uchino Y, Kobayashi E, Saeki N, Yamaura A. Prognostic significance of changes in the internal acoustic meatus caused by vestibular schwannoma. Neurol Med Chir (Tokyo) 2002;42(11):465–470, discussion 470–471

8. Osborn AG, Blaser S, Salzman KL. Rathke cleft cyst. In: Diagnostic Imaging: Brain. Salt Lake City, UT: Amirsys; 2004:II-2-16

9. Tien RD. Sequence of enhancement of various portions of the pituitary gland on gadolinium-enhanced MR images: correlation with regional blood supply. AJR Am J Roentgenol 1992;158(3):651–654

10. Osborn AG, Blaser S, Salzman KL. Intracranial hypotension. In: Diagnostic Imaging: Brain. Salt Lake City, UT: Amirsys; 2004:II-4-22

11. Osborn A, Blaser S, Salzman KL. Diffuse axonal injury (DAI). In: Diagnostic Imaging: Brain. Salt Lake City, UT: Amirsys; 2004:I-2-30

12. Osborn A, Blaser S, Salzman KL. Dandy Walker spectrum. In: Diagnostic Imaging: Brain. Salt Lake City, UT: Amirsys; 2004:I-1-26

13. Osborn A, Blaser S, Salzman KL. Sturge-Weber syndrome. In: Diagnostic Imaging: Brain. Salt Lake City, UT: Amirsys; 2004:I-1-94

14. Redekop GJ. Extracranial carotid and vertebral artery dissection: a review. Can J Neurol Sci 2008;35(2):146–152

15. Osborn A, Blaser S, Salzman KL. Traumatic carotid-cavernous fistula. In: Diagnostic Imaging: Brain. Salt Lake City, UT: Amirsys; 2004:I-2-62

16. McLaughlin N, Villablanca PJ, Jahan R, Martin NA. An infundibu-
    lum of thalamoperforator arteries: importance of angiographic
    images for appropriate diagnosis. Surg Neurol Int 2013;4:44

17. Osborn A, Blaser S, Salzman KL. Multiple sclerosis. In: Diagnos-
    tic Imaging: Brain. Salt Lake City, UT: Amirsys; 2004:I-8–74

18. Nguyen JB, Ahktar N, Delgado PN, Lowe LH. Magnetic resonance
    imaging and proton magnetic resonance spectroscopy of
    intracranial epidermoid tumors. Crit Rev Computed Tomogr
    2004;45(5–6):389–427

19. Bergui M, Zhong J, Bradac GB, Sales S. Diffusion-weight-
    ed images of intracranial cyst-like lesions. Neuroradiology
    2001;43(10):824–829

20. Osborn A, Blaser S, Salzman KL. Cavernous malformation.
    In: Diagnostic Imaging: Brain. Salt Lake City, UT: Amirsys;
    2004:I-5–24

21. Osborn A, Blaser S, Salzman KL. Wilson disease. In: Diagnostic
    Imaging: Brain. Salt Lake City, UT: Amirsys; 2004:I-9–70

22. Osborn A, Blaser S, Salzman KL. Arteriovenous malformation.
    In: Diagnostic Imaging: Brain. Salt Lake City, UT: Amirsys;
    2004:I-5–4

23. Osborn A, Blaser S, Salzman KL. Moyamoya. In: Diagnostic
    Imaging: Brain. Salt Lake City, UT: Amirsys; 2004:I-4–42

24. Osborn A, Blaser S, Salzman KL. Traumatic intracranial
    dissection. In: Diagnostic Imaging: Brain. Salt Lake City, UT:
    Amirsys; 2004:I-2–56

25. Osborn A, Blaser S, Salzman KL. Dural sinus thrombosis.
    In: Diagnostic Imaging: Brain. Salt Lake City, UT: Amirsys;
    2004:I-4–96

26. Tang PH, Chai J, Chan YH, Chng SM, Lim CC. Superior sagittal
    sinus thrombosis: subtle signs on neuroimaging. Ann Acad Med
    Singapore 2008;37(5):397–401

27. Tuna M, Göçer AI, Ozel S, Bağdatoğlu H, Zorludemir S,
    Haciyakupoğlu S. A giant dissecting aneurysm mimicking
    serpentine aneurysm angiographically. Case report and review
    of the literature. Neurosurg Rev 1998;21(4):284–289

28. Osborn A, Blaser S, Salzman KL. Cowden syndrome. In: Diagnos-
    tic Imaging: Brain. Salt Lake City, UT: Amirsys; 2004:I-1–112

29. Cognard C, Gobin YP, Pierot L, et al. Cerebral dural arteriovenous
    fistulas: clinical and angiographic correlation with a revised clas-
    sification of venous drainage. Radiology 1995;194(3):671–680

30. Horská A, Barker PB. Imaging of brain tumors: MR
    spectroscopy and metabolic imaging. Neuroimaging Clin N Am
    2010;20(3):293–310

31. Snelling B, Shah AH, Buttrick S, Benveniste R. The use of MR
    perfusion imaging in the evaluation of tumor progression in
    gliomas. J Korean Neurosurg Soc 2017;60(1):15–20

32. Bouthillier A, van Loveren HR, Keller JT. Segments of the internal carotid artery: a new classification. Neurosurgery 1996;38(3):425–432, discussion 432–433

33. Kilic AK, Kurne AT, Oguz KK, Soylemezoglu F, Karabudak R. Mass lesions in the brain: tumor or multiple sclerosis? Clinical and imaging characteristics and course from a single reference center. Turk Neurosurg 2013;23(6):728–735

34. Rodallec MH, Marteau V, Gerber S, Desmottes L, Zins M. Craniocervical arterial dissection: spectrum of imaging findings and differential diagnosis. Radiographics 2008;28(6):1711–1728

35. Garg RK, Sinha MK. Multiple ring-enhancing lesions of the brain. J Postgrad Med 2010;56(4):307–316

36. Antony J, Hacking C, Jeffree RL. Pachymeningeal enhancement-a comprehensive review of literature. Neurosurg Rev 2015;38(4):649–659

37. Petrella JR, Coleman RE, Doraiswamy PM. Neuroimaging and early diagnosis of Alzheimer disease: a look to the future. Radiology 2003;226(2):315–336

38. Collie DA, Sellar RJ, Zeidler M, Colchester AC, Knight R, Will RG. MRI of Creutzfeldt-Jakob disease: imaging features and recommended MRI protocol. Clin Radiol 2001;56(9):726–739

39. McKiernan EF, O'Brien JT. 7T MRI for neurodegenerative dementias in vivo: a systematic review of the literature. J Neurol Neurosurg Psychiatry 2017. pii: jnnp-2016-315022

40. Gillams AR, Chaddha B, Carter AP. MR appearances of the temporal evolution and resolution of infectious spondylitis. AJR Am J Roentgenol 1996;166(4):903–907

41. Deliganis AV, Baxter AB, Hanson JA, et al. Radiologic spectrum of craniocervical distraction injuries. Radiographics 2000;20(Spec No):S237–S250

42. Iizuka H, Sorimachi Y, Ara T, et al. Relationship between the morphology of the atlanto-occipital joint and the radiographic results in patients with atlanto-axial subluxation due to rheumatoid arthritis. Eur Spine J 2008;17(6):826–830

43. Wolfa CE, Resnick DK. Neurosurgical Operative Atlas: Spine and Peripheral Nerves. New York, NY: Thieme Medical Publishers and the American Association of Neurological Surgeons; 2007

44. Modic MT. Degenerative disorders of the spine. In: Ross JS, Masaryk TJ, eds. Magnetic Resonance Imaging of the Spine. Chicago, IL: Year Book Medical; 1989

45. Greenberg MS. Handbook of Neurosurgery. 8th ed. New York, NY: Thieme Medical Publishers; 2016

46. Lee JK, Amorosa L, Cho SK, Weidenbaum M, Kim Y. Recurrent lumbar disk herniation. J Am Acad Orthop Surg 2010;18(6):327–337

47. Benzel EC. Spine Surgery: Techniques, Complication Avoidance, and Management. 2nd ed. Philadelphia, PA: Churchill Livingstone; 2004

48. DeBehnke DJ, Havel CJ. Utility of prevertebral soft tissue measurements in identifying patients with cervical spine fractures. Ann Emerg Med 1994;24(6):1119–1124

49. Kawaida H, Sakou T, Morizono Y. Vertical settling in rheumatoid arthritis. Diagnostic value of the Ranawat and Redlund-Johnell methods. Clin Orthop Relat Res 1989;(239):128–135

50. Nader R, Sabbagh AJ. Neurosurgery Case Review: Questions and Answers. New York, NY: Thieme Medical Publishers; 2010

51. Kim RY. Extradural spinal cord compression from metastatic tumor. Ala Med 1990;60(1–2):10–15

52. Gilbert RW, Kim JH, Posner JB. Epidural spinal cord compression from metastatic tumor: diagnosis and treatment. Ann Neurol 1978;3(1):40–51

53. Kyoshima K, Akaishi K, Tokushige K, et al. Surgical experience with resection en bloc of intramedullary astrocytomas and ependymomas in the cervical and cervicothoracic region. J Clin Neurosci 2004;11(6):623–628

54. Samartzis D, Gillis CC, Shih P, O'Toole JE, Fessler RG. Intramedullary spinal cord tumors: Part I-Epidemiology, pathophysiology, and diagnosis. Global Spine J 2015;5(5):425–435

55. Asthagiri AR, Helm GA, Sheehan JP. Current concepts in management of meningiomas and schwannomas. Neurol Clin 2007;25(4):1209–1230, xi

56. Sze G, Krol G, Zimmerman RD, Deck MD. Malignant extradural spinal tumors: MR imaging with Gd-DTPA. Radiology 1988;167(1):217–223

57. Mechtler LL, Nandigam K. Spinal cord tumors: new views and future directions. Neurol Clin 2013;31(1):241–268

58. Sa'adah M, Al Shunnar K, Saadah L, Shogan A, Inshasi J, Afifi H. Atypical presentations of conus medullaris and filum terminale myxopapillary ependymomas. J Clin Neurosci 2004;11(3):268–272

59. Dorfer C, Tonn J, Rutka JT. Ependymoma: a heterogeneous tumor of uncertain origin and limited therapeutic options. Handb Clin Neurol 2016;134:417–431

60. Amos B, Agarwal A, Kanekar S. Imaging of multiple myeloma. Hematol Oncol Clin North Am 2016;30(4):843–865

61. Oei L, Koromani F, Rivadeneira F, Zillikens MC, Oei EH. Quantitative imaging methods in osteoporosis. Quant Imaging Med Surg 2016;6(6):680–698

62. Yoshioka K, Niinuma H, Ehara S, Nakajima T, Nakamura M, Kawazoe K. MR angiography and CT angiography of the artery of Adamkiewicz: state of the art. Radiographics 2006;26(suppl 1):S63–S73

63. Abou Al-Shaar H, AbouAl-Shaar I, Al-Kawi MZ. Acute cervical cord infarction in anterior spinal artery territory with acute swelling mimicking myelitis. Neurosciences (Riyadh) 2015;20(4):372–375

64. Kivrak AS, Koc O, Emlik D, Kiresi D, Odev K, Kalkan E. Differential diagnosis of dumbbell lesions associated with spinal neural foraminal widening: imaging features. Eur J Radiol 2009;71(1):29–41

65. Kim H, Kim HS, Moon ES, et al. Scoliosis imaging: what radiologists should know. Radiographics 2010;30(7):1823–1842

66. Langensiepen S, Semler O, Sobottke R, et al. Measuring procedures to determine the Cobb angle in idiopathic scoliosis: a systematic review. Eur Spine J 2013;22(11):2360–2371

Index